REST UNEASY

Critical Issues in Health and Medicine

Edited by Rima D. Apple, University of Wisconsin–Madison, and
Janet Golden, Rutgers University, Camden

Growing criticism of the U.S. healthcare system is coming from consumers, politicians, the media, activists, and healthcare professionals. Critical Issues in Health and Medicine is a collection of books that explores these contemporary dilemmas from a variety of perspectives, among them political, legal, historical, sociological, and comparative, and with attention to crucial dimensions such as race, gender, ethnicity, sexuality, and culture.

For a list of titles in the series, see the last page of the book.

REST UNEASY

Sudden Infant Death Syndrome in Twentieth-Century America

BRITTANY COWGILL

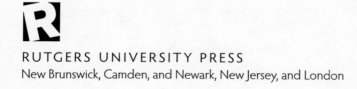

RUTGERS UNIVERSITY PRESS

New Brunswick, Camden, and Newark, New Jersey, and London

Library of Congress Cataloging-in-Publication Data

Names: Cowgill, Brittany, 1986– author.
Title: Rest uneasy : sudden infant death syndrome in twentieth-century America /
Brittany Cowgill.
Description: New Brunswick, New Jersey : Rutgers University Press, [2018] | Series:
Critical issues in health and medicine | Includes bibliographical references and index.
Identifiers: LCCN 2017021380 (print) | LCCN 2017022153 (ebook) | ISBN
9780813588216 (E-pub) | ISBN 9780813588223 (Web PDF) | ISBN 9780813588209
(cloth : alk. paper) | ISBN 9780813588193 (pbk. : alk. paper)
Subjects: | MESH: Sudden Infant Death—etiology | Sudden Infant
Death—prevention & control | Infant Mortality—history | Risk Reduction Behavior
| History, 20th Century | United States
Classification: LCC RJ320.S93 (ebook) | LCC RJ320.S93 (print) | NLM WS 430 |
DDC 618.92/026—dc23
LC record available at https://lccn.loc.gov/2017021380

A British Cataloging-in-Publication record for this book is available from the British
Library.

∞ The paper used in this publication meets the requirements of the American
National Standard for Information Sciences—Permanence of Paper for Printed
Library Materials, ANSI Z39.48–1992.

www.rutgersuniversitypress.org

Manufactured in the United States of America

To Patty

CONTENTS

REST UNEASY

INTRODUCTION: REINTERPRETING SUDDEN INFANT DEATH

Explaining the Unexplainable

In 1915, 10 percent of babies born in America perished before reaching their first birthday. Over the course of the next eight decades, as a result of both public health initiatives and medical advances, infant mortality rates plummeted to less than 1 percent. In 1997, only 0.7 percent of babies died before they turned one.[1] These ongoing gains, combined with the advent of antibiotics, the proliferation of nutritional and electrolyte therapies, and dramatic advances like the polio and diphtheria vaccines, led baby boomers to trust that medical expertise would safeguard their children. But even while more babies were surviving into childhood than ever before, new sources of anxiety about the first year of life were percolating, and parents could not rest easy.[2]

Starting in the early 1960s, American newspapers, magazines, and medical periodicals began publishing reports about the concerning and distressing fate of "crib death." The *New York Times* first carried a reference to the phenomenon in a brief snippet in 1963. Following the headline "Baby Crib Deaths Up," the piece explained the situation: seemingly healthy babies were placed to sleep for the night, and then died. No one knew why. The next year, the paper reported on the full extent of the problem; doctors estimated that anywhere between 10 and 15 thousand crib deaths occurred nationwide each year.[3] This grave "new" concern sharply blunted the sense that modern medicine could eliminate infant mortality.

Americans in the 1960s were living through what they saw as a "golden age of medical research," and that made any sluggish progress disappointing.[4] After the rapid improvements in infant death rates in the first fifty years of the 1900s, the average 1 percent annual decline from 1950 through 1965 appeared "rather modest." Furthermore, the U.S. infant mortality rate was declining slower than that of other industrialized countries. In 1960, amid the rivalrous international climate of the Cold War, the U.S. ranked twelfth in terms of infant mortality.[5] If infant mortality was indeed a "barometer of the health of a nation," as Harvard physician David Rutstein proposed, America was in trouble. Not only was it trailing behind nations ranging from Finland to Czechoslovakia, not all American babies had equal chances of surviving. Infant mortality rates varied drastically by race, income, and education level, and the least privileged American families were disproportionately bearing the burden of the nation's infant fatalities. In the postwar decades, infant mortality became a source of national embarrassment. "Frankly," asserted Rutstein in a 1964 issue of *Reader's Digest*, the "U.S. infant death rate is a national disgrace."[6] The opprobrium conveyed that with American medical capabilities, no baby's death should be unaccounted for. In the nation supposedly at the helm of a "worldwide war on disease," as Lyndon Johnson announced America was in 1965, stagnant improvements in infant mortality were intolerable.[7] Against this backdrop, reports of increasing rates of sudden, unexpected infant deaths—crib deaths—stood out as a flagrant, glaring deficiency.

Saul and Sylvia Goldberg moved to Baltimore in 1954. Saul worked in advertising and Sylvia worked as an X-ray technologist until she decided to stay home after giving birth to her first child, Ann, in 1959. Soon the couple welcomed another daughter, Michele, and in 1963 they brought their third daughter, Suzanne, home. One afternoon, when Suzanne was eight weeks old, Sylvia took Suzanne outside in her carriage. Sylvia went in from the backyard to answer a phone call and returned to a scene that haunted her for the rest of her life. Suzanne was not breathing and would not respond to stimulation or CPR. At the hospital, a doctor told Sylvia that her baby was dead.[8] The Goldbergs were traumatized. Suzanne's passing was as stunning as it was unforeseen, as abrupt as it was incomprehensible. For years, medicine was unable to explain Suzanne's death. In 1969, Saul Goldberg observed that his family's loss was "all the more puzzling because it persists in an era when babies have been made more safe from fatal diseases . . . than ever before . . . It is the very success of modern medicine today that has ironically exposed this serious sudden infant death problem."[9]

That same year, the Goldbergs listened closely at a gathering convened to discuss the problem that had turned their lives upside down and shattered their family. They were witness to the first formal proposed definition of sudden infant death syndrome (SIDS): an infant death "unexpected by history and in which a thorough post-mortem exam fails to demonstrate an adequate cause of death."[10] Parents like Saul and Sylvia learned that SIDS was a diagnosis of exclusion; it existed only once all other possible diagnoses—causes of death—were ruled out. The only recognizable feature of the malady was that the cause of death was unknown.

The Goldbergs became lifelong crusaders against SIDS, devoting themselves to supporting other parents who experienced their same shocking loss. Just after SIDS was defined, Saul Goldberg, speaking to a Senate Appropriations Subcommittee, passionately accentuated the "actual existence" of a problem. He described SIDS as a "mysterious phenomenon which concerns our most precious asset—our babies and their lives," and urged policymakers that "America can no longer sit idly by while millions of hours of manpower and talent which could be put to peaceful and productive purposes are buried forever."[11] Other observers invoked similar rhetoric, comparing SIDS to lung cancer in severity and describing it as a mystery and "the greatest killer" of American infants. (After SIDS statistics started being collected, it turned out that SIDS was the second-greatest killer of American infants, behind congenital anomalies; SIDS was the foremost cause of post-neonatal death, however.)[12] Parents like the Goldbergs experienced the sting of loss twice over—SIDS stole their babies' lives and then wreaked havoc on their families; it was all the worse because it was such an empty diagnosis. As Barry Goldblatt, a father victimized by SIDS, articulated in the mid-1970s, "I find it very tough to accept that it's nothing. It can't just happen . . . it doesn't make sense [and] it's not logical." Diane McCarron, a SIDS mother, echoed the same: "It's very hard to accept that sometimes there just aren't any reasons," she said. "It's a spooky feeling."[13]

CONSTRUCTIONS OF SUDDEN INFANT MORTALITY

SIDS illustrates how diagnoses are "made" and then adapted to new circumstances over time. SIDS is informed by both medicine and society; it is a product of science, of society, and of sadness. It is a dynamic diagnosis that exemplifies the social construction of medicine. To say that SIDS is socially constructed does not deny its authenticity, but the purpose of this work is neither to debate nor determine whether or not SIDS was or is "real." As the renowned historian of medicine Charles Rosenberg explains, "In some ways disease does not exist until we have agreed that it does, by perceiving, naming, and responding to it." "In our culture," Rosenberg continues, "the existence of a disease as *specific* entity is a fundamental aspect of its intellectual and moral legitimacy."[14] SIDS is not an abstraction or a vacant social construction—it is "real" because American society and the American medical establishment decided it was. SIDS is the way in which late-twentieth-century Americans tried to make sense of and cope with a particular loss.[15]

Still, SIDS encapsulates the fluidity of diagnostic medicine. It is well established that American society and organized medicine reconstruct diseases and diagnoses. Indeed, medical historians have illustrated that Americans have a talent for reimagining medical ailments—in recent history, they reconfigured tuberculosis, cholera, polio, fetal alcohol syndrome, cancer, homosexuality, menopause, pregnancy, and plumbism, among many other conditions.[16] Medicine is a complex product of its time, a malleable output fashioned by both science and society. No medical condition is fixed, and so it is with SIDS. Americans conceived of sudden infant death differently over time and according to varying perspectives. Their various approaches, one of which was SIDS, linked sudden infant deaths to all kinds of different causes—biological, anatomical, environmental, and social—and their ideas were consistently shaped by contemporary ideologies about medicine, infant care, technology, and family.

From its inception, the SIDS label served medical and social purposes. Medically, it created a standardized language for doctors to diagnose, record, and research sudden infant deaths, with the aim of finding a solution. Socially, it helped parents cope with the loss of a child by offering them any (if vacuous) explanation for what had happened, by mustering overdue social empathy, and by effecting channels for peer support. Disease always runs on a two-way street; medicine and society interact and affect one another. This is apparent in the case of SIDS. For a medical category, SIDS was profoundly influenced by social considerations. Parents of babies who died suddenly without discernible reason were so distressed by their loss that they accepted a strikingly empty medical label. Physicians, rattled by their own powerlessness to explain or prevent the situation, were also acutely upset by the inexplicable passing of American infants. If the SIDS cause-of-death label could offer parents any relief, physicians were ready and willing to apply it—the foremost experts asserted that the SIDS diagnosis served "counseling purposes" for families. Parents and doctors accepted the SIDS label because it was a welcome and promising alternative. SIDS offered the chance to disengage uncomfortable ideas about parental culpability, and, because it sculpted a "new" problem, SIDS provided an avenue to pursue a solution. Constructing SIDS led to measurable benefits, but, ultimately, fell short of meeting Americans' expectations; the SIDS diagnosis foundered.

Unexpected infant mortality that presented very similarly to SIDS did occur in the past, but it was not actually SIDS. Before they had the SIDS label, Americans understood the physiology and circumstances of sudden infant mortality differently. Sudden infant deaths were thought to be the fault of parents, almost exclusively mothers, and prior to the 1800s westerners interpreted sudden infant death under the pretense of infanticide. In the nineteenth century, they increasingly made sense of sudden infant deaths as "overlaying." The term had been around for centuries; it described when a child died from suffocation from literally being "laid over" by a parent or otherwise from smothering in its bedding materials. In the decades leading up to the twentieth century, European and American medicine ascertained overlaying as a major social problem and described it as almost entirely the fault of mothers. Medical professionals were uniquely bothered by overlaying because they saw it as so straightforward; they distinguished overlaying for how easy it was to explain. Around 1900, other physicians maintained an alternative, anatomical explanation for overlaying, saying that babies died suddenly as the result of oversized thymus glands. Following from this interpretation, medical practitioners tried to treat infants and children with enlarged thymuses by either removing the organ surgically or shrinking it with radiation. Then, in the 1930s, a few American physicians articulated the concept of "accidental mechanical suffocation" and argued that it was a more appropriate way to describe and explain sudden infant deaths.

In the second half of the twentieth century, American physicians and parents worked to banish each of these previous categorical descriptions for sudden infant death—overlaying, enlarged thymuses, and accidental mechanical suffocation—by replacing them with the fresh moniker of Sudden Infant Death Syndrome. They castigated previous frameworks for being both unscientific *and* inhumane. And instead of providing a new explanation to account for why babies died suddenly, SIDS pronounced that there *was no explanation*. Physicians tried, to little avail, to find one. The SIDS diagnosis recast sudden infant deaths as a medical mystery, a problem worthy of professional analysis, public funding, and social support.

The configuration of SIDS did not mark the endpoint in Americans' revisions of sudden infant death. After they coined SIDS, Americans continued to reinterpret its social meanings and medical elements. First, they stressed that SIDS was a freak occurrence that struck normal, healthy babies. SIDS was a parent's worst nightmare; it was an unpreventable, unpredictable tragedy, decidedly not related to smothering or suffocation. Decades of medical research never unearthed a cause for SIDS, but certain findings contributed to more revisions of the problem. After misplaced research in the 1970s indicated that abnormally long breathing pauses might cause SIDS, American medicine recounted SIDS as the result of multiple interacting risk factors, a complex multifaceted event. SIDS babies, rather than being completely well, were perceived to suffer from subtle abnormalities. After it was named in 1969, SIDS was conceived of first as a momentary, unforeseeable catastrophe and then as a composite outcome of various anatomical and environmental risk factors that might be able to be anticipated.

SIDS PARADOXICAL

The term "syndrome" is derived from the Greek words *syn* (together) and *dromos* (running); medically, a syndrome literally signifies "a running together" of symptoms.[17] The *Oxford Dictionary* defines a syndrome as "a group of symptoms that consistently occur together or a condition characterized by a set of associated symptoms." By definition, syndromes are diagnosable based on their symptomology—not their causation. The first characteristic symptom of SIDS is death. In some ways, SIDS is the "perfect" syndrome because it is *only* recognizable by its symptomology—unexplained death—and its definition disallows any source of causation. Strictly speaking, explaining SIDS would be impossible because doing so would invalidate the diagnosis. Explained infant deaths are not SIDS deaths. In a way, then, the late-twentieth-century American project of explaining SIDS was literally an unwinnable battle, because it had as its mission the goal of describing and clarifying SIDS.

SIDS contested American medicine's ability to save and protect children, casting a dark shadow over bedtime and over families' very survival. In a postwar culture where the home and family symbolized the American promise of security, culture and society celebrated parenthood, and especially motherhood. Towards the final years of the baby boom, in a climate characterized by what historian Elaine Tyler May calls "family fever," SIDS emerged as a literal and metaphorical danger.[18] But SIDS did more than imperil the American family—it was a devastating exposure of the limits of American medicine. By the 1970s, Americans' previously steadfast faith in modern medicine as a catchall cure for their ailments was crashing down. Publicity of travesties such as the Tuskegee study, the horrifying effects of diethylstilbestrol, and the thalidomide scandal, alongside powerful feminist critiques of the medical establishment, all shook Americans' long-standing confidence in the medical field to the core. As they became increasingly familiar with disappointments in the medical arena—ranging from rising rates of cancer, to mounting concerns about unanticipated effects of oral contraceptives and hormone replacement therapy, to the disturbing new visibility of environmental diseases—Americans began questioning the value and possibilities of medical care and progress.[19] SIDS was another shortfall, a poignant manifestation of modern medicine's inability to safeguard American lives.

SIDS was a disappointment in other ways as well. One of the most difficult aspects of this history is that sudden infant death, like infant mortality at large, has always affected disadvantaged and minority Americans disproportionately. Dating back to its characterization as overlaying in the 1800s, medicine documented this imbalance repeatedly. Yet sudden infant death's continual associations with underprivileged Americans baffled doctors just as much as the condition itself. Unable to explain the syndrome they were studying, doctors were also powerless to comprehend the correlations they discovered—including the one that SIDS was more likely among families in need. Professional publications frequently mentioned the connection but were at a loss how to combat it.

Furthermore, especially before the 1980s, doctors broached the topic only tentatively because it risked undermining their mission to impress upon Americans that SIDS was as random as being "struck by lightning."[20]

Into the second decade of the twenty-first century, SIDS continued to elude medical explanation and also continued to affect Americans disproportionately. If available evidence does not clearly explain *why* SIDS affected Americans unequally, it does indicate that they were treated unequally after SIDS occurred. Compared to families with more facilities—be they financial, social, or educational—poor and minority families were less likely to receive information on SIDS, less likely to benefit from the support of parent networking, and more likely to endure suspicions about their behaviors.

Misgivings about certain types of parents date far back in the history of sudden infant death. When doctors apprehended sudden infant mortality as overlaying, they were deriding mothers for (presumably) sleeping with their children, working, or consuming intoxicants. Over time, questions about parental culpability migrated; they did not dissipate. In the twentieth century, American parents challenged such misgivings via the SIDS diagnosis. Parent activists tended to be from the middle and upper class, or to have powerful connections that enabled them to effectively express their indignation—at being made into suspects and at the nation's inability to account for their loss. They did not make sudden infant mortality into a problem (medicine was already examining it), but they did play a pivotal role in reshaping the public's perception of it as something that could happen to anyone—even Congressmen, models, and movie stars.[21] Even so, given the characteristics of SIDS, suspicions lingered.

As is the case with many topics, Americans with social and financial assets left more historical evidence than those without access to resources. Medicine left the most visible trail of all. Even though *Rest Uneasy* is primarily an account of SIDS medicine, every family whose life was shattered by SIDS is bound to this story through loss and through fear. It is impossible to comprehensively chronicle their experiences; in capturing how persistently medicine and society let them down, *Rest Uneasy* can only begin to speak to their suffering.

REST UNEASY: A ROADMAP

Despite its remakings, SIDS was always an ambiguous and frustrating medical entity. It was also a personal tragedy and a harrowing social experience. The history of SIDS reflects the condition's two predominant functional objectives in twentieth-century America: to ultimately facilitate a medical explanation and solution for sudden unexpected infant mortality and to support the surviving families of SIDS victims by offering them informed, sympathetic counsel and reducing the stigma of sudden infant death. *Rest Uneasy* is a narrative analysis of this history—it is the story of the SIDS diagnosis and its evolving forms and functionalities.

The following chapters are organized loosely chronologically and thematically. The opening chapter reviews the brief existing historiography of sudden infant death and documents social and medical perceptions of infant mortality in the western world from the late 1800s to the turn of the twentieth century. In the final decades of the nineteenth century, medical practitioners began to publish case reports of infant deaths they described as overlaying. Writers portrayed overlaying episodes as obvious instances of suffocation and unanimously attributed overlaying to parental—maternal—wrongdoing, whether intentional or not. When scientists began to pay attention to and discuss incidents of overlaying in their professional journals, they precipitated a critical interpretive shift: sudden and unexpected infant deaths became a medical issue. The perception of sudden infant death as a medical problem that was the fault of mothers had a lasting influence, and the concept of overlaying colored SIDS even into the twenty-first century.

Chapter 2 moves into the twentieth century and discusses how the SIDS diagnosis came into existence. From roughly 1900 through the 1930s, published medical reports endeavored, with varying levels of vehemence, to unseat two notions: overlaying and the idea that enlarged thymus glands caused sudden infant death. During these decades, medicine found faults in both assessments and attempted to discredit them. A handful of doctors offered a new explanation: "accidental mechanical suffocation." But this premise was short-lived, and actually instigated a new set of challenges to the possibility of suffocation itself. Critics questioned the medical veracity of the notion that babies discovered dead in their cribs had suffocated, arguing that it was an unsophisticated, backwards explanation. They believed it was inaccurate as well as cruel to suggest to parents of deceased infants that their babies had suffocated, and they sought to provide an alternative answer to the problem.

Between 1949 and 1969, scholars contending with these issues organized three crucial conferences on sudden death in infancy. These meetings, assembled by physicians and distraught parents, were crucial moments in the history of SIDS. By 1970, they had produced a "new" diagnosis: the label and working definition for sudden infant death syndrome. The proposal was formally adopted into medical vocabulary, and it helped convert unexpected infant deaths from stigmatized episodes into inexplicable, medically justified losses. Constructing SIDS was a watershed, but naming the disease was only the "first step in organizing against it."[22]

From the early years of the twentieth century through the 1960s, so little medical research was produced on sudden infant death that nearly every published article made a notable contribution to the dawning field. By the 1970s, though, research studies with such highly varying theses and logical perspectives were produced so rapidly as to be perceived as a hindrance. Chapter 3 recounts this flurry of work that followed on the heels of constructing the SIDS diagnosis. Scientific research on SIDS followed ambiguous, erratic, and inconclusive pathways. Although mounting scholarship yielded neither understanding nor solutions, it did uncover the extent to which grieving parents needed relief, information, and assistance. Medicine concerned itself with the devastation SIDS left in its wake and sought to attend to families' needs by communicating with parents.

Medicine's goal of solving SIDS was never fully realized, and its twin mission of aiding affected families was equally persistently stymied. Chapter 4 explores the ways in which a fresh understanding of SIDS, as an outcome of multiple risk factors, failed to serve families. As SIDS' associations with minority and impoverished families became more entrenched, so too did its links with optional behaviors such as smoking. Even further, SIDS was repeatedly examined in conjunction with overt parental transgressions such as abuse or neglect.

Despite its drawbacks, parents and doctors continued to approach SIDS as a personal and public problem, and they worked to force SIDS onto the national agenda and enhance its visibility. Chapter 5 documents the activities, successes, and struggles of SIDS activists and the National SIDS Foundation, the largest SIDS parent network. Its most visible victory was to compel passage of the 1974 SIDS Law, which increased federal funding for SIDS research and mandated that states establish and operate SIDS information and counseling centers to serve SIDS families and to implement programs to educate a variety of health professionals about the tragedy of SIDS. In their efforts to mitigate the experience of SIDS, parent activists shared their stories and supported thousands of Americans who were straining to cope with an unthinkable eternal void in their families.

The parents who participated in the National SIDS Foundation found some measure of solace through their fellowship and activism, but tens of thousands more American parents sought comfort elsewhere. American families in the 1970s and 1980s turned to home monitoring devices in the hopes of protecting their babies. Apnea monitors measured babies' breathing, and sometimes their heartbeats, and sounded an alarm if a baby might be in danger. Chapter 6 unpacks the origins, unfounded medical basis, proliferation, and widespread adoption of electronic breathing monitors to prevent SIDS. Monitoring instruments may have offered parents the façade of safety, but they were a highly problematic and intrusive intervention.

Besides spurring the widespread use of monitors in American homes, the science behind monitoring also distracted scientists' attention. The particular ways in which American physicians understood SIDS prevented them from recognizing and critically analyzing the simple components of safe sleep that scientists determined were highly significant in SIDS starting in the late 1980s. Chapter 7 traces the history of pediatric contentions regarding infant sleeping behaviors as they relate to sudden infant death, and shows how international and interdisciplinary collaborations promoted the kind of "thinking outside the box" that eventually helped professionals realize the only intervention documented to minimize the risk of SIDS.

CONCLUSION

In 1972, reporter Judy Klemesrud interviewed families who had lost a baby to SIDS for a piece in the *New York Times*, and parents' comments reify the kind of unremitting fears SIDS sowed in American homes. After Arthur and Ann Siegal lost their son Danny, in 1966, for example, they chose to pursue two adoptions in the hope that their decision might, if "crib death" was genetic, reduce their chances of suffering the same fate a second time. Judith Choate and her husband, Edward, buried their baby son, Robert, in 1965. They had another child, Christopher, just eleven months later, and Judith said the first year after Christopher was born was "the longest period of my life . . . I had to fight myself from going into his room every five minutes to check on him." Kevin and Mary Ann Deas's eleven-week-old baby, Michael, died in his car seat, right behind them, on their way home from a family vacation—"there was no sound, absolutely *nothing*," Mary Ann recalled. Even when her other son Kevin was two years old, far outside the age range for SIDS, Mary Ann still worried: "I'll go into his room in the middle of the night," she said, "and I'll twitch him, just to see if he is still alive."[23]

Once they became familiar with the threat of sudden infant death syndrome, Americans struggled to come to terms with its slippery and paradoxical nature. Lacking sufficient explanations, they adhered to a wide variety of beliefs and strategies in their often-desperate attempts to clarify, prevent, or recover from devastating loss. But the ambiguity of the information they amassed on SIDS and the tactical interventions they developed to prevent it sent even the most erudite experts and careful parents running to check on their babies during the middle of the night.

1 · "DEATHS OF INFANTS IN BED"[1]

The Historical Origins of SIDS

In 1895, *The Lancet*, one of the world's most prestigious medical publications, published a piece concerned with how to prevent "overlaying." A term that had been around for centuries, overlaying described when a child died from suffocation in bed—smothered either by a parent or family member or by blankets or pillows. The article's author suggested that infants would cease dying from being overlaid as soon as "the careless, the indolent, and the drunken" stopped sleeping in beds with babies.[2] The idea was hardly unique, and in fact was quite a popular one among late-nineteenth-century physicians. Just three years before the *Lancet* article, another physician in Scotland who noticed a preponderance of overlaying cases on the weekends had similarly attributed them to parents' inebriety and ignorance. His colleagues applauded his work.[3] Historically, these articles and the many comparable accounts that stood alongside them are important because they recognized, in a professional medical context, an overlaying category of infant mortality. Doctors at the time—first in Britain and then in the United States—were becoming newly attuned to overlaying as a medical problem, and they considered it one with a very simple solution.

Up until the first decade of the twentieth century, unexpected infant deaths that presented similarly to SIDS were overwhelmingly, and with little dispute, comprehended as overlaying. Americans became familiar with overlaying by way of Britain, whose residents harbored exceptional concerns about infant mortality.[4] From the late 1800s through the early 1900s, ideas about infant mortality moved fluidly across the Atlantic. Reformers, new professionals (such as public health workers and child development experts), and medical journals transmitted observations, ideologies, and policies surrounding infant mortality to and from Europe. As with many areas of reform, Americans emulated and modified European perceptions and responses to the "new" problem of infant mortality. Overlaying was one of their concerns, and it formed the first constellation of cases that professionals later interpreted as SIDS.[5] The published medical discussion of overlaying that took place in British medical journals helped frame the nature of the American discourse, which ultimately followed a similar trajectory.

Contemporary physicians were quite certain as to overlaying's chronic and acute causes, and they confidently advanced what they thought were promising solutions. Overlaying, they said, occurred when a baby suffocated in its bed, usually as a result of its mother, who herself was likely to have been in a compromised state, brought on by intoxication or overtiredness. The best means of prevention, they continued, was to inhibit parents from sleeping with their babies, either by legal coercion or by education and individual imperative. Later physicians challenged these presumptions, but the premise of overlaying never entirely disappeared. Although it would not emerge as a recognizable utterance for decades to come, the seeds of the SIDS diagnosis lay in the early cohort of cases recognized as overlaying. The story of SIDS is, in many ways, one of unsuccessful attempts to distinguish sudden infant death from overlaying and to bury the overlaying notion altogether.

At the turn of the twentieth century, overlaying was a circumstantial problem—it was the unfortunate outcome of a particular environment. Disadvantaged mothers, themselves apt to over-exhaustion or alcohol consumption, who did not provide separate beds for their babies, endangered their children. Based on this rendering, overlaying was completely preventable. Crucially, not only the physical possibility of overlaying had staying power. The phenomenon of overlaying was directly tied to underprivileged, disadvantaged members of society, in both England and the United States. Babies born to lower-class and minority families were understood to be at a higher risk of overlaying because their parents—namely their mothers—were unable to provide adequate care. Lower-class parents were perceived as intemperate, irresponsible, and careless—all of which made them insufficient caretakers and endangered their babies.

One of the many ironies of SIDS is that the label derived from explained deaths. Although it laid the foundation for growing attention to sudden *unexplained* infant mortality, overlaying was plainly explained. In the history of SIDS, the idea of overlaying moved in and out of the spotlight but never wholly dissipated. Americans' aversion to the premise of overlaying first helped provoke the SIDS diagnostic category and then continued to shape SIDS by affecting broader responses to it. The socio-behavioral rubric for overlaying established in the late 1800s was enduring, and it underlies SIDS. The story of how Americans came to perceive the broad category of overlaying as a reasonable way to explain some infant deaths, especially among certain populations, informs the entire history of the SIDS diagnosis.

A NOTE ON METHOD: OVERLAYING IS NOT SIDS

The history of SIDS does not commence with its formal documentation. Sadly, infants have died unexpectedly throughout human history and sudden infant mortality has been a problem much longer than SIDS has existed. Many scholars point to the Biblical story of King Solomon as the first recorded SIDS case, documented as overlaying. In the Book of Kings, two new mothers (both prostitutes) approach King Solomon with a baby and explain that one of their infant sons just died. "And this woman's child died in the night," one recounted, "because she overlaid it." As the story continues, each mother claims the living child as her own. King Solomon resolves the dispute by decreeing that the surviving child be split in half and divided equally, a verdict which prompts the true mother to reveal herself by her willingness to relinquish her baby rather than see it killed. In the end, rightful mother and living child are apparently reunited.[6]

Evidence certainly indicates that well before the mid-1900s, episodes that resemble SIDS did occur. In fact, it appears they occurred relatively often. Church records "repeatedly spoke of the dangers of overlaying," and up through the sixteenth century, European church leaders were constantly "baffled and frustrated ... by the many cases of reputed suffocation, the 'overlaying' or 'overlying' of an infant in bed by its allegedly drunken parents."[7] Often, ecclesiastic statutes prohibited mothers from sleeping in the same bed with their children.[8] Into the early modern period and the Enlightenment, overlaying continued to pose a hazard and mostly fell under the rubric of infanticide.[9] Medical authors have relied on such evidence to show that SIDS, tagged as overlaying, has occurred since ancient times.[10]

Yet it would be misguided to argue definitively that such cases were SIDS. Technically, doing so would be scientifically inaccurate. The SIDS category did not exist before the 1960s. The definition agreed upon also demanded an autopsy as a diagnostic criterion; thus without autopsy the syndrome cannot be established. Furthermore, while cultural context is intrinsically salient to any disease or syndrome, it was especially predominant in the SIDS diagnosis. The cultural meanings associated with SIDS in the second half of the twentieth century were not present before the category came into existence. SIDS is not merely a cultural fabrication, but to describe past "SIDS-like" cases as SIDS would mistakenly dismiss the centrality of contemporary actors and convictions. It would be anachronistic.

In her biography of fetal alcohol syndrome (FAS), Janet Golden states that when FAS was coined in 1973 "it was something new." Golden located "historical sightings"—rather than actual diagnoses—of FAS in the past.[11] This strategy is useful in approaching SIDS. When the syndrome was named in the 1960s, it represented a novel and particular way of medically (not) explaining the sudden death of an infant; it also conveyed a new and carefully crafted social message. Prior to this, historical actors described and labeled sudden infant deaths in various ways, but none of those ways were SIDS. Contemporary mechanisms of identifying and explaining infant deaths that ultimately might correspond with the SIDS definition are enormously telling. The "historical sightings" approach intends to pay those incarnations their due.

The mechanisms by which professionals and parents delineated sudden infant deaths before SIDS was formulated informed the SIDS diagnosis in powerful ways. The predominant ways of construing sudden infant deaths before SIDS were overlaying, status thymicolymphaticus, and accidental mechanical suffocation. Although it is impossible to interpret any of these paradigms as SIDS, each is essential to the history of SIDS. Somewhat peculiarly, none of these devices included the notion of inexplicability. This is one of the most striking aspects of the history of SIDS: the diagnosis—which depends upon a victim's death being unexplained—originally sprouted from a conglomeration of cases professionals considered patently explainable. Medical frameworks may have encompassed a certain enigmatic quality, but anatomically doctors considered sudden infant death cases relatively straightforward. Historical sightings of SIDS are at odds with the modern conception of SIDS in a fundamental way: they were explained. This divergence appears incongruous at first glance, but it makes more sense in historical context.

The transitions leading to the notion that a sizable portion of sudden infant deaths were actually unexplainable began with heightened social and medical attention to overlaying in the late 1800s. There are brief glimpses of overlaying figures from the mid-1800s, and Americans were witnesses to well-documented social indignation regarding overlaying in Britain. Hence, although Americans were relatively quiet about overlaying before the twentieth century, they were familiar with the problem. Their initial exposure to overlaying, and its perceived causes, laid the foundation for a pursuit for answers that continues into the twenty-first century. That overlaying was primarily documented among lower-class or minority families is highly significant. Class- and race-based correlations not only continued through succeeding renditions of sudden infant death but also contributed to the enduring propensity to insinuate that parents were at fault.

"HISTORICAL SIGHTINGS" OF SIDS

Some of the first concentrated reports of overlaying emanate from nineteenth-century slave owners; invested as they were in property records, they diligently documented infant mortality. Apparent suffocation was a significant source of controllable infant mortality among enslaved populations. According to the 1850 census, 9.3 percent of infant slave deaths resulted from suffocation (compared to 1.2 percent of white infant deaths).[12] Most contemporaries supposed that infant slave suffocations resulted from infanticide and neglect, but slave infant deaths recorded as overlaying, smothering, or suffocation in bed actually shared much in common with SIDS.

Indeed, qualitative and quantitative evidence indicates that a majority of overlaying and accidental suffocation deaths among slave babies in the antebellum South were similar to SIDS. In his investigation of 202 reports of smothering, suffocation, and overlaying in Virginia between 1853 and 1860, Todd Savitt found a remarkable congruence with modern SIDS cases, including significant epidemiological similarities. Most tellingly, the peak ages (two to four months) and the seasonal distribution of case frequency (prevalence in the winter) aligned.[13] Michael Johnson similarly demonstrated that smothered slave baby cases from the antebellum era conformed to SIDS epidemiology. Between 1790 and 1860, more than sixty thousand infant slave deaths were attributed to smothering. At the time, owners typically condemned slave mothers as careless, reasoning that mothers accidentally smothered their babies. Yet the circumstantial parallels to SIDS are striking: most deaths occurred during sleeping hours, in beds, among infants who were not noticeably ill beforehand, within the two-to-four-month age bracket, and during the winter months.[14]

Additionally, slave infants were much more likely—nine times more likely—to have died from suffocation than free infants. In 1860, of the reported 2,129 infant suffocation deaths in the nation, 94 percent transpired in slave states. Research produced in the 1970s indicated that SIDS was more likely to occur in underprivileged and minority homes, among young mothers, and among women who had lower levels of prenatal care. Johnson drew a direct comparison between the tendency for SIDS to strike disadvantaged families and the tendency for suffocation to strike slave families, whose "disadvantaged" status could hardly be questioned. Even more, smothering death rates were highest in those geographic regions that demanded the most labor of female slaves. Smothering rates also fell steeply after Emancipation, even accounting for reporting omissions and errors. For Johnson, the inferior living conditions and intensive labor requirements of young pregnant enslaved women constituted "the most promising explanation for the high incidence of SIDS among slave infants."[15]

Other historians have upheld this basic argument. In 1985, building the case that slave mothers were deeply connected to their identities as mothers, Deborah Gray White pointed to Savitt's and Johnson's research as evidence in defense of slave mothers' dedication to their children. Rejecting contemporary accusations that slave mothers whose babies suffocated were homicidal, neglectful, or careless, White maintained that these mothers were victims of SIDS.[16] Ariane Kemkes backed these same conclusions. Kemkes studied Federal Mortality Schedule data from 1850 through 1880 in the southern United States with the specific objective to "empirically investigate whether 19th century infant deaths conventionally attributed to smothering or overlaying follow known SIDS trajectories." She determined that circumstantial evidence (again, especially the parallels in seasonality and age) mirrored the hallmarks of SIDS: "smothering/overlaying deaths . . . mimic the clinical features of SIDS," she concluded.[17] These studies present a compelling case that, at least in the corporeal sense, Americans perceived deaths that very closely resemble modern SIDS.

It is difficult to continue to track sudden infant death in the second half of the nineteenth century because it presented under a host of different monikers. Although most fell under the rubric of respiratory failure, a great diversity of labels existed. Indeed, later pathologists repeatedly remarked that the cornucopia of labels employed obscured the prevalence and constitution of sudden infant death. In addition, through most of the 1800s, individual states and cities kept their own vital statistics, and the result was a haphazard, incomplete system. No truly comprehensive birth or deaths records exist.[18]

It is clear from the available figures, though, that in the second half of the nineteenth century, suffocation deaths and deaths from unknown causes—two frequently used proxies for sudden infant death—were common among American babies. Moreover, these categories of death beset babies to a much greater extent than any other age group in society. In 1870, more than 60 percent of deaths from "unknown causes" (almost 10,500) happened among babies under the age of one, and no other age group experienced anywhere near this number of deaths from unknown causes (the next closest bracket, one-year-olds, accounted for just 7 percent of deaths from unknown causes). The same trend exists regarding suffocation deaths. In 1870, 74 percent of suffocation deaths recorded happened to infants under one year old.[19] In 1880, nearly 67 percent of suffocation deaths occurred in babies under one year; in 1890, just over 57 percent of suffocation deaths were among babies.[20] Since overlaying was not a discrete category, it is of course impossible to know whether these cases were regarded as overlaying, but the facts that so many babies were thought to have died from two umbrella categories that often incorporated overlaying, and that the overwhelming majority of those deaths happened in the first twelve months of life, help begin to contextualize the problem of overlaying.

THE PROBLEM OF INFANT MORTALITY

Americans left much more evidence attesting to their growing unease about infant mortality at large—and mothers' responsibilities to prevent it—than about overlaying specifically. The emergence of infant mortality as a discernable problem was a critical precondition for a discourse on sudden infant death. By the early twentieth century, functional changes in the professionalization and standardization of vital records allowed the government to begin systematically chronicling annual mortality statistics, and Americans were confronted with alarmingly high infant mortality rates.[21]

Just before the turn of the century, infant mortality varied significantly by geographic location, but it hovered at average rates between 100 and 150 deaths per thousand live births (10 to 15 percent).[22] (In 2013, the U.S. infant mortality rate was 5.9 deaths per thousand live births, or 0.6 percent.[23]) Statistically speaking, a baby's chances of surviving into childhood hinged on location. In 1885, for example, the infant mortality rate in New York City was 247.8 deaths per thousand live births (24.7 percent); in Portland, Oregon, it was 87.2 (8.7 percent); and in Charleston, North Carolina, it was 322.7 (32.3 percent).[24] From 1900 to 1902, the mortality rate for babies under the age of one was over 12 percent.[25]

Statistics like this illustrate that up through the late nineteenth century, American families were forced to accept an upsetting level of infant and childhood mortality as normal. As scholar Rosie Findlay explains, "The precariousness of children's existence was the rule not the exception, and infant mortality was seen as an unfortunate but natural part of the lifecycle."[26] At least through the middle of the 1800s, Americans considered infancy a vulnerable time period, analogous to the modern conception of old age as a period in the life cycle when morbidity and mortality are expected.[27] Although families were "resigned to the possibility of imminent infant death and to the realization that there was little or nothing they could do to prevent it," the loss of a baby was still a deeply sorrowful experience. Parents mostly "suffered in relative silence." Additionally, given their religious convictions and the prevalence of infant mortality, parents who lost babies were "less likely to demand an explanation for their loss."[28]

Towards the later years of the 1800s, however, the likelihood of infant mortality began to fluctuate, and by the twentieth century a major transformation was well underway. Childhood continued to be a time of vulnerability, but its meanings shifted measurably. As the premium placed on young lives elevated even more, adults started to perceive children as individuals with unique personalities and childhood as an important and meaningful time of growth and development.[29] During the Progressive Era, Americans bestowed upon children and babies unprecedented value. The rise of the field of pediatrics as a formal medical specialty in the 1880s coincided with this sentimental appreciation of children and childhood.[30] Children's bodies and health, now seen as different from those of adults, became deserving of special focus and attention.

Simultaneously, women's roles as mothers became even more entrenched. Society esteemed women as elemental caregivers.[31] Women's role in American society was motherhood; child-rearing "constituted a woman's principal reason for existing."[32] Furthermore, becoming a mother was the primary mechanism for women to "find their identity and life fulfillment."[33] By the turn of the century, women's separate sphere, encompassed by domesticity and motherhood, was so firmly established that it actually became a powerful mechanism for women's advancement.[34] Paired together, the ascendance of childhood and the elevated reverence towards motherhood made women's child-rearing duties all the more serious. Infant and childhood survival—facilitated by mothers—became increasingly urgent matters.[35]

In this setting, the death of a child assumed dramatically new meaning as a personal, familial, and social tragedy. Childhood mortality transformed from anticipated to painfully abnormal; far from ordinary, a child's death became the most harrowing and unbearable kind of loss. The emotional sorrow associated with losing a child magnified to such a great extent that consolation literature directed towards bereaved parents became a dominant literary theme and genre.[36] By 1900, "mothers' attitudes toward infant death had undergone a sea change. No longer was the loss of a child to be viewed passively as the will of God or to be endured silently in the privacy of the home. Instead, women in communities throughout the United States made the nation's high infant mortality a matter of serious public, political concern."[37] Childhood and infant fatalities emerged as losses "to be battled with science and reason."[38] Women and women's groups forced infant mortality onto the national agenda as a pressing public problem. Parents' private losses swelled to become society's losses and a matter of great concern to the public. This novel interpretation urged that childhood deaths were preventable and that both society and parents were responsible for children's survival.[39] In opposition to the ubiquity of infant mortality in the previous century, historian Jacqueline Wolf explains, the notion that infant deaths could be prevented was a "revolutionary concept." It completely altered how Americans perceived infant mortality and also amplified the role of medicine in parenting.[40]

These transformations contributed to the construction of infant mortality as a categorical social and medical problem. As it became a national dilemma, Progressives took up infant health as one of their most noble and urgent reform causes. They focused their efforts on babies more than older children because they saw infants as especially vulnerable to outside influences. Using data collection and publicity campaigns, Progressives worked to alert Americans that infant mortality was a serious, extensive problem. As the renowned pediatrician

L. Emmett Holt explained, learning "the facts of infant mortality" was the first step in preventing it.[41] Indeed, a major purpose of the American Association for the Study and Prevention of Infant Mortality, formed in in 1909, was to convince the public "not only that a tremendous number of infants died each year, but that many of those deaths could and should be prevented."[42]

Reformers' strategies for prevention shifted over time, but they eventually approached infant mortality as "a problem of motherhood"—an ideology that profoundly and lastingly influenced American conceptions of and approaches to infant mortality.[43] George Newman's classic 1906 publication *Infant Mortality: A Social Problem* captured the underlying sentiment. Newman contended that a mother's ability to care for her baby was the predominant factor in her infant's overall health; the roots of infant mortality lay in mothering.[44]

Implicit in this world view was the conviction that quality of maternal care correlated with infant health. Progressive programs promulgated the notion that every infant's survival and development hinged on its mother's attentiveness to and implementation of scientific medical parenting advice. Determined to improve "mothers' abilities to carry, bear, and rear healthy infants," reformers developed an educational strategy emphasizing maternal instruction.[45] Expectant and new mothers became the most crucial students of infant health. Infant care manuals, stressing that "good mothering required scientific knowledge applied with care," proliferated.[46] Their content conveyed that "a child's health depended mainly on maternal dedication and appropriate medical treatment."[47] In 1914, the Children's Bureau, created to "investigate and report . . . upon all matters pertaining to the welfare of children and child life among all classes," started publishing *Infant Care*, an advice book on infant-rearing rooted in science. It was available free of charge and was the most popular free national guidebook ever published.[48] Through materials like this, American women learned that their own activities, successes, and failures as mothers could influence, either positively or negatively, their children's survival.

American mothers in the 1900s were thus distinct from their predecessors in the 1800s in their understanding of infant deaths as preventable and in their underlying belief that society should share in the task of providing for their children's security and survival.[49] Rima Apple has dubbed the partnership between mothering and medicine "scientific motherhood." The notion of scientific motherhood rested on the idea that mothers' best source for advice in raising healthy children lay within the medical realm. The most skilled, effective mothers relied on physicians and medicine in their everyday parenting habits and decisions. Implicit in scientific motherhood, Apple explains, "was the expectation that modern science would result in more healthy children."[50]

The adoption of infant mortality as a barometer of public health and the cardinal belief that medicine and skillful mothering were necessary to raise healthy babies signaled unprecedented awareness to infant mortality. Reformers success-fully engendered a "virtual explosion of public concern over infant mortality" in the early decades of the twentieth century, and their efforts resulted in dramatic improvements.[51] Over the course of the 1900s, infant mortality in the United States declined dramatically (from 1915 to 1997, rates dropped more than 90 percent, from 100 infant deaths per thousand live births to just 7.2 per thou-sand), but the first quarter of the century was unquestionably the most impact-ful period.[52] By 1930, more than half of the total declines in infant mortality for the twentieth century had already been accomplished.[53] Early twentieth-century Americans lived through the most protracted improvements to the infant mor-tality rate in the nation's history.

The historical construction of infant mortality in general—as a critical mea-sure of public health, as a meaningful personal and social loss, and as a medical problem with medical solutions—ultimately made it much more likely that pro-fessionals would look for and scrutinize uncharacteristic or anomalous causes of infant mortality, such as overlaying. And as infant health campaigns actual-ized appreciable declines in infant mortality rates, in the words of historian Christian Warren, a "decline in epidemiological background noise" resulted, and instances of overlaying presented one category of infant death that could be easily removed.[54]

OVERLAYING IN MEDICAL PERSPECTIVE: BRITAIN AND THE U.S.

Amid heightened international responsiveness to infant mortality, physicians, first in Britain and then in the United States, lent their attention to overlaying. Much as it was for infant deaths in general, the broad sweep of the nineteenth century was a crucial phase of transition in the handling of unexpected and sud-den infant deaths. During this era, physicians began to select and treat episodes of sudden unexpected infant death as subjects of medical inquiry.[55] Progressive-era ideologies moved back and forth across the Atlantic in an exceptional transnational exchange. Americans borrowed all sorts of reform initiatives and strategies from industrialized European nations, ranging from city planning to public schools and sewage to welfare systems. The notion of infant mortality and the ensuing infant welfare movement together comprised one of many issues Americans appropriated from Europe.[56] Most of the earliest professional discus-sions regarding unexpected infant deaths occurred in Europe, and their content and attitudinal considerations transferred to the twentieth-century American medical landscape. Because the overlaying conversation in Britain directly informed parallel conversations in the United States, it is worthwhile to take a brief trip across the Atlantic to ascertain British conceptions of overlaying.

London drew special criticism for its "shamefully high" rates of overlaying, and in the late nineteenth century, British physicians were highly attuned to cases in which babies seemed to pass away inexplicably.[57] In the 1890s, there were more than fifteen thousand recorded cases of overlaying in England and Wales, with 1,774 occurring in 1900 alone. In London, the average annual number of cases was 600.[58] Various sectors decried these numbers and pointed to overlaying as a circumstance of the industrial working class—and especially of inebriate parents—that typically transpired on weekend nights.[59] In *Infant Mortality*, George Newman observed that overlaying, like infant mortality writ large, was a common problem in the "wake of urbanization—that is, high density of population in town—combined with industrial and social conditions." Summarizing other noteworthy features, Newman stated, "Suffocation in bed occurs mostly amongst the youngest infants, is more frequent in winter than in summer, is highest in the poorer districts, and usually more than twice as high on Saturday night and Sunday morning than any other night in the week." The cause, he proffered, is "more probably due to neglect or alcoholism."[60]

Physicians saw overlaying as parents'—mothers'—fault. A report published in *The Lancet* in 1843 explained the case of a "remarkably healthy" infant found deceased in its crib. The author, without hesitation, attributed the death to the child's over-exhausted mother. Although she was a "sober" and "industrious" woman, she had most likely "interfere[d], to a greater or less extent, with the free respiration of the child." This conclusion is especially interesting because when the mother woke up, her child actually lay awake next to her—it was only some time later, while it was napping alone, that the baby was discovered dead. In this instance, the writing physician was so wed to the overlaying framework whereby a mother accidentally suffocated her child that he applied it to a situation in which it made no sense. (The editor did include his response that the "proof of the child having been 'overlain' is exceedingly incomplete.")[61] In a similar situation in the late 1880s, another contributor to *The Lancet* pondered the deaths of two babies. He opined that their deaths could "hardly be wondered at" since they were sleeping in the same bed with two other persons: they must have been overlaid.[62] The immediacy of these conjectures demonstrates how overlaying was typically presumed when a child was discovered deceased in a bed. *Cassell's Book of the Household* exclaimed that "infants who sleep with grown-up people are so often overlaid and suffocated, that there is no doubt of the danger of the practice."[63]

In 1858, city officials in London began to record suffocation deaths separately to distinguish them from deaths by hanging. Within just two decades, one physician noticed that almost all the recorded suffocation deaths were in children under the age of one. (Although the same was true in the United States, no physicians remarked on it.) Based on the victims' youth, physician W. H.

Willcox concluded that it was "obvious that [the deaths] were almost solely due to 'suffocation in bed' or 'overlaying.'" Willcox thought parents were responsible for most of the deaths but also reflected that other children or even cats might cause some. The main factors at hand in these cases, Willcox explained, could be "briefly summed up in the broad terms 'Ignorance and Vice.'"[64]

Willcox was not alone in his opinions. Many commentators adopted incriminating perspectives and associated overlaying cases with particular social groups—the poor, young mothers, illegitimate children, and alcohol users. Such persons were criticized for engaging in behaviors—not-so-subtly attributed to either their ignorance or their vice—that were construed as causative in otherwise unexpected infant mortalities. Importantly, these same groups were later correlated with increased SIDS risk in the 1970s and 1980s.

In the context of a vigilant temperance movement that spanned the Atlantic Ocean and demonized alcohol as the "monster evil" in society, the common finding that overlaying occurred more than twice as often on Saturdays than any other night of the week alarmed observers.[65] In an oft-cited 1892 article, Charles Templeman, a police surgeon in Dundee, Scotland, documented a high correlation between sudden, unexpected infant deaths and weekend nights, poverty, and intoxication.[66] Templeman personally examined 258 overlaying cases (of a total of 399 reported) over the ten years between 1882 and 1891. Almost all of the cases occurred, he said, among the industrial working classes, where parents were often "of dissipated and dissolute habits." One hundred eighteen of the cases (about 45 percent) transpired on a weekend night, a coincidence Templeman called "more than an accidental one." After analysis, Templeman's report asserted that the main causes producing "this great mortality from overlaying" were: "1. Ignorance and carelessness of mothers; 2. drunkenness; 3. overcrowding; and 4. according to some observers, illegitimacy and the life insurance of infants." Templeman was most outraged about numbers 1 and 2 on his list. "The only explanation" for the weekend overlaying rates, he said, was "no doubt that, receiving their week's wages on Saturday, many of the lower classes, among whom these cases are so common, indulge freely in drink, and go to bed more or less intoxicated." As Templeman described it, the drinking habits of the industrial working class were downright malicious, playing "a very prominent part in producing this frightful mortality."[67] Shortly thereafter, D. L. Thomas also observed that in the Limehouse district of London's East End, overlaying occurred "much oftener on some days than on others": weekend days.[68] The city coroner for Manchester likewise explained that infant suffocation deaths were "the usual thing during the week-end."[69] Writing in 1869, Mrs. M. A. Baines wrote that suffocation in bed was a common cause of death among infants. The "so-called 'accidents,'" she said, "which are often surrounded by an unpleasant atmosphere of doubt," mostly occurred on Saturday nights, when parents were in either "a semi-intoxicated or wholly senseless condition." Baines argued that such gross negligence should be criminalized and made punishable by imprisonment; "to admit the plea of drunkenness as an excuse for such wanton neglect," she stated, "is really giving indirect encouragement to immorality and crime."[70]

Through overlaying, these examiners claimed, careless, drunken female caretakers posed a danger to the babies they supervised.[71] Willcox considered "drunkenness of the parents" to be "a very important factor" in recorded cases of suffocation in bed. As he described, an intoxicated mother exposed her baby to the risk of overlaying twofold: first by inadvertently smothering it while sleeping, and second by passing along alcohol to her baby through her milk and rendering it "unable to struggle sufficiently to arouse the drunken parents overlying it."[72] Speaking of suffocation-in-bed deaths, an anonymous contributor to *The Lancet* explained that "in the 'mean streets,' . . . most of these deaths occur from the mothers being more or less drunk and too stupid or too tired to notice that the child they have with them in bed is being suffocated."[73]

These accounts illustrate that medicine sustained society's gendered expectations of women as sober caregivers. Social concerns about men's alcohol consumption manifested in the temperance movement (orchestrated by women); in medicine, physicians were troubled by women's alcohol consumption. Mothers were the foremost physical and moral guardians of the nation's children, and drinking mothers posed a special danger. In a diatribe against female insobriety, William Westcott, an English coroner who later gained notoriety as one of the founders of a secretive magical order that studied the occult, recapitulated the prevailing interpretation of overlaying: "The poorest women of London are the most drunken; the overlaying of infants is most common among the poorest, and we may safely say that parental intemperance is the cause of many such deaths. The drunken woman is a reckless, depraved, dissolute being, with only half a mind and no conscience, who goes stupidly to bed with her baby in her arms when she is drunk, quite careless of the consequences."[74]

In 1924, D. R. Gibson pled the same case, saying that infant deaths correlated strongly with alcohol consumption. Although Gibson's colleagues challenged his claim with lively discussion, in part their criticism stemmed from their association of alcoholism with men much more so than with women, the primary caretakers of infants. An alcoholic father was one thing, but "an intemperate mother," Dr. Spinks exclaimed, "was a calamity." The connectivity between overlaying and drinking was so entrenched that overlaying was cited as a social cost of drinking.[75]

British physicians proffered suggestions to reduce the numbers of infants ostensibly dying from suffocation by overlaying. Their proposals convey that medical contemporaries considered overlaying deaths to be needless, preventable losses. Most authors insisted that families amend their sleeping customs such that babies and children sleep separately from their parents. Solitary sleeping was discussed as such an easy solution to the problem of overlaying that the advice inherently condemned parents. Doctors editorialized that parents who slept with their children had no excuse for their irresponsible, selfish behavior. Speaking to the Lexington and Fayette County Medical Society in Lexington, Kentucky, Henry Enos Tuley insisted that "every newborn baby should be provided with a bassinet, unrockable cradle or crib, and under no circumstances allowed to sleep with its mother." Tuley praised the "excellent" French legislation that prohibited parents from sharing beds with their babies for its ability to "prevent the accident of overlaying the child, which is a possibility to be reckoned with."[76] Even if parents could not afford a crib, one author wrote, "a box, a basket—in short, any one of twenty simple contrivances—might form an extemporised crib in cases where a cradle or cot-bed is not obtainable."[77] Another physician suggested that families unable to purchase a cot could use "a drawer placed on two chairs, an orange box, or a clothes' basket."[78] With such simple alternatives widely available even to families with severe financial restrictions, sleeping with a child posed an "unnecessary risk to human life, with no corresponding advantage, except self-indulgence."[79] If by merely adjusting their bedtime habits parents had the power to protect their children, those who lost children were entirely culpable.

The hypothesis that separate sleeping would eradicate overlaying was so widely accepted that some physicians considered joint parent-child sleeping criminal. To enact broad cultural change, one solution favored instituting penal codes against sharing a bed with a child younger than two years of age.[80] Even for those who shied away from directly charging parents with murder, many argued that going to bed with a child, especially if alcohol was involved, constituted "criminal recklessness" and deserved legal consequences.[81] D. L. Thomas suggested "it be made compulsory that an infant of a certain age should not sleep with the parents, but have a separate cot by the side of the bed, even if it be an old box, which can be made comfortable."[82] Others pointed to Germany, where "overlaying of an infant may be brought [to court] as 'death from carelessness,' and is punishable by three years imprisonment."[83] Physicians who encouraged legal provisions on sleeping arrangements to minimize overlaying uniformly communicated that parents—either purposefully or not—were the primary cause of their own children's deaths.

Tangent to legal doctrines intended to alter sleeping practices, interested medical professionals touted education as an avenue to reduce overlaying. Part of the problem, in their estimation, was that parents were oblivious to the severity of the issue. If parents were taught the dangers of sleeping with their children, as well as of excessive drinking, overlaying could be prevented, physicians said. Beyond legal redress, Willcox advocated that "health visitors" call on

mothers in "crowded districts" to deliver "tactful and kindly advice." He also proposed that school-age girls be taught about overlaying so "when the time arrives
that they themselves become Mothers it will be impossible for such accidents to
happen to their children. Being forewarned they will be fore-armed."[84] Summarizing his approach, Willcox anticipated that "the gradual removal of ignorance
and carelessness of parents, and the awakening to a sense of their responsibilities,
are bound to be followed by the disappearance of deaths from this essentially
preventable cause."[85] William Westcott begged English temperance organizations, charities, and the clergy to take up the mantle of education. "Poor mothers," he urged, "need to be supplied with cradles; they need to be taught that to
overlay a baby is a disgrace, and that to go to sleep with a young infant in the
mother's bed is to court disaster. As to the drunken woman, she should at any
rate be taught that when intoxicated it is a crime to go to sleep with a baby at
the breast."[86]

At the same time, midwifery and nursing guidebooks advised preventing
mothers from sharing beds with their babies for fear of overlaying.[87] "It takes
little to suffocate a child," one warned.[88] Mothers' manuals and physicians' texts
urged the same. "The baby must sleep alone . . . Many a child when sleeping with
its mother or nurse has been suffocated by 'overlaying,'" Henry Arthur Allbutt
cautioned in *Every Mother's Handbook*.[89] In *The Modern Physician*, Andrew Wilson, perturbed by the "astonishing" number of overlaying cases brought about
by "careless or intoxicated mothers," recommended that children sleep in separate beds adjacent to their mothers.[90]

Although most accounts plainly regarded the dominance of weekend cases
to be a consequence of overindulgence in alcohol, a handful attributed it to parents' exhaustion, built up over the course of the work week. Without challenging
the notion that parents caused overlaying, the coroner of London, F. J. Waldo,
defended parents' intelligence and intentions against accusations of ignorance
or maliciousness. "Instead of criminality," Waldo wrote, "in the majority of these
cases . . . suffocation of children was more often due to the desire of the mother
for the welfare of her child." Waldo gave parents the benefit of the doubt, believing that in "nearly all suffocation cases the parents had the clearest character for
sobriety and anxiety for the welfare of their children." He contended that the
preponderance of weekend suffocation deaths was the outcome of overtired
mothers, enervated by their routine responsibilities rather than of intoxication
or recklessness.[91] Interestingly, other British professionals hinted at the confusion surrounding the causes of overlaying when they admitted the difficulty
of "proving anything" in overlaying cases. Medico-legal texts remarked that in
apparent overlaying cases, examiners often found "nothing to positively show
the cause of death."[92] Instead, diagnoses had to emanate "from a consideration
of the collateral circumstances attending death."[93]

In the second half of the 1800s, Americans perceived overlaying—conditioned as a subset of infanticide—as a uniquely British problem, yet they were still conscious of its toll. Indeed, it appears that Americans increasingly began to pay attention to overlaying as a categorical problem precisely because of what they read about overlaying in Britain. On balance, American medicine imitated British impressions of overlaying, and American physicians read what British physicians read. Citing British examples, they reported that overlaying occurred to an "astonishing" degree, predominantly on weekend nights, that it stemmed from parental drunkenness, and that "the failure to provide cradles or cots" for babies was a foundational component.[94]

American pieces on overlaying essentially rebroadcast British pieces on overlaying. U.S. medical journals mostly maintained British ideas that overlaying was rooted in parents' alcohol consumption, negligence, and poverty. Moreover, existing evidence reveals that the class-based confines of overlaying were virtually unchallenged. In 1869, in the *Chicago Medical Examiner*, George Elliot Jr. explained that a mother who slept with her baby left the child vulnerable to accidents such as smothering and overlaying.[95] In the *Tri-State Medical Journal* in 1896, R. C. Blackmer identified overlaying as a frequent outcome of adults and babies sleeping together, especially if adults had consumed intoxicants.[96] Misbehavior was presumed to the extent that righteousness was worthy of comment. In a presentation for the Massachusetts Medico-Legal Society, medical examiner Oliver Howe described two sudden infant death cases, one of which he attributed to suffocation from a pillow and the other to overlaying. In the overlaying case, he made a special point to note his observation that "both parents had a great fondness for their children and grieved deeply over this unfortunate event."[97]

These patterns persisted into the early twentieth century, as U.S. medical publications continued to detail the British overlaying crisis.[98] At an annual meeting of the American Medical Association in 1908, pediatrician Edwin Graham claimed that the "prevalence of drinking among the poor on [Saturday] night is proverbial." Graham deduced that intoxicated mothers were accidentally smothering their children in their sleep, and advocated for "rigid" inquests of overlaying to help eradicate infanticide.[99] Similarly, in a 1912 pediatric text, Edmund Cautley referenced the recurrent overlaying dilemma in Britain and described it as "an avoidable cause of death [that] must be ascribed to carelessness, reckless indifference, or culpable neglect, almost amounting to manslaughter or murder." He pointed to intoxication and "the lack of a cot or cradle for the child" as the two most significant factors, opining that children should be strictly prohibited from sleeping with their parents until they reached the age of two.[100] The same year, out of Boston, the *Scientific Temperance Journal* published content from the anti-alcohol exhibit at the International Congress on Hygiene implicating Saturday-night binge drinking in the British overlaying crisis.[101]

Although some U.S. physicians, to a certain extent, considered overlaying anomalous in the United States, others conveyed that it was a pervasive but overlooked problem. Discrete statistics are scant, and even states that did document overlaying cases reported small numbers. Around the turn of the century, for example, the Rhode Island State Board of Health's annual reports noted a handful of cases per year.[102] This likely explains why the Massachusetts Medico-Legal Society, in 1898, detailed overlaying as "a very common form of death among infants in the cities of England" but "comparatively rare in this country."[103] Yet practicing physicians alluded to overlaying as a more prevalent problem that often flew under the radar. Two New York physicians, in 1890, gauged "the accidental suffocation of infants in bed by bed-clothing and by 'overlaying' a very common occurrence among the lower classes."[104] Into the 1900s, American physicians increasingly took up overlaying as a perturbing, "very common" occurrence.[105] Some American writers employed the notion of "accidental suffocation," one cause of which could be overlaying by a drunken (or epileptic) adult.[106] Other sources suggest that labels such as "unknown," "respiratory disease," or "pneumonia" may have been used for causes of death in lieu of overlaying.[107] In a 1904 piece, one American physician, instancing London's overlaying statistics, wrote that "though all medical men in practice among the poor are frequently brought into contact with cases of overlain infants, it is doubtful many are aware of the enormous mortality of this cause." He went on to explain that most cases were probably accidental, but that mothers "may be the principal cause" sometimes, and observed that the largest number of overlaying deaths transpired on Saturday nights. He recommended that "tactful female visitors" pay visits to mothers and "advise the use of cots" for babies.[108]

Just as medical writings primarily espoused the British interpretation of overlaying, lay publications similarly discussed the predicament. In the second half of the nineteenth century, American periodicals ranging from the *Christian Advocate and Journal* to *The Round Table* to the *New York Observer and Chronicle* reported on the overlaying problem in London. In 1865, when the London *Spectator* published a piece propounding that overlaying deaths were "deliberate" and alleged that some twelve thousand mothers in London alone "must have murdered a child," American publications covered the account almost word for word.[109] Accounts that periodically freckled death notices and local news briefs in papers also assigned mothers fault.[110] U.S. descriptions maintained the British interpretation that overlaying was a morality issue—an evil rooted in intemperance, irresponsibility, and illegitimacy. Pieces presumed that many cases were purposeful, not accidental.[111]

CONCLUSION

At of the turn of the twentieth century there was a recognizable, if small, assemblage of doctors contemplating the problem of overlaying. By 1910, overlaying was included in some medical texts as a subset of the relatively "new" problem of infant mortality. Medical interest in overlaying during the decades surrounding the turn of the century—a period of monumental change in virtually every aspect of life—signaled major shifts in the ways professionals, and ultimately parents, approached sudden infant deaths. Physicians' interpretations, which stressed class and parental culpability and also insisted that a simple preventative solution existed, fundamentally shaped, if not facilitated, the materialization of SIDS.

These scattered reports and commentary, from both Britain and the United States, shed light on some of the most challenging and uncomfortable themes that later embroiled SIDS. The turn-of-the-century professional conversation about overlaying recognized it as a special kind of case and revealed a distinctive discomfort with overlaying. Professionals parceled out and interpreted overlaying separately from other causes of infant mortality. "These deaths of infants in bed," William Westcott explained, "form a class of cases which differ from almost all others."[112]

The original simplicity of overlaying and its perceived associations with "inferior" populations shadowed the evolution of sudden infant mortality throughout the entire twentieth century. Westcott and his contemporaries initially distinguished overlaying based on the fact that they saw it as *preventable*—it was a circumstantial transgression that befell subordinate populations. Especially compared to infant deaths resulting from infectious and congenital disease, suffocation by overlaying presented as easily avoidable. Admonishing parents for bringing about the premature deaths of their children by suffocating them in their beds, physicians consistently expressed frustration over what they viewed as unnecessary losses. Their mentality projected into the future. Indeed, the commentary regarding overlaying highlights the deep roots of blame and guilt surrounding sudden or unexpected infant deaths. The original category of infant mortality that later yielded SIDS—overlaying—was fettered to accusations of parental irresponsibility or ineptitude that abated but were never fully displaced.

Later generations of physicians were unsatisfied with this interpretation. They went on to reappraise the problem and began to offer alternative explanations for overlaying incidents. The first major challenge to the notion of overlaying came by way of a theory that located a precise cause (an oversized thymus gland) for infant deaths. This anatomical hypothesis, and those that succeeded it, only partly supplanted the overlaying category. Alongside new postulates about "these deaths of infants in bed," the *possibility* of overlaying, and all the accusatory abstractions it conjured, remained very much intact.

2 · CAUSE OF DEATH: SIDS

In late 1949, a small group of physicians gathered at the Federal Security Building in Washington, DC, for a single-day convention. Dr. Katherine Bain, director of research for the U.S. Children's Bureau, commenced the meeting by identifying the problem they had come to discuss. "The story is usually this," she explained: "an infant, in apparent good health and usually between the ages of 2 and 5 months, is put to bed . . . Several hours later the infant is found dead . . . The physician, the coroner, or the medical examiner confronted with such a case assumes that the infant has smothered, and without an autopsy, or at most a very sketchy one, signs the infant out as 'accidental mechanical suffocation.'"[1] Decades earlier, doctors delineated this "story" as overlaying.[2] In 1949, Bain and her colleagues dismissed not just overlaying but also two subsequent depictions of the "story" (oversized thymus glands and accidental suffocation) as untenable explanations for these disconcerting deaths of babies. Medicine, they agreed, needed to "start from scratch."[3]

A small group of professionals undertook to do just that, and two decades later they were describing similar episodes with a new moniker: sudden infant death syndrome. The first formal definition of SIDS, proposed in 1969, explained the syndrome as an infant death "unexpected by history and in which a thorough post-mortem exam fails to demonstrate an adequate cause of death."[4] As a diagnosis of exclusion, its only certain marker was that death resulted from the unknown.

At the turn of the century, medicine's conception of "deaths of infants in bed" as overlaying held that the problem was easily explainable and easily preventable. Over the next fifty years, scholars gradually challenged those notions and helped forge the SIDS construction, which was implicitly *un*explainable and *un*preventable. From the historical account of overlaying, doctors crafted new explanations for sudden infant death. In the mid-nineteenth century, they described it as an anatomical defect, the consequence of an oversized thymus. In the 1930s, physicians fashioned a separate rendition, one strikingly akin to overlaying: "accidental mechanical suffocation." Sudden infant death syndrome was the next appellation. SIDS did not apprehend a new problem, but it did embody a fresh approach. It represented a medical reappraisal of "deaths of infants in bed" as inexplicable and also reflected a crucial social reconfiguration. Where overlaying was a mishap born of negligence, ignorance, or misconduct, sudden infant death was a tragedy whose surviving victims deserved respect and empathy.

The transitions in nomenclature between overlaying and SIDS show the continuity of certain beliefs about sudden infant deaths. In particular, misgivings about parental wrongdoing and suffocation held steady through different interpretations of sudden infant death. In addition, the basic notion of the SIDS configuration—inexplicability—framed a paradox that stymied medical progress. How could Americans come to grips with a medical condition defined by the unknown?

In his book *How We Die*, the acclaimed surgeon and writer Sherwin Nuland wrote that "putting a name to a demon helps to decrease its fearsomeness."[5] In 1970, a *Washington Post* article reported that the "biggest breakthrough" in studying sudden infant death was "to identify the mysterious child killer and give it a name."[6] Yet SIDS medicine was constantly inhibited by its paradoxical nature; doctors' medical task was to explain the patently unexplainable. And for all its novelty, the conception of SIDS clearly drew from its past, betraying its origins in overlaying. In "naming the demon" of SIDS, Americans initiated a new set of parental fears and anxieties, one delineated by worries, suspicions, and dead ends.

THE THYMUS THEORY OF SUDDEN INFANT DEATH

At the dawn of the twentieth century, the notion of overlaying coexisted with another way of explaining sudden infant death: the thymus theory. The thymus is a small organ that functions in the body's immune system. Located beneath the breastbone near the neck, it extends across the windpipe.[7] In the past, doctors were aware the gland existed but uncertain as to its purpose—they called it an "organ of mystery."[8]

Starting in the 1800s, a number of physicians contended that abnormally enlarged thymuses were causing sudden deaths in children by pushing up against their tracheas and suffocating them. In 1889, Vienna physician Arnold Paltauf coined the concept of status thymicolymphaticus to convey the physical state of having an enlarged thymus. Paltauf provided no exact measurements explaining what constituted "enlarged" (nor did other contemporary pathologists). Not thoroughly convinced that physical pressure from the thymus alone was enough to cause death, Paltauf described a constitutional disorder.[9] An oversized thymus did press against the airway, he said, as well as other nearby organs. Paltauf theorized that the cumulative pressure could produce a host of problematic respiratory symptoms and breathing difficulties. Having a lymphatic constitution or being in a lymphatic state could be lethal. The danger, according to Paltauf, was that an enlarged thymus could leave patients vulnerable, predisposing them to sudden death if they experienced any number of subtle triggers, like surprise, fright, or stress. By modern standards, Paltauf's work was "at best, anecdotal," but it ignited a sizable literature. Respected medical minds accepted status thymicolymphaticus as real, and professionals published over eight hundred articles on it by 1922.[10]

Physicians and historians have wrestled with the question of how status thymicolymphaticus—subsequently exposed as "medical mythology"—gained such wide acceptance.[11] There is no singular explanation, but historian Ann Dally and cardiologist Warren Guntheroth offer some insight. Dally argues that status thymicolymphaticus was "invented . . . to fill a gap" in the mid-late 1800s. She and Guntheroth emphasize the capacity for nineteenth-century scientific medicine to catalogue "new" diseases by fabrication. Dally points to labels such as "ovariomania," "hystero-epilepsy," and "railway spine" as contemporary diagnostic inventions of convenience, and ties the rise of status thymicolymphaticus to the growing popularity of chloroform in the second half of the 1800s. Occasionally, when physicians administered the anesthetic, younger patients died suddenly. Dally suggests that doctors who experienced this were "inclined to think that there must be . . . something wrong with the patient that had not been detected"; status thymicolymphaticus offered a precise pathological explanation for such deaths. Guntheroth adds that pathologists may have been "simply uncomfortable admitting ignorance of the cause of death." He also posits that they may have had a morally "loftier motive"—to defend female caretakers against charges of murder.[12] "Whether through the weakness of medical science or through the strength of the pathologists' convictions," Guntheroth writes, Paltauf's theory "fell on fertile grounds." The "elegant unfounded diagnosis" endured.[13]

Its treatments were harmful. One option was a thymectomy, a surgical procedure that removed the thymus altogether. The operation was "imperative" for children—and even more so for babies—who presented with respiratory symptoms attributed to an enlarged thymus.[14] Thymectomies corresponded with the nineteenth-century surgical trend of removing organs whose functionality evaded medical knowledge or appeared to cause patients' symptoms. Yet the procedure had such high mortality rates—one in three according to one study—that it was untenable.[15]

After it was developed, the more prevalent solution to the apparent problem of an enlarged thymus in the late 1800s was radiation. Doctors used X-ray technology to shrink children's thymus glands and hopefully alleviate the symptoms making them susceptible to sudden death.[16] After the first successful case report in 1907, almost every medical textbook recommended X-ray therapy for over-sized thymuses.[17] The protocol was "preventative medicine." In 1924, physicians at the University of Michigan "immediately" treated infant patients diagnosed with enlarged thymus glands with X-rays. The therapy (one treatment per week for three consecutive weeks) was standard hospital practice.[18] A Boston physician in 1934 explained that it was "common procedure" to X-ray *all* newborn babies to ascertain whether they had an enlarged thymus and then, if necessary, administer further X-ray treatments "with the expectation that sudden death may be prevented."[19]

In the 1930s, the thymus theory became a point of contention. Timing had thwarted investigators' attempts to evaluate the theory's basic premise. Still fledgling fields, both pediatrics and radiology had yet to establish basic anatomical norms, especially for newborns and infants. The parameters for a "normal" thymus in a child or baby were based on incomplete knowledge. In the early 1900s, scattered studies began to signal that those ideas were flawed. Physicians realized that what had been recorded as pathologically large thymuses were in fact normal in size, while the "normal" thymuses in controls had actually been rather small. Thymus glands, like most lymphatic tissue, it turns out, mature backwards, shrinking rather than growing from infancy to childhood.[20] These details clashed with the hypothesis that oversized thymuses were responsible for the deaths of infants, but the theory was buried only gradually.

Professional doubts escalated in the 1930s. As Thomas Cone explained, the more researchers tried to "pinpoint the pathogenesis" of status thymicolymphaticus, the more "nebulous" it became.[21] In Britain, medical professors in the 1920s were so concerned about how frequently enlarged thymuses were cited as a cause of death that they compelled the Medical Research Council to investigate. In its preliminary report, the committee of pathologists concluded that normal thymus glands varied greatly in size. It announced that "*there is no evidence to show that there is any connection between the presence of a large glandular thymus and death from unexpected or trivial causes.*" Another large analysis in 1927 called the status thymicolymphaticus diagnosis "largely nonsense" and said that it had "no more value than affirmative evidence in cases of witchcraft [and] . . . ought to be abandoned." When the British Medical Council released its final report in 1931, it conveyed that the diagnosis was a charade, concluding that "there is no evidence that so-called status thymico-lymphaticus has any existence as a pathological entity."[22] In 1932 Dr. Edith Boyd of Minneapolis composed a lengthy article to rectify the misconception that prominent thymus glands could lead to deaths in infants, asserting that thymic size was unrelated to sudden death in infancy.[23] That same year, though, in the same journal, a feature article stated that scholarship on the role of the thymus in sudden death was highly inconsistent and that medical opinion was still divided. "While probably rare," author Edward Campbell said, "death from pressure of an enlarged thymus does occur."[24]

Ten years later, status thymicolymphaticus was still a source of disagreement. One physician described medical knowledge of the thymus as "a gradual progression of confusing details."[25] Although the thymus theory was not decisively disproved, it was becoming unhinged by the end of the 1940s. Physicians who rejected that infants dying suddenly and unexpectedly even possessed oversized thymuses pushed their colleagues to cease radiation therapy and turn their attention elsewhere. A reasonable first step, urged Canadian physicians Alton Goldbloom and F. W. Wiglesworth, would be to perform rigorous autopsies on relevant cases, which, they speculated, would "reveal not one but a multiplicity of causes of sudden death."[26] Such pleas were bolstered at mid-century by new evidence on the dangers of treating "enlarged" thymuses.

Physicians knew by 1910 that X-ray exposure could contribute to the development of cancer; it is unclear why they overlooked this threat in babies and children irradiated for status thymicolymphaticus. In 1949, two doctors from Cincinnati published an eye-opening case report: their five-year-old patient, treated for a large thymus with X-ray as a newborn, had developed cancer. The next year, an article published in *Cancer* reported that children who had received radiation therapy to shrink their thymuses were one hundred times more likely to develop thyroid cancer than children spared from the treatment. Even though by the middle of the 1950s, "the unusual incidence of cancer in those who had been irradiated was widely known and discussed," the "possible significance of the cancer evidence took some time to penetrate." In later decades, when alternative theories and prospective treatments for sudden infant death burgeoned, physicians often recollected the iatrogenic illness that resulted from treating status thymicolymphaticus—a condition that "as far as doctors are concerned . . . does not exist and . . . never did exist"—as a cautionary device.[27]

ACCIDENTAL MECHANICAL SUFFOCATION (AMS)

While the validity of the thymus theory diminished, suffocation crept into position as the prevailing explanation for sudden infant death. As pathologist Bruce Beckwith bluntly described, "with the decline of the thymic theory, blame again descended upon those caring for the dead infant."[28] Beginning in the 1930s, the prospect of "accidental mechanical suffocation" (AMS) started to eclipse the thymus theory as the focal point in research.

This broad designation of suffocation—AMS—subsumed the overlaying label. When professionals repackaged overlaying under the premise of AMS, they accounted for multiple kinds of suffocation in bed. AMS encompassed overlaying, suffocation by bedclothes, and suffocation in bed.

The depiction of AMS precipitated critical interpretative shifts. Physicians conversing about AMS debated the merits of suffocation itself as a credible hypothesis, and regardless of their persuasions, they were all on the same mission. They sought ways to explain and label sudden infant death that were anatomically accurate and more considerate of parents. While still acknowledging overlaying as a hazard, the AMS label did challenge presumptions about parental wrongdoing. It also moved sudden infant death even more resolutely into the medical realm as both a scientific and a social issue.

One of the first practitioners to reflect on the issue was Sidney Farber. Prior to his widely recognized work on children's cancer in the postwar era (which gained him an appellation as the father of modern chemotherapy), Farber published an article on infant deaths from streptococcus infections in the *New England Journal of Medicine*.[29] Describing his study, Farber summarized that the typical case was a child "said to have been perfectly well until the sudden onset of the fatal illness." The strep infection could act so quickly that it left only traces of its presence at autopsy. "The streptococcus may cause death with such rapidity," Farber wrote in 1934, "that its killing effect may be compared to that of powerful chemical poison." Two patients stood out to Farber. Both had been "found dead a short time after having been put to bed apparently in good health." Both were diagnosed—misdiagnosed, Farber thought—as suffocation. Neither underwent an autopsy. Skeptical, Farber consulted Massachusetts's death records. For 1932, he found seventy-six recordings of "thymic death" and forty-eight recordings of "accidental mechanical suffocation."[30] They were the two predominant explanations for sudden infant deaths.

To Farber, both labels were problematic. Based on contemporary research showing that supposedly "pathologically large" thymus glands were actually normal, Farber dismissed thymic death as an unjustified explanation. The label might offer "an easy way out in distressing incidents of sudden death," Farber said, but it was "misinformation," and pathologists should discontinue its use.[31] He considered the suffocation label equally fallacious, and combatted it as an inappropriate outgrowth of accidents formerly defined as overlaying. He clarified that overlaying did sometimes occur, but that the concept failed to account for situations in which infants were found *alone*, without "any evidence of foul play or of accident." "It seems logical," Farber suggested, that suffocation not be diagnosed "merely upon the basis of a story of sudden unexpected death and observations on the outside of the body." Reflecting the contemporary supremacy of the body over the environment in disease etiology, Farber called for thorough anatomical postmortems in all suspected cases.[32]

Around the same time, William M. Gafafer, a senior statistician with the U.S. Public Health Service, published a series analyzing national statistics on fatal accidents in childhood. One of his pieces looked exclusively at AMS; among babies less than one year old, it was the leading cause of death by a substantial margin. In 1930, of the 2,405 babies who died accidentally, 35 percent (849) suffocated. Suffocation killed four times as many babies as the next leading cause of death (burns).[33] Startled, Gafafer set out to determine the nation's accidental suffocation rates in previous years. From 1925 to 1932, accidental causes of death accounted for 1,921 of the total 121,366 infant deaths; of those, suffocation accounted for 687 deaths—about 37 percent of the accidental deaths and about 1.6 percent of all the deaths. Although his data only accounted for race in the Southeast, in that region blacks suffered between two and three times higher rates of AMS compared to any other area of the country and compared to whites in the same area.[34] Gafafer's display of evidence confirmed what Farber had found to be true in Massachusetts: AMS was a problem.

Farber's and Gafafer's work drew attention to the extent of AMS during the exact time when status thymicolymphaticus was coming under critical scrutiny. As the thymus theory retreated further out of the picture, AMS moved to the foreground in medical literature. In the 1940s, researchers gradually expanded on the details Farber and Gafafer reported. At first, they underscored the scope of AMS cases. By the end of the decade, professionals were either defending or refuting the legitimacy of AMS, and suffocation in general, as accurate ways to explain sudden infant deaths.

In 1944, an article in the *Journal of Pediatrics* stirred the debate. Harold Abramson, lead epidemiologist for the Division of Maternity and Newborn Services of the Bureau of Preventable Diseases in New York City, was appalled by the scale of AMS. He said it was an understudied, "sadly neglected" issue. The number of AMS infant deaths had risen notably over the preceding decade. In 1933, there were 692 cases nationwide; in 1942, there were 1,333. Abramson defined AMS as the "occlusion of the external openings (nose and mouth) to the air passages by some object so that smothering occurs by obstructive cutting off of air supply." He implicitly endorsed the suffocation aspect of the label as accurate, and insisted that the problem, especially because it was largely preventable, demanded public and medical attention. "Vigorous efforts," Abramson said, "should be made by public health agencies to acquaint parents, nurses, physicians, and others concerned with the care of infants with the hazards to which these babies are unwittingly exposed."[35]

In the hopes of working towards a remedy, Abramson conducted a review study of 139 cases (between 1939 and 1943) and identified significant commonalities. He found that AMS typically happened before babies turned six months, mostly when they were between two and three months old. More victims were male, and more babies succumbed during the winter (November through January). Fifteen percent of Abramson's case pool was black, and "in most instances the families were of the lower income groups." Sixty-eight percent of babies were found facedown, compared to only 17 percent found lying on their backs. AMS occurred in cribs, beds, and carriages, and was correlated with blankets and coverings, mattresses, pillows, or parents' bodies.[36]

For Abramson, the circumstantial evidence was clear: AMS was synonymous with smothering. Abramson argued that suffocation was the recognizable mechanism of death *and* that it occurred accidentally. He saw AMS as preventable—parents could preempt accidental suffocations by removing the objects that caused them. Abramson recommended caretakers fashion clear sleeping spaces for babies.[37] Other scientists concurred that AMS was a problem, but for the most part rejected Abramson's environmental appraisal of its causes. Even the few scholars who were sympathetic to the premises behind Abramson's ideas—that oxygen deprivation was at the heart of these cases—underscored that a healthy baby would "resist *strenuously* any attempt to smother him."[38] Indeed, researchers over the next four decades constantly pointed to Abramson's interpretations as emblematic of the very notions they aspired to dispel.

Right on the heels of Abramson's piece, for example, Paul Woolley, a pediatrician in Portland, Oregon, criticized the entire understanding of AMS. Woolley seconded Abramson's concerns about the prevalence of episodes *recorded* as AMS, but he saw a different problem. Instead of suffocation, Woolley thought something entirely else was at play. His commentary contained an anatomical component, but Woolley's opposition to AMS stemmed primarily from his sympathies for parents struggling to cope with the sudden death of their child.

Woolley agreed with Abramson that the reported numbers of babies dying from AMS were striking. "It is difficult to read a city newspaper over an extended period of time," he observed, "and not be impressed by the frequency with which infants appear to be asphyxiated in their beds." But Woolley thought the AMS description was all wrong—and that it was misleading doctors and parents. "A distressingly large number of babies die without noticeable predisposing cause," he explained, "but is the primary premise correct, that all reported as having suffocated actually died from simple occlusion of air passages by bedding, sleeping attire, or other mechanical means?"[39]

For Woolley, the answer was "no." He argued that the suffocation explanation was based more on "folklore" than scientific observation (an ironic stance given the flimsy nature of his own evidence), and that the evidence for AMS simply did not add up. Observing the frequency of deaths in minority and economically disadvantaged families—a correlation Abramson and Gafafer both noted—Woolley commented that "crowding and poor living standards" were more likely to play a role than was mechanical suffocation.[40] Moreover, he faulted AMS for what it supposed about families: "we should be overly critical of a diagnosis which saddles the family with the entire blame for the death of their babies; for having allowed him to smother." Instead, said Woolley, doctors should assuage parents' worries and "leave the family with a clear conscience." He even reasoned that the thymus theory was preferable to AMS specifically because it "implied no negligence."[41] Woolley's concerns about parents' guilt were significant in motivating him to challenge the accuracy of the AMS diagnosis.

To make his case, Woolley vaguely recounted an earlier project in which he and a colleague analyzed infants' breathing while covering their faces with various bedding materials. The infants successfully maneuvered around every obstacle posed, he reported, with the sole exception of a tightly-pulled rubber sheet. Ordinary bedding materials caused babies "no discomfort until sufficient time had elapsed for heat and humidity to come into play." Woolley also said he was unable to induce anoxemia (reduced blood-oxygen levels) "by having the subjects sleep with nose and mouth closely approximated to mattresses and pillows." Every baby, he proclaimed, even "the smallest," could roll to secure an airway.[42]

Woolley left no record of specific methodologies or measurements, and gave no indication as to the numbers and ages of his subjects. His article was more of an editorial than an analytic scientific study. As multiple commentators assessed in the 1980s and 1990s, Woolley's conclusions were based on shoddy evidence by all modern standards.[43] Building from his subjective observations, Woolley urged that suffocation be reserved only "for instances when actual deprivation of oxygen by mechanical means can be proved." If evidence was unclear, Woolley hesitantly suggested that "perhaps we should be pushed so far as to admit that we are ignorant of the cause of death, thereby saving the family the stigma of having allowed their baby to smother in the bedclothes."[44]

Despite its theoretical nature, researchers pointed to Woolley's paper for decades as manifest proof that normal infants in normal sleeping environments simply could not be suffocated. In a 1967 review of the world literature, Marie Valdes-Dapena, an expert known for her objectivity, cited Woolley's work as an "experiment" that "established the fact that a well child—even a newborn—cannot be suffocated by ordinary bed clothing."[45] Twenty years later, in the *Journal of Pediatric Nursing*, Susan Swoiskin informed readers that Woolley had "showed that it is impossible to smother a baby with bed clothes."[46] Although Woolley's descriptions were nowhere near scientific evidence, his narrative persuaded a multitude of researchers that suffocation in bed was a careless explanation for the sudden death of a healthy baby.[47]

In 1945, W. H. Davison, a coroner in Birmingham, England, reiterated the lack of concerted medical attention paid to sudden unexpected infant death, in Britain and the United States. Like Woolley, he rejected suffocation as unrealistic; unlike Woolley, he presented actual anatomical details to support his stance.

Davison reviewed a series of 318 asphyxia-related infant deaths from 1938 to 1944. "Quite a number," he observed, "were discovered in circumstances that suggested suffocation (such as with their faces pressed into pillows). Yet Davison, after performing autopsies, found the explanation wanting. "My experience," he shared, "is that doctors who . . . honestly believed that a child had been suffocated by mechanical means have frequently expressed their surprise on attending the post-mortem examination, which showed that death was not due to these causes but to other factors."[48]

Of the 318 cases studied, 108 transpired in bed with a parent or another person. Davison found, though, that autopsies showed visible evidence of mechanical asphyxia (suffocation) in only 18 of those 108 "in-bed" cases. Among the remaining 210 cases in which babies were discovered alone, just six babies showed visible evidence of having suffocated.[49] Davison's data convinced him that doctors needed to look more closely when infants died from what looked to be suffocation. Circumstantial evidence alone was inadequate; autopsies uncovered the truth.

Davison's logic extended beyond scientific accuracy. Autopsies were necessary, he elaborated, "both from the point of view of correct statistical information and in some cases to relieve the mother from mental torture or reproach." For grieving parents, he explained, "the relief . . . is often very apparent when informed that the death was due to circumstances beyond their control." From both a medical and a humane approach, postmortem exams were "indispensable as part of the routine investigation in every case where suffocation is considered a likely cause of death."[50]

These physicians were all practicing in the World War II era, when doctors were highly esteemed. Physicians delivered medical treatment, arbitrated medical science, and guarded patients. They frequently concealed or withheld information from patients to "protect" them. In line with the traditional ethics in medicine stretching as far back as Hippocrates, doctors would often "keep bad news to themselves." Many physicians believed that as caretakers and healers they were qualified and responsible for determining the appropriate level of information to disclose to patients. As historian David Rothman explains, this judgment was "borne not only of paternalism . . . but [also] of a confidence that doctors were capable of substituting their judgment for that of their patients, able to spare them pain because they intuited their patients' wishes."[51] Physicians such as Woolley and Davison expressed sincere concerns for the emotional health and well-being of parents who lost a baby. Both men were confident their perspective was anatomically precise, but it is also possible that their interests in recasting AMS under different labels stemmed partly from professional medical paternalism and the convention of "protecting" patients by modifying information perceived as harmful or unnecessary.

Regardless, their work redirected attention towards an infective description, and in the 1940s the forecast for curing infections had never looked better. Medicine was churning out "magic bullet" solutions like Salvarsan (to treat syphilis), sulfanilamide (used to treat strep), penicillin (a revolutionary antibiotic used to treat a variety of infections), and streptomycin (an antibiotic used to treat tuberculosis). After the middle of the century, polio vaccines similarly taught that infections could be swiftly conquered with fierce medical investigation. The 1940s and 1950s were the heyday of what Allan Brandt and Martha Gardner describe as the "paradigm of biomedicine"—diseases were located, singled out, and then treated.[52] This find-isolate-eliminate approach had been successful with some of the nation's most visible medical maladies. In the context of these triumphs, the proposition that sudden infant deaths mostly resulted from infection held the tantalizing promise of a new magic bullet.

At the time, no one forwarded an infection theory of sudden infant death more assertively than Jacob Werne and his wife Irene Garrow, both pathologists in New York City.[53] In 1947, they published "Sudden Death of Infants Allegedly Due to Mechanical Suffocation" in the *American Journal of Public Health*. The paper, as its title implies, directly refuted the suffocation theory. Werne and Garrow announced that healthy infants died suddenly and inexplicably with "regularity" in larger cities, and case reports were swelling nationwide. In 1942, the *Statistical Bulletin* of the Metropolitan Life Insurance Company pointed to smothering as "the greatest hazard encountered during infancy." Between 1934 and 1944, AMS cases increased by 57 percent.[54]

In New York City, where Werne and Garrow worked, it was standard protocol to refer any sudden, unexpected, or otherwise unusual death to the medical examiner's office. Over a span of fifteen years, the couple had autopsied 167 infants found deceased in a crib, carriage, or bed, whose deaths would have been "ordinarily certified" as AMS. Werne and Garrow found no evidence of suffocation. Rather, 43 autopsies revealed that a fatal disease (such as mastoiditis, congenital heart disease, or bronchopneumonia) had caused death. The remaining 124 cases were still unexplained after a gross autopsy, so Werne and Garrow performed additional microscopic study. Without exception, they found signs of inflammation in babies' respiratory tracts, as well as other lesions. They determined that 31 deaths were linked to violence and that the other 93 cases were best explained as "fulminating [sudden and severe] respiratory disease."[55]

Werne and Garrow reviewed another 67 incidents that occurred "under circumstances in which there could be no possible allegation of smothering . . . but in whom smothering is ordinarily alleged." (They excluded smothering as a possibility in these cases based on the fact that parent witnesses observed the events.) The results corroborated their conclusions: the majority cause of death was acute respiratory disease. From their perspective, the problem was fundamentally of the body; they never even mentioned race or demography. As Werne and Garrow summarized, "The evidence we have assembled indicates that accidental mechanical suffocation is hardly an acceptable explanation for sudden death during infancy." Among alleged AMS cases, "as a rule," they asserted, diligent postmortem investigations confirmed a different cause of death: acute respiratory disease.[56]

The false explanation of AMS, they postulated, was "based on a misinterpretation by the layman" and persisted simply because it was convenient. AMS, Werne and Garrow warned, was a weighty error. It contributed to "the feeling of culpable negligence experienced by the mother or other person in attendance" and added "considerably to the intensity of these tragedies." The "proper approach to this problem," the pair advised, "requires that failure to find a cause of death be readily admitted and honestly recorded; and not concealed under such listing of our mortality tables as accidental mechanical suffocation and status thymicolymphaticus." Werne and Garrow left absolutely no doubt as to their stance: "List No. 182, accidental mechanical suffocation (of the *International List of Causes of Death*), is erroneous."[57]

Werne and Garrow's research was exceptionally impactful. It presented a serious scientific challenge to the notion that AMS was an acceptable way to explain a particular type of infant death, and subsequent projects continued to explore its plausibility. Most authors castigated AMS and threw a wrench in the very possibility of suffocation. But sustained presumptions that healthy infants found dead had either been suffocated or were victims of some sort of "foul play" did not die out.[58] Indeed, the continuation of these ideas fueled the "anti-suffocationists." Some practitioners still believed that parents, and especially mothers, were implicated. Commenting on accidental infant suffocation in England in 1948, for example, Letitia Fairfield explained that "one point leaps to the eye; the practices which experience shows to be dangerous are nearly all due to lack of personal care of the baby—of 'mothering' in the old-fashioned sense."[59] The matters of suffocation and the parental role in "causing" it have never been fully resolved. Both questions have bedeviled the SIDS diagnosis since before its inception. But emerging scholarship disputing AMS in the 1940s, in the words of historian Todd Savitt, "marked the start of a new era in thinking about sudden unexplained infant deaths."[60]

STARTING FROM SCRATCH: THE AMS CRITICS CONVENE

That "new era in thinking" commenced with Katherine Bain and her colleagues' impulse to "start from scratch" at the end of their 1949 Conference on Sudden Death in Infancy. The group quickly agreed that sudden infant deaths recorded as AMS were not actually the result of suffocation.[61]

Measuring AMS was problematic. Where available, national numbers were not comprehensive or reliable. W. Thurber Fales, a public health physician from Baltimore, was unable to deliver his planned presentation, "AMS Incidence in Cities," because he had such difficulty amassing statistics from urban centers. He recommended implementing a program to investigate "the whole group of sudden, unexpected deaths among infants"—not only AMS cases. Amassing data, echoed pathologist Paul Cannon, "would be the first thing to do."[62]

Especially given that they barely had tabs on the problem, those present wondered what to tell American parents. They decided that families needed to know AMS was a misapprehension. It had destructive social ramifications, triggered guilt, and sometimes provoked familial divisions. Sending a uniform message to the public that AMS was inaccurate could alleviate "the damage done to parents who must live on and have a sense of blame for something they could not have avoided." Discussants treated "the psychologic trauma" in families who experienced AMS as an urgent matter. They strategized to propagate the idea that "considered medical opinion indicates that suffocation is not the usual explanation of these [AMS] deaths."[63]

In unanimously negating AMS, these conversations crept towards the possibility that at least some unexpected infant deaths were *unexplained*. Those present straddled the fence on the matter of explicability—they collectively expressed confidence that an autopsy and postmortem investigation tended to reveal some cause of death (most often, respiratory disease), but they also started to flirt with the admission that in some cases they were unsure what was going on. Farber summarized this stance when he said that pathologists had well established that "there is no such thing as mechanical suffocation, [and] an adequate cause of death can be found in post-mortem examinations, [but] that there are probably a great many other conditions which are responsible for unexpected death which have nothing to do with suffocation."[64] The problem was, no one knew what they were. Everyone agreed that suffocation be discarded, and most favored the alternative explanation of respiratory disease, but it still only applied to a fraction of cases. Respiratory infection could not uniformly replace the AMS framework. What else was going on?

Concluding the meeting, Bain outlined a data collection strategy that partly came to fruition by the 1960s. She imagined a study in which a handful of cities enlisted coroners or medical examiners to refer cases to pediatric pathologists for autopsy exams and epidemiologic review. One central office would collect and analyze the materials. She and her colleagues moved to create the Commission for the Study of Unexpected Death During Infancy. They specifically opted to leave out the word "prevention" from the commission's title for fear that it might give a false impression. "The sense of the meeting," Farber summed up, "is that we will study first and then prevent."[65] This became the mantra for the next two decades, during which the "study" venture unfolded and ultimately culminated in the circumscribing of a new condition, one that was plagued from the beginning by the notion of suffocation.

STUDY FIRST

The meeting at the Federal Building in 1949 represented a certain break from the past. All present dispelled AMS as a misdiagnosis, and concurred that the problem of unexpected death in infancy was extensive. Although most of them had definite ideas about the next best plausible explanation, they decided to step back and evaluate before getting ahead of themselves.

First, they took preliminary steps to remove AMS from medical and lay minds. The Children's Bureau worked to spread the word to parents in publications like *The Child, Today's Health* (the American Medical Association's magazine for the public), and *McCall's*. With titles such as "Babies Don't Smother," pieces conveyed that suffocation was off the mark. Recounting interviews with mothers whose babies' deaths were wrongly documented as AMS, they stressed that parents were not at fault. They derided the idea of smothering as "superstition" that "wrecked . . . family happiness."[66] They also, however, in line with researchers' persuasions about respiratory disease, warned parents to be attentive to signs of infection and take common cold symptoms seriously. "A sick baby should be looked at every two hours or so day and night . . . At any time, he might take a turn for the worse."[67] A précis in the *Journal of the American Medical Association* updated physicians and reiterated the clear notion that smothering and suffocation were slipshod explanations for a widespread problem.[68]

Arguably the most important outcome of the conference, however, was that the U.S. Public Health Service agreed to bankroll four studies in different locations, just as Bain had envisioned. Medical examiners in Boston (Richard Ford), Baltimore (Russell Fisher), Cleveland (Lester Adelson), and New York (Jacob Werne and Irene Garrow) were enlisted to conduct investigations into sudden infant death. Their work was planned to start in 1950. In Boston, Ford apparently met so many legal obstacles that he never launched a study. In Baltimore, Fisher decided his results were too inconclusive to pursue publication.[69] Werne and Garrow sustained the work they had already started in New York City. They published preliminary results, reiterating their stance that AMS was completely "unsupported" as a mechanism of death, but their study was discontinued abruptly after Werne's career disintegrated in the aftermath of an indictment for professional misconduct.[70] After New York ended its participation in the study, only Cleveland was left standing.

Lester Adelson cultivated an abiding interest in sudden infant death early in his medical career. He attended undergraduate at Harvard University before completing his medical degree at Tufts College Medical School in 1939, and served as a physician with the Air Force during World War II. When he returned to the United States, Adelson completed a pathology residency at Hartford Hospital in Connecticut and then a fellowship in legal medicine at Harvard.[71] A leader in the young field of forensic pathology, Adelson also became a passionate advocate for families, once describing the medical examiner as "the family physician amongst the bereaved."[72]

As a medical student at Tufts, Adelson witnessed a single case of sudden infant death, interpreted to him at the time as "smothering in bedclothes." Later, Adelson intimated that this episode—and its dissatisfying explanation—touched him. Although at first he scarcely encountered this "very special kind of tragedy," Adelson began to regularly observe cases after he accepted a job in 1950 as a medical examiner in Cleveland, Ohio. His dedication to sorting out sudden infant death—a phenomenon he saw as "a scientific, medical, legal, and humanitarian problem all wrapped into one"—ultimately earned Adelson unofficial status as one of the founders of its modern field of research.[73]

In many ways, Adelson's impressions reflect the major transition that occurred in the 1950s: he stressed inexplicability. Even after years of dedicated research, Adelson conceded, often and willingly, that he remained clueless about the causes of sudden infant death. "I can make some kind of sense out of putrefied bodies from Lake Erie, incinerated hulks from fires, sudden coronary deaths without 'new' anatomic changes which I can demonstrate, multiple gunshot homicides, etc. etc.," he wrote to Page Hudson, chief medical examiner at the University of North Carolina at Chapel Hill, "but the answer to [sudden unexpected infant death] continues to elude my best efforts."[74]

In 1956, Adelson and his colleague Eleanor Kinney, a scientist at Western Reserve University, published the results of the only successfully completed study funded by the 1950 Public Health Service grant. Printed in *Pediatrics*, the official journal of the American Academy of Pediatrics, the piece surely encountered a sizable audience of professional readers. Adelson and Kinney compared findings from 126 children who died without any apparent cause (between the ages of ten days and twenty-four months) to a small set of sixteen control cases consisting of children who had died "rapidly as a result of violence." In each case, Adelson and Kinney performed an autopsy, observed the death scene, and interviewed parents. They "carefully appraised the socio-economic level of the family, the mother's intelligence and integrity, and her ability to care for the child and to recognize symptoms." Families, Adelson and Kinney reported, "welcome[d] the chance to speak with informed professionals about their child's death."[75]

Unsure of little else, both authors rejected suffocation: "mechanical asphyxia by bedclothes is not a serious consideration." Adelson and Kinney found no alternative etiological leads but noted that many children had exhibited cold-like symptoms in the days before they died: coughing, sneezing, runny noses, fussy behavior, lack of appetite, or spitting up. The pattern was strange and prevalent enough to warrant mention, but the symptoms were always so minor that they failed to worry adults. Though this finding perplexed them, Adelson and Kinney still clarified that their research "disclosed no clinical syndrome which should alert parent or physician to the prospect of sudden and unexpected death."[76]

The study established new standard methods. Autopsies became the crux of serious investigations into sudden infant death. Conducting home visits was another innovation. Home interviews enabled researchers to collect data, offer information, and console parents. Adelson's study denoted routine factors of consideration: race, class, sex, timing, age, season, pathological autopsy results, and home quality. Importantly, Adelson and Kinney discussed their methodology as a public health delivery mechanism: "proper dissemination of . . . information to the parents of dead infants and to the general public has practically eliminated the notion in this area that these deaths are accidental. Thus a real dividend of reassurance and peace of mind has been contributed to the community."[77] Even though his work involved assessing parents, the implied message here, and one Adelson would later articulate much more explicitly, was that responsible medical study could, if nothing else, help parents recover from their loss.

Adelson's work emerged in the context of growing medical acknowledgement of sudden unexplained infant mortality. By the end of the 1950s, Adelson and others had refined the medical case against suffocation, and their work signaled two discursive shifts. First, armed with more evidence, researchers increasingly detailed unexpected infant fatalities as both medical and social predicaments. Authors—in the U.S. and in some other industrialized western countries like Britain and Australia—made special note of the negative psychological implications associated with "inaccurate and distressing" death certificate labels.[78] Their critique of suffocation swelled from anatomical to personal. Not only was suffocation a misnomer that failed to capture the "true nature" of unexpected infant deaths, it was also stigmatizing.[79] Pathologists contended that the label "accidental suffocation" had harmful consequences—its use could "amount to a life sentence of self-reproach for the parents."[80]

Second, physicians started to admit more openly that they had no idea what was going on. George Carroll, a pathologist in Richmond, captured this concession in the mid-1950s; he explained that "the overall picture . . . seems to indicate some type of unknown process is attacking these children."[81] Clear labeling, he said, even if it was ambiguous, was superior to trendy but spurious labels "which may or may not be accurate."[82] "I feel it is far better to make a diagnosis of 'unknown natural,'" Carroll said, "which tells us we do not know, than it is to state that these children suffocate, strangulate, aspirate vomitus, or die of interstitial pneumonitis."[83]

THE CONFERENCE ON CAUSES OF
SUDDEN DEATH IN INFANTS, 1963

By 1960, numerous professionals agreed that some cases of sudden unexplained infant death formed a special category of mortality and had nothing to do with accidental suffocation.[84] They saw these deaths as medically strange and uniquely devastating, and families agreed. In September 1963 the National Institute of Child Health and Human Development sponsored a small conference on sudden death in infancy in Seattle, featuring speakers from the United States and Britain. In attendance were several medical professionals—mostly pediatricians and pathologists—as well as parents. The meeting marked the first concerted attempt since the 1949 conference to bring together documented information, evidence, and perspectives relevant to sudden infant deaths.

While they rejected flawed labels like "thymic death," "pneumonia," "suffocation," or "smothering," researchers in different locations and across fields employed varying labels, including sudden unexpected death, crib death, and cot death. For uniformity, the convention adopted the term "sudden death syndrome" (SDS) to encompass all such labels. At the time, most SDS inquiries were either epidemiological, gathering facts and figures, or etiological, testing hypothetical theories of causation. Those present in Seattle in 1963 were disappointed with the "miniscule" epidemiological data that existed on a problem "of a comparable order of magnitude to the number of adults who die from carcinoma of the lung."[85] Still, they agreed on some basics. All babies seemed vulnerable, and the rate of about two or three deaths per thousand live births seemed consistent across the Atlantic. Researchers could find no familial or genetic associations. Although the precise time span of highest risk would still be further refined, researchers knew most cases occurred before six months of age.

Pathologically, two findings were especially consistent and intriguing. Both pointed to some type of respiratory explanation. Pulmonary edema, a buildup of fluid in the air pockets of the lungs, was present in many cases at autopsy. Additionally, pathologists located petechiae (pronounced peh-tee-key-eye), tiny reddish dots indicative of localized bleeding, in the lungs and thymus glands (which, they pointed out, were normal in size) of many SDS victims. Pathologists agreed that these two findings were at least characteristic of, if not specific to, SDS.

Most presenters in Seattle had explored SDS's associations with certain populations; their conclusions emphasized that babies across all socioeconomic groups were vulnerable. Although studies documented increased incidence among lower-class and black infants, cases still occurred among upper-class white families. Marie Valdes-Dapena, a pediatric pathologist in Philadelphia who quickly earned a reputation as one of the nation's preeminent sudden infant death experts, interpreted a series of studies conducted in the Philadelphia area. One incorporated a detailed follow-up home survey that enabled investigators to assess socioeconomic status and create an epidemiological map of SDS deaths. There was a clear preponderance of cases in the most heavily populated, impoverished residential sectors of the city. "It is apparent," Valdes-Dapena conveyed, "that there is indeed a tendency for the sudden deaths to cluster in what might be called our poorer neighborhoods, or slums."[86]

Various hypotheses generated robust conversation throughout the conference proceedings. One attractive explanation was that infants hypersensitive to cow's milk might experience anaphylactic reactions that ultimately caused death. The idea was that if cow's milk somehow entered the lungs of an infant with hypersensitivity, he could aspirate, choke, and die. Robin Coombs, an experimenter at the University of Cambridge, tested this theory on guinea pigs and baboons with mixed results. Its simplicity made this a particularly appealing notion. Yet few infants were solely breastfed, and researchers experienced great difficulty ascertaining exact feeding patterns. Even breastfed babies might occasionally receive a bottle, and the milk infants consumed varied markedly by location. Furthermore, this was incompatible with the clear age bracket of vulnerability—why would an infant suddenly become vulnerable to cow's milk around two months of age? Professionals wondered about this, as well as the proposition that viral infections might cause SDS.[87]

Another focal point of discussion was whether infants who died suddenly were suffering from a single identifiable problem. Alternatively, multiple types of causation could lead to the same result. This possibility was daunting—as Warren Guntheroth explained, multiple numerous pathways could mean that every theory discussed might be correct. The "endlessly debatable" query was tabled.[88]

Attendants emphasized the special psychological trauma and grief associated with SDS. Those present in Seattle, both professional and lay, had all been moved by the emotional problems wrought by SDS—they hardly needed further convincing. Instead, the lack of such an appreciation among Americans *absent* from the conference needed to be rectified. The public's general unawareness of SDS posed an impediment to recovery; most families were unfamiliar with even the possibility of their situation before they found themselves trying to cope with it. Yet familiarity offered little protection. Lester Adelson possessed an intimate knowledge of SDS, its biological and anatomical facets, and its inexplicable nature, but awareness did not exempt him from palpable fears. Adelson often ran to confirm his own children's quiet breath in the middle of the night.

As he put it, "My pathologic experience was roosting in my own home, a kind of poetic injustice."[89]

The occasional likeness between the "medical mystery" of crib death and the atrocity of infanticide continued to harry parents and researchers. It was an uncomfortable matter. Pathologists made clear that not every instance in which a child was found dead in its crib was necessarily SDS. Adelson shared a quintessential case: a child was brought in "with the monotonous story that he was found dead in his crib in the morning after being perfectly well the previous evening." Some findings at autopsy were normal, but there was also evidence of brain damage that indicated violence. After further questioning, the baby's father ultimately admitted he had been drinking, played with the child, and then "tossed him into his crib" at bedtime. The baby never woke up.[90] Adelson's case recounted that abuse could present similarly to SDS.

By the close of the 1963 conference, the thymus theory, long in decline, was put to rest. Adelson deemed status thymicolymphaticus a "prime piece of medical gobbledygook. It is polysyllabic, has Latin endings, and sounds impressive. It merely serves to confuse the issue."[91] He jettisoned the suffocation theory equally as forcefully. "*I do not believe that a healthy child can smother in its bedclothes,*" Adelson emphasized, "and I think this erroneous notion should be eliminated once and for all from medical thinking."[92] Most of his colleagues agreed, but there were nagging doubts. Francis Camps presented a study carried out by two colleagues in London who located an association of SDS with "a history of respiratory symptoms, the use of soft pillows and mattresses, [and] having the mouth and nose covered by bedding." The 170 babies in the study were "significantly" more likely to be found with their mouth or nose covered by bedding, and in bed with other people, than control children. The evidence raised questions about suffocation, but the study was cited infrequently until the late 1980s, when doctors began rethinking these issues.[93] Instead, the 1963 conference brought into stark relief the scarcity and ambivalence of information on sudden infant deaths. As Adelson wryly suggested, the conference, if nothing else, "should help crystallize . . . ignorance."[94]

THE SUDDEN INFANT DEATH STUDY PROTOCOL

Two investigations in the 1960s reflected the ambitions from the 1963 conference and cemented the mold for studies of sudden infant death. Both used similar methods and emphasized parallel concerns. Investigators streamlined data collection. They stressed the significance of autopsies and demonstrated a commitment to communicating with families. They modeled the systematic case review process that became standard protocol for studying sudden infant mortality. The first was a follow-up study in Cleveland. Adelson and his colleagues conducted a ten-year analysis of over one thousand cases of sudden infant death. It was the largest and most comprehensive study to date. The second, a smaller near-replica of that work, took place in the Seattle area.

Abraham Bergman, J. Bruce Beckwith, and C. George Ray investigated all 119 reported cases of sudden death in infancy between 1965 and 1967 in King County, Washington, and compared their data against a control group consisting of every baby born in the county during the trial period. All bodies were brought to a central location. Beckwith, a pathologist with special training in pediatrics, performed almost every autopsy exam personally within twenty-four hours and applied accurate terminology on death certificates. He interpreted the "unexplained" cases, for the first time, as "sudden infant death syndrome." Beckwith himself called parents to discuss autopsy results and followed up with formal letters of condolence and written information. Within a few more days, the program nurse, specially trained to handle sudden infant death cases, contacted the family and made plans to visit in person. She provided additional information, answered questions, discussed therapy and peer support contacts, and collected demographic and incidental information for review.[95]

The Cleveland and King County studies were similar in purpose, methodology, and findings. Eager to shed new light on the problem, the premise in both locales was to find every case, perform an autopsy, and study it thoroughly. The result was an epidemiological portrait that was soon largely corroborated by others who launched comparable projects around the world. The average rate was approximately three cases per thousand live births. Investigators found slightly higher representation in males (although in Seattle this only held true for the white population). More deaths occurred during the winter, and the peak incidence age was three months. Seattle researchers observed that premature infants had elevated rates of death compared to full-term babies and stressed that most deaths corresponded with sleeping hours. They considered their study's 100 percent association with sleep highly significant, "implicating sleep as a necessary component" in SIDS.[96]

Data on demographic distribution were problematic. As Bergman described, there was an apparent "predominance of SIDS among lower socioeconomic class families as measured by income, occupation, status of housing, and class of neighborhood." Statistics revealed glaring racial discrepancies. In Cleveland, rates for whites measured at 2.39 per thousand compared to 5.85 per thousand in non-whites. In Seattle, the incidence was 1.82 for white babies and 5.1 for nonwhite babies. Other researchers documented similar differences. In poorer areas, rates could be as high as ten infant deaths per thousand live births.[97] Yet investigators remained skeptical that race, in itself, was a risk factor—economic groupings appeared far more stable than racial ones. The finding that racial discrepancies were subsidiary to economic ones suggested, in Adelson's words, "that factors of infant care and development affected by economic status play an important role in the occurrence of sudden, unexpected infant death."[98] Researchers like Adelson were invested in dispelling suspicion of parents, but their findings brought up new questions about parents' roles in sudden infant death. Even while these physicians were working against the suffocation hypothesis, it is difficult to imagine that the consistent association of sudden infant death with lower-class and minority families had nothing to do with perpetual misgivings about parents who lost babies to sudden infant death. And despite emerging recognition of class- and race-based associations, sudden infant death was still a universal possibility. No child could be counted as immune.

THE SECOND INTERNATIONAL CONFERENCE ON CAUSES OF SUDDEN DEATH IN INFANTS, 1969

Six years later, in early February of one of the most chaotic years in U.S. history, forty-three Americans gathered at the Rosario Hotel off the coast of Seattle to reassess sudden infant death. Joining the 1963 conference alumni were additional physicians from the U.S., Ireland, Czechoslovakia, and Canada as well as parents.[99] The brief assemblage produced the first formal definition of the modern notion of SIDS. The most substantial exchanges at the 1969 conference pertained to broader concepts, categories of causation, and questions. Physicians continued to cultivate the seeds of questions that would dominate SIDS research and activism for the next two decades, fine-tuning a series of disputes whose outlines they literally built into the very origins of the conception of SIDS. The polarities and paradoxes that bubbled up in 1969 became deeply and powerfully entrenched in SIDS as both a medical entity and a social experience.

Reflecting on the years since their 1963 gathering, researchers congratulated one another on two overarching accomplishments. First, they felt sudden infant death had gained recognition as a legitimate arena for concerted academic study. Before 1963, Marie Valdes-Dapena explained, "There were believers and there were non-believers in the existence of anything like 'sudden death syndrome.'" Now, she said, the notion and study of such a phenomenon was "respectable."[100] Second, by stressing the paucity of intelligence, the 1963 conference had stimulated research. Since 1963, several data collection projects had begun and multiple articles evaluating hypotheses had been published. Discussants had much more material with which to work.

Exploring terminology, participants stressed the need for a uniform label with a clear definition. They well understood that an exact, standard naming device was crucial for medical research. They also knew such a designation would have meaningful social implications. "A good title for this entity," J. Bruce Beckwith opined, "should be short and euphonious, sufficiently descriptive to prevent confusion with other types of sudden death, and readily comprehensible for lay persons." Many practitioners continued to use "sudden death syndrome," the favored terminology from 1963, and Beckwith suggested incorporating the word "infant" to enhance the term's clarity for laypeople. (He also noted that the initials used to abbreviate sudden death syndrome, S.D.S., were "at the present time popularly used for a militant student group" and might engender confusion surrounding the issue.[101]) Inversely, Beckwith argued against including "unexplained" in the label, as he thought it would interfere with families' abilities to understand and cope with their loss. In the future, Beckwith anticipated that more refined scientific information could conflict with the idea that the syndrome was "unexplained." In the end, Beckwith's proposal of sudden infant death syndrome, or S.I.D.S., stuck. (The abbreviation was originally pronounced as the individual letters rather than the common modern pronunciation as the word "sids.") Participants agreed SIDS was a more appropriate label than sudden unexplained death (SUD), crib death, sudden unexplained death syndrome (SUDS), and King's syndrome (named for King County).[102]

If its title would carry the most weight socially, the syndrome's signifying details were most salient medically. The Seattle research team's own definition was a blueprint: "the sudden death of any infant or young child, which is unexpected by history, and in which a thorough post-mortem examination fails to demonstrate an adequate cause for death."[103] There were obvious ambiguities in this definition, foremost of which was the question of what actions constituted "demonstrating an adequate cause for death." Pathologists settled on a baseline list of procedures to rule out explained deaths, naming gross autopsy examinations as paramount. Attendants adopted the Seattle description, and professional medicine indexed the same language as the formal SIDS definition in the coming years. Employed more for lack of any better ideas than for metaphorical sturdiness, the SIDS label and definition encapsulated the frustrating incomprehensibility of the phenomenon they represented.

Epidemiological data circa 1969 was remarkably more plentiful and more pronounced than that of 1963. Since 1963, multiple studies had successfully amassed (seemingly) relevant and relatively consistent statistical information on sudden death in infancy. In 1969, proceedings stressed the regularity of epidemiological findings related to age, socioeconomic status, race, seasonality, sex, weight, prematurity, and sleep.[104] A clear majority of SIDS cases struck lower or middle class families, and it was almost twice as likely to victimize black families.[105] The epidemiology appeared "fairly well defined" and "amazingly uniform" around the globe.[106] One presenter exclaimed that it was "amazing how the data from the various countries are so similar."[107] But the close matrix of findings only accounted for Western industrialized societies, and also failed to sufficiently advise physicians what was happening.

Epidemiologists working on a syndrome without a definition were at an obvious disadvantage, but this was especially so with sudden infant death syndrome. In the 1960s, not only did the condition lack a definition and diagnostic criteria, there was also enormous variability in recording patterns geographically and over time. Some coroners or medical examiners continued to use the label "mechanical suffocation"; others might favor "pneumonia," "natural causes," or "respiratory infection." Investigations were hampered by the fact that they could only be conducted retrospectively, a brand of scientific analysis that suffers from a number of flaws. It was difficult to obtain valid control groups, and the proverbial "chicken-or-egg" question nagged at researchers. Were noteworthy findings related to SIDS? If so, were they a cause or a result of death? Added to these issues were even more challenging questions about the singularity of any given factor. Categories such as race, socioeconomic status, birth weight, parity, or maternal age (among many others) were listed separately, but it was almost absurd to attempt to evaluate each one's independent effects.[108] Despite the field's contributions, epidemiological study had undeniable limitations. Since by 1969 an epidemiological template already existed, professionals worried that additional similarly structured studies would be redundant. "I don't see any point in doing more large-scale epidemiologic field studies," Abraham Bergman divulged. "The field of epidemiology has only a limited amount to offer the understanding of Sudden Infant Death Syndrome. We shouldn't try to squeeze too much out of the turnip."[109]

Anatomists and virologists were equally ill-equipped. Pathologists demanded that autopsy examinations be standardized. They saw dissection as the most significant medium for understanding how bodily malfunction led to SIDS.[110] Others were unsure about whether SIDS actually resulted from a physical breakdown. Were SIDS babies completely healthy? Or were they unwell? Virologists made the case that infection was involved. C. George Ray, for example, thought viruses might be "inciting agents" that could potentially start a series of events leading to SIDS; common viruses could be lethal, then, but only to a small minority of vulnerable babies. Charles Gardner, from Oregon, agreed. He speculated that almost all forty infants in his 1967 study, having been exposed to "large numbers of people" within one week of their deaths, might have come in contact with viruses. Carol Brandt concurred—viruses could function as a "triggering mechanism" for SIDS, although perhaps not a direct cause.[111]

Across disciplines, there were even larger uncertainties about causation: did SIDS result from a single, identifiable cause or was it the culmination of multiple factors acting in concert? The question, raised in 1963, remained unresolved. Bergman suggested that SIDS was a "conditional probability phenomenon." By this, he meant that SIDS resulted when an infant was predisposed to various different risks that all co-occurred, effectively acting to "'trip the switch' and throw the infant into the 'final common pathway.'" He illustrated the general scenario by comparing it to an overloaded electrical outlet that blew a fuse—all the plugs contributed to the blown fuse differently, and it would be impossible to predict when the fuse would go out and which particular electrical conduit was the main cause in tripping it. In part, this discussion owed to a more extensive and abstract conversation ongoing in medicine about the nature and origins of disease in general. Frederic Robbins explained as much when he noted that the group's task was part of a "process which is broader than the concerns of this particular conference, namely, realization that the disease (and I don't care what disease you are talking about) is not simply a matter of *a* specific etiologic factor, or causing *a* specific universal result. We are only now beginning to learn how to think in terms of eligibility and conditional probability factors in relation to all diseases."[112]

From debates about health, illness, and causation, speculations about reversibility were not a far reach. If SIDS was the final result of a series of "triggers," could the process be interrupted or reversed? Could it be entirely prevented in the first place?[113] Almost every researcher present had encountered a case that appeared as if SIDS was interrupted. A case from a Canadian study was typical: a child had stopped breathing and was successfully revived by its father, but physicians could locate no cause for the event. Was this a case of revived SIDS? Bergman posited that since sleep altered babies' autonomic control, "probably many sleeping infants come close to the trigger all the time—the process must be reversible up to a certain point. This is suggested by the 'near misses.'" The ensuing dialogue regarding the logistical propensity of "abortive crib death" or "near miss" cases became even more divisive after it was wed almost exclusively to apnea monitor therapy starting in the 1970s.[114]

Crafting the outlines of these debates—whether SIDS babies were healthy or ill, whether SIDS was caused by a single or multiple factors, and whether SIDS could be preempted or reversed—contributed to the most significant outcome of the 1969 meeting. The discussions, disagreements, proposals, and rejections that occurred in Seattle recognized and configured a new condition, "a real disease every bit as much as cancer is a disease."[115] By the close of the 1960s, the problem of sudden unexplained infant mortality had a name and a definition: sudden infant death syndrome, an infant death unanticipated by history and in which a thorough postmortem exam fails to demonstrate an adequate cause of death.

CONCLUSION

American medicine grew increasingly attentive to sudden unexpected infant deaths as a discrete phenomenon in the first half of the twentieth century; physicians in succeeding generations approached the problem from varying angles, ultimately categorizing SIDS in 1969. Especially for parents who had suffered the loss of a child, the production of formal terminology to signify their experiences was deeply meaningful. In naming SIDS, Americans at the 1969 conference formally agreed that it existed.

In reality, the "new" diagnosis was only a new beginning. Even after Americans designated sudden unexplained infant mortality "SIDS," its nature and meaning remained far from absolute. The SIDS diagnosis did not necessarily quickly or simply bestow legitimacy, much less solutions. In many ways, naming SIDS heightened the fearsomeness of sudden unexplained infant death, stiffening Americans' resolve to conquer it. They carried SIDS through morgues and laboratories, civic centers, hospitals, and homes, constantly working to overcome the syndrome. But dealing with "a disease whose first and only symptom is death" was not easy.[116]

3 · THE THEORY OF THE MONTH CLUB
Conducting Research on SIDS

After it was designated in 1969, SIDS remained caught in diagnostic limbo for some time. Transmitting the puzzle of SIDS to the larger medical community was a challenge. In a 1970 issue of *The Lancet*, one writer asked the question bluntly: "*is* it [SIDS] a real disease and *is* there a syndrome?"[1] In 1973, participants in a series of Congressional hearings *on SIDS* debated whether SIDS was even a "definite disease."[2] Through the 1980s, doctors maligned SIDS as a "waste-basket term" or a "diagnostic dustbin," and parents and professionals alike felt the need to avow that SIDS was a "real disease."[3] Nonetheless, organized medicine did accept SIDS, if slowly. In 1975 SIDS gained a place in the ninth edition of the bible of disease taxonomy, the *International Classification of Diseases,* and shortly thereafter the Centers for Disease Control began recording SIDS statistics.[4]

The two 1960s conferences on unexplained infant death helped "make" SIDS and also professed that it was an urgent research endeavor. Documenting SIDS converted sudden infant mortality from a topic of scattered medical inquiry into a more coherent and "worthy" medical dilemma. In 1974, reporter Nicholas Wade wrote in *Science* that SIDS research had "recently become rather more fashionable," and he was certainly right.[5] In 1963, core medical journals carried no articles on sudden infant death; in 1979, they published seventy. This rash of research coincided with the nation's lowest infant mortality rate ever recorded: 18.2 deaths per thousand live births.[6] During the 1970s, infant mortality plummeted by 35 percent, the largest proportional reduction in any decade in U.S. history.[7] Amid this drop, SIDS emerged as one of the leading causes of infant death. Doctors undertook to combat this source of mortality, but the first scientific forays into SIDS research were characterized by dead ends.

In the twenty years after it was defined, SIDS prompted a profusion of research characterized by such rapid turnover that veteran scientists often facetiously referred to the SIDS "theory of the month club." SIDS baffled American doctors and remained obscure. Their task was hamstrung by the enigma of SIDS, as every promising theory of causation threatened—if it was accurate—to undo SIDS itself. If medicine solved SIDS, the category would become obsolete. The search for causation therefore inadvertently encroached on the simultaneous campaigns to uphold SIDS' legitimacy and advocate for families.

More than a medical mystery, though, SIDS was a comprehensive human problem. As medicine continued to falter in its scientific venture, it focused on the SIDS family as the only arena in which it could offer anything demonstrably productive. Medical professionals had begun thinking about the psychological fallout from sudden infant death decades prior. Building on earlier initiatives, doctors studying SIDS prioritized humanitarian measures designed to serve families and revise social patterns. Researchers who incorporated parents' needs into their study protocols helped establish that SIDS made victims out of whole families. Their work gave rise to formal academic attentiveness to the psychological effects of SIDS as a unique trauma.

SIDS scholarship was continuously stymied by the condition's own contradictions, and professionals struggled to balance the goal of etiological discovery with their desire to protect and support affected families. Physicians played a role in provoking a broader understanding of SIDS, and did work to address SIDS families' mental health, but ultimately their research came up short. Medically, the history of SIDS research is a story of a foundering.

MEDICAL THEORIES ON SIDS

In the post-WWII era, the federal government doled out unprecedented amounts of money in the medical arena—dollars went to hospital building, medical schools, laboratory research, and clinical studies. Healthcare became one of the country's top industries. In the two decades after 1950, the size of the medical workforce more than tripled (to 3.9 million workers) and health spending skyrocketed from $12.7 billion to $71.6 billion.[8] In this climate of growth, SIDS research did benefit, although advances related to SIDS paled in comparison to more conspicuous health sectors. The National Institute for Child Health and Human Development (NICHD) had helped support the 1963 and the 1969 conferences in Seattle, both of which were central to establishing SIDS and stimulating research. After the 1969 meeting yielded the SIDS definition, the NICHD began increasing its contributions. In 1970, it gave $34,000 to research targeting SIDS. By 1973, that tally had increased to $604,000.[9]

Medical study produced an increasingly uniform depiction of SIDS. Recurrent findings and patterns paved the way for a spectrum of interpretations, ranging from simple to complex and biological to environmental. Recall that most SIDS infants were discovered in places associated with sleep, hence the popular contemporary terminology of "crib death." Most babies died between two and four months old, during the winter. SIDS occurred more often in males and in premature or low-birth-weight babies. It was not uncommon for parents to find their babies cold, bruised, or stiff, with frothy or bloody fluid covering their faces, circumstances that understandably magnified parents' trauma. These and many other factors weighed by epidemiologists—altitudinal location, temperature, time of day, age, birth weight, head circumference, blood type—became potential candidates for causation.

Earlier explanations for unexpected infant death—overlaying, enlarged thymus glands, and accidental mechanical suffocation—had been certain. The new "non-explanation" of SIDS was fundamentally uncertain. SIDS research bred plentiful hypotheses, all of which hinged on the notion of inexplicability. The breadth and creativity of medical suspicions had few limits; scientists and doctors intended to investigate every feasible realm. Some of their theoretical proposals were less conscientious than others—one doctor wryly likened attempting to locate the cause of SIDS to "trying to catch a handful of smoke"—and most theories cycled from prominence to defeat quickly.[10] The overwhelming number of proposed theories for SIDS reflect longstanding professional discomforts with the puzzle of sudden infant death. One critical question was whether SIDS resulted from a singular entity or from multiple varying causes.[11] Researchers were keen to the former of these possibilities, but they quickly conceded that the latter was more likely. In addition, the plethora of explanations offered portrays that medicine's fluctuating approaches to SIDS continued to come up against the premise of suffocation.

As the cow's milk allergy proposition was slowly discredited (multiple studies reported no significant correlation between feeding habits in SIDS and control infants), many physicians became captivated by viral hypotheses. Boiled down, viral theories suggested that respiratory infection could cause a child to suffocate by blocking its airway. SIDS parents frequently reported that their infants had experienced some kind of infection or cold, albeit mild, in the days or weeks preceding death. Furthermore, at autopsy, pathologists continued to locate petechiae in babies' lungs. These findings hinted that some kind of airway obstruction, occasioned by viral infection, was a reasonable idea.[12]

The most outspoken proponents of a viral hypothesis saw themselves as continuing and contributing to a long line of estimable research begun by Jacob Werne and Irene Garrow back in the 1940s. They thought viruses were the "cause" of SIDS and thus implied that SIDS was a misnomer. By 1980, this viewpoint was no longer treated as credible.[13] In part, this was due to a lack of evidence. But it was also because the contention that SIDS resulted from a specific, identifiable virus (such as pneumonia) so blatantly exposed the paradoxical nature of the diagnosis.[14] If a virus caused SIDS, SIDS was not an unexplained problem. Additionally, if sudden infant death proceeded from a virus, medicine could test for and treat the virus to prevent deaths. Unqualified, viral theories flew in the face of the fundamental substance of the SIDS definition as a completely unknown, unpreventable event. Of course, these tensions were not unique to viral hypotheses—every potential hypothesis butted heads with the dominant message that SIDS was inexplicable and unpreventable on some level. Viral causation simply magnified the dilemma because it often pointed to distinctive diseases and also implied parents may have missed visible signs of illness. This category of medical inquiry highlights the profound problems associated with studying an essentially irreconcilable medical condition.

Researchers had plenty of other ideas to investigate. No correlation was off limits. They published articles exploring whether SIDS was related to vitamin deficiencies, metabolic abnormalities, enzyme performance, botulism poisoning, hormone levels, infant vocal acoustics, and crying patterns.[15] More hypotheses stemmed from contemporary medical revelations on external sources of disease causation. In the 1960s and 1970s, environmental hazards, maligned medical "cures," and cigarette smoke shared the center stage in academic medicine. The growth of the environmental movement as well as catastrophes that brought to light the harmful effects of substances such as thalidomide and lead additives taught that some environmental and prescriptive substances could be dangerous. Following suit, many studies considered whether such exposures might be causative in SIDS, but evidence consistently failed to identify associations.[16]

An episode in Tennessee at the end of the 1970s surrounding a possible link with the diphtheria-tetanus-pertussis (DTP) inoculation prompted a SIDS "vaccine scare." Eight SIDS babies (out of a sample of 77 SIDS babies) died within one week of receiving the shot; four of the deaths occurred within twenty-four hours of inoculation. (The vaccine was typically administered to infants during the peak window of risk for SIDS when babies were two to four months old.) In response, the Tennessee Health Department placed a hold on the vaccination lot connected to the deaths and launched an investigation. The manufacturer, Wyeth Laboratories, agreed to withdraw all 100,000 remaining unused doses. Almost that many doses had already been administered.[17] The state review in Tennessee compared the vaccination histories from SIDS cases against controls over the previous few years. It found no statistically significant variation between both groups' DTP records, but noted a "temporal association" between the vaccination lot in question and SIDS.[18]

The "P" in DTP was a whole-cell vaccination (meaning that it included inactivated whole cells of the infecting bacteria) that inoculated against pertussis, or whooping cough. The inciting bacteria, *Bordetella pertussis*, was isolated in 1906, and already by the 1930s a host of varying pertussis vaccines were in use across the nation. They differed in success rates, but all of them contained trace amounts of toxins.[19] In the 1960s, vaccination was in its glory days, and DTP started to be widely administered. But reports of brain damage and neurological reactions to the shot surfaced; even manufacturers acknowledged that the inoculation sometimes caused adverse reactions.[20]

Parents grew concerned, and their fears magnified in the next decade as Americans began to doubt the consummate vaccine. After a national campaign to vaccinate Americans against a seemingly deadly strain of the flu in the mid-1970s backfired—the impending flu epidemic never materialized and instead numerous serious iatrogenic reactions were reported—Americans started to grow skeptical of vaccines. As historian Elena Conis summarizes, the flu vaccine episode "was widely mocked in the press and led to confusion, doubt, and consternation."[21] In 1978, the Food and Drug Administration started requiring that parents whose children received vaccinations funded by federal dollars sign a statement detailing the risks of immunization. Parents now had to confront an "important information statement" telling them that the almighty vaccine, medicine's most heroic triumph, might be dangerous.[22]

As a result of the DTP situation in Tennessee, the Centers for Disease Control conducted a multicenter epidemiological review. It failed to link the vaccine with SIDS. In fact, researchers showed the opposite. More SIDS babies had *not* received the DTP shot, suggesting that if anything the vaccine was protective against SIDS. But in the context of a society singing a "chorus of criticism" against the DTP shots, the association did not die easily.[23] In 1982, physician Gerald Fenichel brushed aside concerns about the link, complaining that DTP "had been blamed for 'almost everything.'" "It was just as possible," he remarked, "to relate crib death to wearing diapers."[24]

But given the climate, Americans stayed wary. In 1982, NBC aired a widely viewed documentary called *DPT: Vaccine Roulette* (the inoculation is sometimes branded DPT). The broadcast weaved together testimony from lawyers, science researchers, and health professionals as well as parents to convey the shocking message that pertussis vaccines could cause brain damage. Although scholars characterize *Vaccine Roulette* as "a devastating piece of muckraking," it made an indelible mark. After the film aired, lawsuits soared. Within just a few years, about 220 suits were underway, all alleging that the pertussis vaccine had inflicted harm on a child. Disturbed parents banded together, forming a group with the clever name of Dissatisfied Parents Together—DPT. When a controversial book, *DPT: Shot in the Dark*, hit the press in 1985, warning parents about the hazards of supposedly life-saving immunizations, it was just another source of consternation.[25]

Babies received their first and second (of three total) doses of DTP during the peak risk period for SIDS. It is not surprising that the initial studies after the SIDS deaths in Tennessee confirmed that "many SIDS cases occur after immunization in temporal association."[26] Soon, controlled studies confirmed that DTP was not causative, but the continuation of the DTP controversy makes plain just how frightened American parents were. Moreover, this situation marks a fascinating moment in the history of SIDS. Research located a correlation—between SIDS and DTP inoculation. The timing of DTP administration made the association look like a confounding factor, a fluke in the data. But the legacy of public doubts about the pertussis vaccine and the palpable outcry over vaccines in general at the time forced science to critically investigate the correlation. In the end, the original hunch—that the connection was based on pretense—turned out to be right. But other correlations that appeared similarly coincidental—such as most babies being discovered on their stomachs—did not generate such swift scrutiny. The climate of suspicion surrounding vaccination forced science to reconcile with the DTP association, where others drifted out of view without controversy.

Parallel to vaccination, refined awareness of the harms associated with tobacco smoke, and even secondhand smoke exposure, led SIDS investigators to examine parental smoking and drug habits. By the 1970s, studies indicated that mothers of SIDS babies were more likely to have smoked during and after their pregnancies, and that SIDS parents smoked "more heavily" compared to controls.[27] It is interesting that simultaneously, new smoking trends were becoming apparent: cigarette smoking became more highly associated with disadvantaged Americans. As of 1980, breaking with historical usage rates, blacks were more likely to smoke than whites, and working-class Americans were more likely to smoke than middle- or upper-class Americans.[28]

By the early 1980s, nearly every study reported a correlation between SIDS and maternal smoking. Cigarette smoking was one of the strongest correlating factors with SIDS; babies whose mothers smoked while they were in utero were between two and four times more likely to die from SIDS.[29] These findings met with mounting publicity about the permeability of the uterine wall and the extent to which prenatal exposures, ranging from rubella to alcohol, might pose dangers to developing fetuses.[30] The connection between tobacco and SIDS contributed to the growing body of evidence that smoking was deleterious to the healthy development of human fetuses. In 1964, the landmark surgeon general's report on the dangers of smoking included a note that mothers who smoked gave birth to babies with lower weights. Follow-up reports further publicized the hazards of maternal smoking, noting observed connections with SIDS. In 1979, the surgeon general specifically implicated smoking during pregnancy in SIDS.[31]

These verdicts compelled research into other substance exposures. Uproar over the so-called crack epidemic in the 1980s—fueled by crack's presence in impoverished minority urban areas—led to a surge of medical research and media reporting on whether pregnant users of cocaine were impairing their unborn children.[32] Studies indicated that users were putting their children at an increased risk for SIDS. One analysis concluded that infants born to women who used cocaine were at a five to ten times higher risk of dying from SIDS compared to the average infant.[33] A major study conducted in Los Angeles in the 1980s reported that substance-abusing mothers' babies had much higher rates of SIDS—8.87 per thousand live births—in comparison to a control group with rates of just 1.22 per thousand live births. A large-scale epidemiologic study backed by the NICHD further indicated that SIDS risk doubled with illicit prenatal drug use.[34] Projects exploring the possible role of in utero drug exposure on SIDS worked to control for confounding factors, but still noted that study populations tended to flow from the lower classes, seek little to no prenatal care, and give birth to lower-weight babies, all of which were documented SIDS associations.

APNEA

Of the correlative findings in SIDS research, the association with sleep was nearly universal. Expectedly, it generated a substantial amount of conjectures, and researchers turned to contemporary sleep science for help. The field was a product of the 1950s and grew out of a fascination with a single condition—the "Pickwickian syndrome." In 1956, a case report in the *American Journal of Medicine* described a patient with symptoms that approximated those of a character in Charles Dickens' *The Posthumous Papers of the Pickwick Club*. Both subject and character were obese and excessively tired. The 1950s patient also experienced hypoventilation (slow breathing) when awake, had an elevated red blood cell count due to hypoxemia (low levels of oxygen in the blood), and had high blood pressure and signs of heart disease. Investigators traced these ailments to breathing problems—namely the lack of breathing—during sleep. The Pickwickian syndrome was a precursor to the condition that became known as sleep apnea, in which breathing ceases repeatedly and unpredictably during sleep.[35] By the 1960s, sleep apnea, in all kinds of patient populations, constituted its own category for study in the thriving field of sleep medicine.[36]

Newly established professional societies, journals, and sleep clinics proclaimed that sleep science was a serious branch of medicine. By the middle of the decade, the first sleep disorders clinic opened at Stanford University in California and professionals founded the Association for the Psychophysiological Study of Sleep. Soon sleep study centers existed across the country, surveying and treating slumbering patients. They studied sleeping phases, cycles, and patterns and insisted that sleep was an important factor in personal health. As researchers charted the boundaries of their new specialty, identifiable disorders like sleep apnea, narcolepsy, and restless leg syndrome received concerted attention. Sleep apnea was officially added to the *International Classifications of Disease* in 1964, about a decade before SIDS.[37] The sleep apnea and SIDS diagnoses grew into adolescence during the same era.

Sleep apnea presented SIDS researchers with a curious possibility. At the 1963 conference in Seattle, pediatric cardiologist Warren Guntheroth had proposed that sleep apnea might be a culprit in unexplained infant deaths. His brainstorm resurfaced from time to time over the next ten years.[38] Alfred Steinschneider, a physician at Upstate Medical Center in Syracuse, New York, had been following SIDS since the 1960s. He attended both 1960s Seattle conferences and was immersed in ongoing "theory of the month" research. In 1972, *Pediatrics* published an article of his titled "Prolonged Apnea and the Sudden Infant Death Syndrome: Clinical and Laboratory Observations." The paper nudged the entire SIDS field onto a different course.

Steinschneider's article reported on five infant patients from three separate families.[39] The study employed sleep laboratory observation using an electronic breathing monitor to reveal that all five babies experienced frequent periods of brief apnea while they were asleep. Most of their apneas measured short in duration (two seconds or less) and were "self-limited" in nature, meaning the babies began breathing again on their own. But Steinschneider also noted a disturbing number of prolonged apnea episodes. The prolonged apneas, at least fifteen seconds in length, were associated with cyanosis, a symptomatic condition in which the skin becomes discolored (usually bluish) due to lack of oxygen to the blood. Some of the events were severe enough to warrant "vigorous resuscitation efforts."[40]

Steinschneider treated his infant patients with continued electronic monitoring, first in the hospital and then in their homes. The monitors were set to trigger an alarm after fifteen seconds of inactivity to alert the attention of a nurse or a parent. Ultimately, two of the infants in the study—siblings—died; their deaths were attributed to SIDS. Steinschneider hypothesized that "prolonged apnea, a concomitant of sleep, is part of the final physiologic pathway culminating in SIDS." Furthermore, he suggested that "infants at risk might be identified prior to the final tragic event."[41] These were exciting prospects for anyone concerned with SIDS. If sleep apnea was a possible cause of SIDS, identifying and managing sleep apnea could reduce SIDS.

In time, Steinschneider's conclusions were debunked. His study was riddled with methodological problems and scholars have since excoriated his entire investigation. For example, he treated all five of his patients in a carefully controlled environment maintained at the "ambient" temperature of 90 degrees Fahrenheit—despite available evidence that such elevated temperatures increased the frequency of sleep apnea in infants. Most damning is the fact that in 1995 the two siblings who died in his study were determined to have been victims of infanticide.[42] Notwithstanding flaws recognizable from the vantage of hindsight, the reality in 1972 was that a sizable community of researchers, parents, and physicians were ready and willing to observe the apnea theory of SIDS causation and experiment with potential solutions. When it was published, Steinschneider's article offered a seemingly concrete and promising new direction for research. Indeed, it would be difficult to overstate the extent to which the apnea theory guided SIDS research. From 1974 to 1996, Steinschneider's article was quoted more times—404—than any other paper on SIDS.[43]

In the wake of this piece, infant sleep research became a newly urgent and distinguished field. Babies' lives could be at stake. With the daunting possibility that infant apnea could be fatal, scholars began working to better understand infant sleep apnea. Researchers delineated different types and categories of episodes. "The apneic spells of infancy are not all of the same nature," articulated neurologist Ruthmary Deuel, and "some are amenable to prevention and treatment."[44] Ascertaining which spells could be prevented or treated was a tricky endeavor, especially layered over doctors' broader uncertainties about "abnormal" breathing in babies. While apnea in general might have been "normal" or "common" in infants, prolonged apneas seemed rare (and therefore, suggestive of "clinical abnormality") and had the most potential to exert harmful effects on sleeping babies.[45] They deprived babies' bodies of oxygen for longer periods of time and stood to impede healthy neurological and physical development. Given Steinschneider's research, there was also direct speculation that prolonged apneas could cause death. A number of case reports and clinical trials suggested that infants could be saved if prolonged apneas were interrupted in time or if swift resuscitation was provided. "Careful surveillance during sleep until at least 8 to 10 months of age in children with history of repeated and prolonged apnea may prove to be life-saving," one Kansas physician wrote.[46] Researchers further acknowledged that apneic episodes could themselves affect babies differently—not all infants coped with apnea equally.[47] The same infant could even respond to similar apneas variably over time.[48]

Prolonged apnea was hardly a smoking gun. Even so, the concept that certain babies might have some identifiable abnormality contributed to a major revision underway in the broader currents of SIDS research. In the 1960s, researchers almost universally argued that SIDS babies were physiologically "normal."

Gradually through the 1970s, clinical evidence increasingly persuaded research-ers that SIDS babies, rather than being "normal," were somehow different.[49] Steinschneider's apnea theory bolstered this turn.

SIDS MANAGEMENT IN THE U.S.: "A DISGRACE"

The year 1972 was momentous in the world of SIDS research. The same year that Steinschneider's work came out in *Pediatrics*, a major project took stock of what was happening around the country when SIDS occurred. Its results were disappointing, and even though Abraham Bergman, the project's chief archi-tect, admitted that it was "not, strictly speaking, a 'scientific' study," it became a principal piece of evidence showcasing how poorly the country handled SIDS.[50] Broadly speaking, the project was a national survey of SIDS management proto-cols, assessing professional responses to SIDS. It investigated a handful of urban sites and procured data on autopsy statistics, death certificate procedures, and standard conventions for communicating with parents. No one was pleased with its findings. The study's final report exclaimed that there was "a consider-able lack of knowledge about crib death among public health and safety officials" and directly linked that shortcoming to a "lack of sensitivity to the needs of bereaved parents."[51]

In the summer of 1972, Bergman hired twenty graduate students and ran a one-week training session in Seattle. He brought the students up to speed on SIDS science, taught them about the psychological devastation that beset affected families, and had them practice interviewing one another. After com-pleting the crash course, the graduates spread out in pairs to document the han-dling of SIDS cases in a sample of 148 counties across the country. They spoke with death investigators, health professionals, and 421 SIDS families.[52] Their launching point was learning about autopsy customs.

Autopsy findings were the some of the most highly valued sources of infor-mation for SIDS. Babies' corpses were literal bodies of knowledge; they car-ried with them the potential to help medicine better comprehend cases and to help parents better come to terms with their loss. Since by definition patholo-gists could only list SIDS as a cause of death after ruling out all other possible causes through an autopsy, the procedure was essential for accurately record-ing SIDS deaths. Technically, autopsies were supposed to be performed in any case of sudden death (regardless of age), but numerous obstacles stood in the way of making SIDS autopsies routine, not the least of which was funding.[53] Beginning in the mid-1960s, autopsies became less habitual and less popular among the general population, SIDS aside. Hospital pathologists were disap-pointed about dwindling rates: one thin-slice sample showed that 41 percent of bodies were autopsied in 1964, while only 21.7 percent were in 1975. By 1981, that rate would drop even further, to just 15 percent. In part, these reductions stemmed from the fact that autopsies were costly for hospitals (ranging from $250 to $300 per case) and the public was increasingly ambivalent towards the procedure. Autopsies also were no longer a sole and integral source of general medical education—dissection procedures of deceased bodies were no longer the major mechanism for observing and learning about human anatomy. But they were the major mechanism for learning about and diagnosing SIDS, and Bergman's student investigators did not return with great news about the procedure's applications to sudden infant mortality.[54]

Autopsies were only performed in 74 percent of cases. Of those, just 39 percent of families learned their child's autopsy results within one week. Another 13 percent heard within one month; 10 percent heard within three months; 3 percent heard later than three months; and 9 percent of families never learned the autopsy results. Half of parents did not feel they were ever given an adequate explanation of what had happened to their child, and one third said their child's death certificate deviated from the verbally communicated cause of death.[55] Professionals used a "bewildering array of terminology" to convey SIDS on death certificates. Some investigators eschewed SIDS entirely, listing separate diseases (such as pneumonia) as causes of death.[56] These findings replicated those from an independent study conducted during the previous year, which found that health officials used at least sixteen different terms to convey SIDS on death certificates.[57] A retrospective review in 1973 further highlighted the confusion surrounding death-coding protocol for "unexpected" verses "unexplained" infant deaths. Authors concluded that professionals "poorly elicited, incompletely provided, and often inappropriately classified" information regarding sudden and unexpected infant deaths.[58] Bergman was appalled: "the management of sudden infant deaths (SIDS) in the United States is a disgrace," he told a reporter for the L.A. Times.[59]

SYMPATHIZING WITH SIDS FAMILIES: THE EVOLUTION OF HOME VISITATION

Bergman's work was indicative of a crucial shift in SIDS research; it showcased how and why professional medicine in the U.S. approached sudden infant death as a twofold problem. An obvious goal of standardizing and regulating the reporting procedures for SIDS cases was to accumulate data for medical investigation. Yet studies also candidly aimed to humanize SIDS as an experience—to replace reproach, miscommunication, and blame directed at grieving parents with sympathy, open communication, and support. A few of the early epidemiological surveys, which set the de facto templates for evaluations of SIDS, illustrate that protocols evolved to address social concerns, focusing on communication with parents. Over time, researchers refined visitation initiatives and also articulated an increasingly humanistic rationale for including them. Methods from Los Angeles, Cleveland, and Seattle illustrate how SIDS studies progressively fused humanitarian ideals with scientific ambition.

In 1957, the Los Angeles County Board of Supervisors recruited pathologist Theodore Curphey to spearhead its new medical examiner's office. Curphey had an impatient confidence in scientific medicine. He immediately fought to modernize and professionalize his department, making enemies in the process. In a 1958 piece reflecting on his appointment, an *L.A. Times* editorial described Curphey as "curt, rude, tactless . . . [and] arrogant."[60] Brash or not, Curphey was unswerving in his commitment to scientific rigor, and neither interpersonal conflict nor legal obstacles deterred him. When his policy amendments stipulating more thorough autopsies landed him squarely in the middle of a grand jury investigation for professional misconduct, Curphey reportedly "greeted the investigation 'with delight.'"[61] Curphey was determined to apply the scientific method to death investigation broadly; he saw in sudden infant deaths a challenge and "a great opportunity . . . for advancing knowledge in this area of medical responsibility to the community."[62]

Shortly after his appointment, Curphey started collecting case summaries of sudden infant deaths throughout the county. These reports shed light on how Curphey's office handled sudden, unexplained infant deaths throughout L.A. County (but not how the office responded to SIDS, since it had yet to be designated). Each one described an instance of sudden infant death and offered details about the baby, its family, its health, and its death. Curphey collected these surveys for several years, retaining the series in his personal files. (L.A. County received between three and four hundred cases annually.)[63] His motivations were scientific, but the procedures incorporated a rudimentary version of what later became routine home visits.

Curphey's project enlisted public health nurses and physicians to visit and interview parents who lost a child suddenly and unexpectedly, in their own homes.[64] The team members were willing to make multiple attempts to reach parents and families they were unable to locate immediately, often asking neighbors as to families' whereabouts, returning to homes repeatedly, and placing numerous phone calls. Curphey and his colleagues sought information about each case; their visits were a scientific measure, enacted to advance medical knowledge rather than to allay parents' concerns.[65] Still, the interaction established a new point of communication between health professionals and families, and later SIDS researchers used that encounter for different purposes.

Collectively, the hundreds of episode synopses Curphey's office assembled offer insight into the circumstances Curphey and his peers considered significant to the problem of sudden infant mortality. Each file included a referral form posing questions regarding all kinds of information. What were the child's basic living conditions? What was the family like? How were his parents' health habits? What was the baby like? Did he suffer from any defects or injuries? What vaccinations did he receive? When did he visit the doctor? What was his feeding history? How was he discovered deceased? The items of import went on.[66] Most reports documented a baby's and its family's health prior to the event of death, and took careful note of any evidence of contagious or communicable disease. The visits were distinctly intended to amass data—not to console families or offer information.

In contrast, head researchers in Cleveland and Seattle focused deliberately on exploiting home visits as a chance to sympathize with and inform parents from the outset. Where Curphey had discharged health professionals to parents' homes to extract information, Lester Adelson, Bruce Beckwith, and Abraham Bergman discharged health professionals to exchange information. The home visit became an encounter in which communication flowed two ways, and visitors were there as much for parents as for science. In Cleveland and Seattle, physicians explicitly retooled the home visit to serve research *and* families.

In both locales, researchers promptly informed parents of autopsy diagnoses, offered consolation, and provided relevant informative literature. These customs, specifically effected for the benefit of families, became fundamental protocols for SIDS research. The acts of performing and reporting autopsies generated opportunities for medical professionals to communicate with parents of SIDS babies. Adelson and his colleagues in Cleveland and the physicians working in Seattle used those channels to inform and reassure parents they were not at fault. This simple measure was pioneered in Cleveland and then refined and expanded in Seattle. In Cleveland, Adelson regarded communicative measures as important for a family's well-being, but in Seattle a family's well-being became the principal reason to enact similar measures. The Seattle team stressed expedience. Pediatric pathologist J. Bruce Beckwith called parents personally to convey their child's autopsy results. The Washington Children's Hospital quickly mailed families written information on SIDS, emphasizing that it was unpredictable and unpreventable. Margaret Pomeroy, the public health nurse (PHN) who worked with the Seattle project, explained that parents often waited "on edge" to hear about their child's autopsy and went "over and over in their minds all the things that might have caused the death." Many parents indicated that the SIDS diagnosis eased their grief; it offered a cause of death, however indistinct. The only couple in the Seattle study that declined an autopsy later regretted it, telling Pomeroy "now we'll never know for sure."[67]

The PHN played a lead role by performing home visits with SIDS families. Within a week after an event, she contacted the family to set up a time to visit—ideally, both parents would be present. As Pomeroy explained, the calls were originally borrowed from Cleveland as a strategy for epidemiological study, but they almost immediately assumed a therapeutic role that subsumed that original intent. She began each visit with an offer for parents to first ask questions before she inquired about the circumstances of their baby's death.[68] Parents, many of whom thought their child had smothered, relished the chance to speak with an informed professional. As Pomeroy explained, her critical task was to dispel such false assumptions.[69] Her interactions with SIDS families convinced Pomeroy that home visits were of the utmost importance. In arguing that the home visit was an indispensable feature of studying SIDS, Pomeroy underscored the needs of "parent victims." The sentiment she captured in this phrase permeated the SIDS literature to the extent that parents themselves, and whole families, were equated with SIDS patients. The concept signaled an entire off-shoot of SIDS research.

THE EFFECTS OF SIDS

Pomeroy's exact concerns helped establish the task of ministering to families' psychological health as one of the most important and achievable goals. As Beckwith explained, "part of the syndrome of sudden infant death is the reaction of the person caring for the infant at the time." Responding to SIDS families—not just SIDS babies—became a necessity in the medical management of sudden unexplained infant death.[70] If they could do nothing else, doctors could at least aid suffering families. "For the practicing physician," said expert Marie Valdes-Dapena, "currently the single most important aspect of the matter is the care of the stricken family."[71] Her colleagues underwrote Valdes-Dapena's assertion by including familial notification, home visits, and psychological referrals in their research procedures. They expressed that even though they were unable to prevent SIDS, they were capable of helping grieving families.[72] In 1978, *New York Times* health correspondent Jane Brody explained that "while it may not yet be possible to prevent SIDS . . . much can be done to prevent the emotional battering of the family that commonly follows a sudden infant death."[73] Nurses trained to counsel families after SIDS learned the mantra, "you can't save the kid but *you can save the family*."[74]

The notion that SIDS victimized entire families expanded the very concept of SIDS. "SIDS kills families," Dr. Frederick Mandell of Boston Children's Hospital declared. "It never ends. It doesn't go away."[75] Individuals who expressed this view measured SIDS' toll not by the thousands, in terms of SIDS deaths, but by the hundreds of thousands, in terms of survivors. Many practitioners considered their responsibility to care for parents equally as important as (besides more feasible than) caring for babies. When SIDS occurred, the doctor's role extended "far beyond the period immediately after death."[76] Especially as researchers continued to stumble in their attempts to explain why SIDS happened, some physicians thought the field should redirect its entire focus to the task of "prevent[ing] the crippling guilt reactions in the parents."[77] In 1972, the American Academy of Pediatrics (AAP) informed its ranks that SIDS parents "need counsel and support . . . especially when they begin to wonder what they did wrong."[78] In the aftermath of SIDS, doctors became counselors.[79] These goals were further emphasized after parents reported that insensitive responses from professionals could and did deepen and prolong their grief. The use of confusing medical jargon, discrepancies between death certificates and personal communications about the cause of death, and premature advice about having more children could all impact a SIDS family's recovery.[80]

The concept that the SIDS family deserved medical attention sparked investigations into the effects of SIDS. The dedication to the SIDS family might be attributed to a somewhat defeatist attitude about whether medicine would be able to clarify SIDS reasonably quickly. It also stemmed from mounting social and scholarly attention to death itself and to bereavement. In 1944, Eric Lindemann had studied the survivors and relatives of survivors of a fire in a Boston nightclub. He detailed "acute grief syndrome" as a "psychic disorder" that could happen even to people with no prior psychiatric problems. The centerpiece in his approach to recovery was counseling, and his work started a conversation about the differences between "normal" and "abnormal" grief reactions. Psychologists and psychiatrists became more interested in studying how individuals react and respond to crises and death. In the 1950s and 1960s, most American psychiatrists agreed it was possible to avoid psychiatric pathology following a crisis; they suggested that individual, internal characteristics and resources were crucial in averting negative outcomes. In 1969 psychiatrist Elisabeth Kübler-Ross published *On Death and Dying*. The book was very successful and went through multiple editions; in it, Kübler-Ross outlined five stages of grief (denial, isolation, bargaining, depression, and acceptance). With Kübler-Ross's description of the five stages, grief started to become the central mechanism in psychiatry's approach to coping with trauma or loss. In the 1970s and 1980s, grief therapy and counseling became much more popular.[81] The impulse to attend to survivors of SIDS was one manifestation of these types of considerations.

Multiple studies documented the initial presence of shock and denial among parents, mirroring the first of the five stages Kübler-Ross identified.[82] Guilt was the chief concern of medical scholarship devoted to remediating the psychological effects of SIDS. Parents confirmed that guilt was "almost inevitable and universal followings SIDS."[83] Researchers around the country concurred that SIDS was "one of the most traumatic clinical events that a family may ever experience."[84] They regarded SIDS as a unique source of grief, even among childhood deaths, that wreaked personal and familial havoc. Compared to the anticipated loss of a child, the sudden death of a child deprived parents of time to "psychologically prepare."[85] As a result, SIDS families were unable to undergo "the mitigating factor of anticipatory grief."[86] The negative attitudinal changes associated with the tragic experience of SIDS were also considered more likely to be "permanent and . . . affect all subsequent behavior."[87] SIDS was a nightmarish trauma; parents who experienced it were completely unprepared. It was "like being struck by lightning on a sunny day."[88]

SIDS researchers and activists from the 1970s onward clearly understood SIDS as a major life crisis. Medical literature described SIDS as a "psychological trauma" that was "profound and destructive to a family unit."[89] In one study, more than 10 percent of parents who experienced the loss of a baby suffered from clinically diagnosable post-traumatic stress disorder, even up to eighteen years after the death.[90] As they became more customary, nurses' reports from home visits illumined the full extent of SIDS parents' maladjustment. They suffered serious, long-lasting psychosomatic symptoms. Anger and guilt, Margaret Pomeroy observed, were virtually "universal and all-pervasive."[91] Many parents suffered from anorexia, insomnia, "time confusion," and depression. Their physical symptoms of grief were so palpable that some parents felt as if they were "losing their minds."[92] Some experienced suicidal ideations for years after their child's death, and many underwent crippling losses of self-esteem in their ability to function as parents.[93] Many reports expressed concern that SIDS was associated with marital separation and divorce.[94] In a 1979 presentation, a SIDS center in Wisconsin summarized that SIDS could "result in family disintegration, divorce, alcoholism, overprotectiveness for or withdrawal from surviving children and social alienation."[95]

Parents' testimonies continually authenticated professional reports that SIDS wreaked havoc on families, although many were at a loss to finds words that captured their suffering. Jennifer and Ken Wilkinson discovered their daughter, Larkin, "dead in her bassinet" the day after Christmas. "To hold the cold stiff body of your infant offspring is to see in one unexpected blow your future chapter deleted," Jennifer recounted. "The longer term repercussions from such an event are endless." Sherry and Ronn Waller, a couple from Texas who lost their son Blake just before Thanksgiving, explained, "We actually contemplated suicide to join our son, we were so lost. We sank to the depths of despair and hopelessness."[96] Parents divulged that their sudden and unexpected losses shook their marriages (sometimes to the point of separation), instigated geographic relocations to "escape," and crippled their abilities to make decisions about reproduction and family planning. Although there are no statistics on the divorce rates among SIDS parents, commentators and parents frequently referred to elevated rates of separation as one of SIDS' auxiliary tolls. They pointed to the ubiquitous problem of guilt, the host of negative psychosomatic symptoms, and perceived gendered grieving patterns all as contributing factors in fracturing marriages.[97]

Numerous pieces commented that men and women grieved differently. According to such judgments, fathers were more likely to "suffer in silence" while mothers preferred to talk to someone.[98] Some nurses thought mothers were especially likely to "torture themselves" over the death.[99] Descriptions of common female responses were much more emotive and included crying, talking about feelings, and a stronger inclination to discuss what happened. Descriptions of typical male reactions to SIDS included clamming up, growing distant, trying to forget the death, and a general aversion to talking about it.[100] One interesting, though small, study exclusively looked at fathers' reactions to SIDS. Based on their analysis of twenty-eight SIDS fathers, the authors suggested fathers were more stoic and pragmatic than mothers and that they tended to cope by busying themselves, mostly in arenas outside their homes such as graduate classes, extra work, or consuming hobbies. Compared to their partners, SIDS fathers were more overtly angry and aggressive, and many of the men in the sample conveyed "thinly disguised statements of blame toward the mother."[101] A small-scale study of six SIDS families undergoing therapy confirmed those conclusions: fathers "sought diversion . . . and displaced their guilt and anger through either denial of the death or covert blaming of their wives for some omission in caring for the child."[102]

Gendered grieving patterns were even built into didactic materials training first responders how to handle SIDS in the 1970s and '80s. Instructors explained, for example, that "fathers tend to become withdrawn and deeply engrossed in their work or a hobby." Meanwhile, "as a rule, mothers are at home in a house filled with memories, nightmares, and long hours for thinking."[103] The presumption that mothers were at home was obviously biased, but it also carried class-based assumptions and disregarded working women's experiences. These stereotypes frustrated first responders. In evaluation forms, one EMT commented that "a man would also feel or cope with the death of a baby in the same way a woman would."[104] Another suggested that this lesson "seemed to be perpetuating the myth that men are incapable of having the same emotional feelings as women. I see no reason for this . . . Men have a great deal of social pressure to act in certain ways just as women have pressures and social training to react a different way."[105]

For both genders, medical literature emphasized the emotional repercussions associated with sudden infant death at least as routinely as it described SIDS, and it advised all doctors to be sensitive towards parents.[106] Doctors treated the intense grief and adjustment problems associated with SIDS as both acute and chronic health issues. As Eileen Hasselmeyer, the NICHD administrator responsible for strategizing the nation's approach to SIDS, emphasized to health professionals, "We need to understand the impact of infant death on the family unit, not just SIDS itself."[107]

CONCLUSION

By the 1980s, it was clear that SIDS was an even more messy diagnosis than anyone originally thought. Heightened research generated an abundance of theories, and the pace of study had accelerated so quickly that it became nearly impossible to keep up with. As one theory after another fell short of credibility, even the most promising propositions ultimately proved misdirected. The plethora of "misguided" theories, Bruce Beckwith quipped, turned the theory of the month club into the "theory of the week" club.[108] In 1985, one doctor asked to summarize his knowledge of SIDS replied, "I know many things, but not anything of much importance."[109]

Others clearly felt the same way: SIDS was a "wide open problem."[110] As their efforts to explain SIDS were repeatedly frustrated, doctors increasingly turned their attention to the social aspects of the unsolvable diagnosis. They recommended routine home visits after SIDS cases, and urged that those encounters benefit parents. With a more thorough understanding of the prolonged ways in which SIDS impacted families, physicians became more and more adamant that the diagnosis "should be humanistically oriented."[111] Some of them even delivered the SIDS diagnosis to families precisely "for operations or counseling purposes," or for "charity"—even when it was not official.[112] This type of empathy did help to mitigate the tragedy of SIDS, yet it also cast doubts on the diagnosis's authenticity.

It is hard to feel any sense of satisfaction with the labyrinth that mid-century SIDS medical research produced. The so-called SIDS theory of the month club illustrates how the growing web of SIDS research spun from the 1960s through the 1980s saturated an already-hazy diagnosis with further ambiguity and doubt. Research returns on SIDS came by fits and starts, and modern medicine did not discover any solution. Furthermore, even though medicine endeavored to alleviate the stigma and suffering associated with SIDS, hints of overlaying lingered. On the brink of defeat, medicine continued to recondition the SIDS diagnosis, and in so doing reintroduced unwanted allusions to parental culpability in fresh ways. The joint ventures of solving SIDS and of segregating it from the notion of overlaying proved as beguiling as pulling the sword from the stone.

4 · RISKY BABIES

Just as medicine failed to discern what was happening to SIDS babies, it also failed to stamp out SIDS' ties to suffocation and infanticide. The physicians who partook in constructing SIDS pronounced that SIDS babies were normal. In the 1970s, those lines of thinking fractured; by 1985, medicine's concept of SIDS had "change[d] 180 degrees."[1] Based on the specious possibility that SIDS babies exhibited abnormal breathing patterns while they slept, physicians began to consider that SIDS babies were not entirely normal. They further reasoned that SIDS was a multifactorial, as opposed to singular, anomaly.[2] Following these revisions, organized medicine reconceived SIDS under a new rubric as the aggregate result of numerous interacting factors, some of which derived from simple demographics. In the wake of the apnea theory, medicine redevised SIDS as the outcome of multiple irregularities.

When researchers started to seriously consider the possibility that SIDS babies were abnormal, they opened a metaphorical Pandora's box of contradictions. "New" lines of inquiry returned attention to ideas researchers had been trying to dispel: overlaying, infanticide, suffocation, and the general notion that SIDS deaths were preventable. On top of this, when medicine subscribed to the schema of multiple causality, it unintentionally sustained challenges to the utility and accuracy of the SIDS diagnosis. If SIDS resulted from numerous causes, could it endure as a valid diagnosis? Was the "disease of theories" real? Transitioning to thinking about SIDS in the context of risk factors did ultimately, inadvertently, contribute to tangible gains, but it also served to raise eyebrows about the SIDS diagnosis and the people it struck. It introduced new challenges to SIDS' legitimacy. In 1991, an emergency room physician from Texas Tech University cast aside political correctness as he wondered about the label. "Who are we protecting?" he asked; "Who are we trying to help? More to the point, who are we kidding?"[3]

ANOTHER FRAMEWORK FOR SIDS

Researchers in the 1960s had latched onto correlations as potential causes, attempting to assess whether any given one could explain SIDS. By the 1980s, they prized correlative findings as potential risk factors, and worked to measure the extent to which associations *contributed* to SIDS. Much of what they found corresponded with disparities across social groups. No piece of information was irrelevant—even the smallest details might turn out to be key pieces to the puzzle. In theory, investigators could not afford to ignore anything. In hindsight, though, they gave precedence to certain auspicious elements while dismissing factors long thought to be inapposite.

Richard Naeye's work, conducted at the Hershey Medical Center of the University of Pennsylvania during the 1970s, was representative of this new approach to SIDS research whereby SIDS babies were perceived as "abnormal." Naeye, a medical examiner with ample experience in SIDS pathology, studied autopsy reports of 114 SIDS victims. His postmortem comparative analysis of SIDS with control infants indicated that SIDS babies had some (he found seven) identifiable abnormalities, all of which were related to hypoxia (oxygen shortages) in bodily tissue. This conclusion—that at autopsy, the bodies of SIDS infants showed signs of chronic oxygen deprivation—lent credence to the apnea hypothesis by connecting chronic oxygen shortages (which could result from apnea) to SIDS. Furthermore, Naeye's findings indicated that SIDS researchers needed to set down assumptions that SIDS babies were normal and healthy and instead grapple with the proposition that victims were in fact anatomically or functionally abnormal.[4] Naeye's work effectively cemented this major conceptual shift: SIDS babies were not "normal" after all.[5]

This apparent revelation constituted nothing short of a sea change.[6] "SIDS babies," Marie Valdes-Dapena reflected in 1976, "are different . . . We can see it under a microscope. And there is evidence they were marked from birth, even in utero, before birth."[7] The reassessment provided a cognitive link uniting SIDS with the sleep apnea hypothesis and formed the basis for studies and clinical trials that emerged through the 1970s and 1980s. Amid this revision to the SIDS framework, investigators began looking for longer-term causation where they had once focused on identifying acute causes of death.[8] They also started to look more favorably on the notion of multiple causality.[9] The idea that SIDS probably included numerous disease pathways began to supplant that of single causality. "It seems valid at this point in history," said Bruce Beckwith in 1973, "to adopt the attitude of the 'lumpers.'"[10]

By 1980, most invested researchers agreed that SIDS had several etiological explanations. As one group of pediatricians described, "the elusiveness of this disease suggests that a constellation of *minor* alterations, each of which alone cannot explain death, interacts to produce vulnerability to SIDS."[11] Accord-ing to this view, SIDS babies were exposed to one or many prenatal influences that somehow predisposed them to SIDS. If a susceptible baby was subjected to some external or internal "trigger," such as an upper-respiratory infection or a choking event, he could become overwhelmed and die.[12] Researchers described SIDS as a "mixed bag" or a blanket diagnosis that might literally consist of differ-ent "subgroups of deaths from different causes."[13]

Stemming from both of these significant changes in perspective—that SIDS affected abnormal babies and that it resulted from multiple conditional factors—the next plausible steps seemed to be to identify abnormalities com-mon to SIDS babies and then construct a profile delineating the high-risk patient.[14] At this moment, medicine appeared deceptively equipped to unravel the SIDS puzzle. It was armed with a new arena for specific, measurable investi-gation (sleep apnea) and a novel underlying belief that it was possible to identify abnormalities related to SIDS deaths—risk factors. The risk factor framework became the hub of SIDS research in the 1980s.

Doctors and scientists stepped back and revisited the epidemiological corre-lations identified decades earlier with new vigor and fresh perspective, updating the SIDS profile. Some items from the 1960s remained—the timing with sleep, higher winter rates, higher male rates, and frequent evidence of mild upper respi-ratory tract infections (colds). Researchers accentuated that SIDS was more likely to occur in younger, unmarried mothers with lower levels of education and lower socioeconomic status. It was associated with prematurity, low birth weight, low levels of prenatal care, and maternal drug use, all of which were linked to lower-class populations.[15] Anecdotally, such ties were reminiscent of the indigent women accused of overlaying in the nineteenth century. With this "refined" epidemiological sketch in the twentieth century, researchers moved forward with preliminary attempts to predict the most vulnerable babies.

A research project in Sheffield, England, attempted to do just this, and it encapsulated the risk factor approach to SIDS. The research team, which pub-lished its initial analysis in *The Lancet* in 1983, studied a subject group of 452 babies born from 1973 through 1979. Using epidemiological studies and ret-rospective case review, the researchers devised a scoring rubric intended to measure and predict a baby's risk of dying unexpectedly without cause. The Sheffield Birth Scoring System numerically quantified a child's overall risk pro-file for SIDS. After all the babies born into the study group were scored, the top 14 percent were deemed "high risk." The authors wanted to evaluate the accu-racy of their system as a predictive mechanism for SIDS, but since they thought it was unethical to restrain their study of a high-risk population to mere obser-vation, they implemented a visitation program to potentially benefit the high-risk babies.[16]

Health professionals called and sometimes visited in person to check in on the high-risk babies every two weeks, and then gradually every month, until the babies turned six months old. The authors admitted that it was problematic to assess the outcomes of this simple intervention without any control group, but they documented lower mortality rates than they expected. Instead of the antici-pated fifty-four SIDS deaths, only twenty-nine occurred. The authors deduced that their intervention program was at least partly to thank for the modest reduc-tion in mortality. "The extra care given to the high-risk infants appears to have saved almost as many lives as are saved by paediatric cancer therapy," they said. They pledged to continue working to improve their scoring system and avowed "that the incidence of . . . [SIDS] can be reduced."[17] In a follow-up study pub-lished five years later, the lead authors stood by their results. They scored 85,000 babies before they were one month old, circumscribed a high-risk group of approximately 9,350 babies, and theorized that health visitations could reduce SIDS mortality within the high-risk group by about 25 percent.[18]

These outcomes were more than enough to push other investigators to try for replication and to develop alternative risk assessment techniques. Their results were not encouraging. Studies that used the Sheffield Birth Scoring System found it had little predictive value. Two teams sought to evaluate whether any of Richard Naeye's findings might form the basis for a different scoring system, but they found insufficient statistical significance for clinical screening use. Using measurements from his own sleep apnea laboratory, Alfred Steinschneider developed an index he termed the Prolonged Sleep Apnea 4 (PSA_4); it too had numerous weaknesses. In a review of the field published in 1980, Marie Valdes-Dapena illustrated that predictive systems suffered from obscenely high false-positive rates, ranging from 90 percent to more than 99 percent. She offered the obvious reflection that "a screening test with that many false-positives cannot be used practically."[19]

A multi-center study begun in the late 1970s deepened the conviction that pinpointing risk factors might be able to further medicine's understanding of SIDS, and also signified a shift towards prenatal care as an important risk com-ponent. The project, supported by the National Institute of Child Health and Human Development (NICHD), compared some 800 SIDS deaths against two sets of control babies. Three independent pathologists blindly autopsied every case. The study strengthened the premise that certain families were at risk; its results corroborated not only that SIDS babies were different but also that their mothers were somehow different. SIDS victims "exhibited retardation of growth and development prior to birth," explained Valdes-Dapena, "confirming earlier impressions that the seeds of SIDS are planted during intra-uterine life." With an eye towards prenatal factors, Valdes-Dapena described that "although anybody's baby can succumb to crib death, there are certain types of mothers who are more at risk than others." Which mothers? "Above all else," Valdes-Dapena clarified, "it is clear that SIDS occurs most frequently in lower socio-economic groups. Around the world—in every nation—it is the children of those mothers who are most deprived, socially and economically, who are most susceptible."[20] Mothers whose babies died from SIDS were less likely to have finished high school or had prenatal checkups compared to controls. Teenage mothers were especially vulnerable. Most fell into other risk categories: they were disadvantaged financially, smoked, had fewer years of schooling, and had less access to prenatal care.[21] When the final results of the NICHD-funded study came out, they indicated incontrovertibly that a "disproportionate number of mothers of SIDS subjects are typically multiparous, nonwhite, poor, smokers of lower socioeconomic status, who receive late or no prenatal care in spite of a high frequency of pregnancy problems and deliver a small preterm infant."[22] Given these results, doctors were increasingly convinced that prenatal care might be the linchpin in curbing SIDS.[23]

At the time, conceiving of SIDS in terms of risk factors looked promising—a glimmer of hope in a field mired in the unknown. But in many ways, it was replete with problems. As one critic pointed out, the concept of risk factors may have become "fashionable" in medicine over the course of the 1970s, but its meanings and implications were far from uniform—the concept was "used and abused."[24] Perhaps nowhere did this play out more clearly than in the case of SIDS.

RISKY FAMILIES

The risk factor framework for SIDS forced scientists to confront the diagnosis's murky associations with lower-class and minority families. Since the 1960s, countless publications reported that a disproportionate number of cases occurred in lower class brackets and among blacks.[25] Study after study produced the same conclusion: SIDS struck black families more frequently than white ones. Rates were highest among Native Americans, Alaskan Natives, and poor blacks, and lowest among Asian Americans.[26] Analyses painted racial disparities in SIDS rates as ancillary to socioeconomic inequalities, but the affiliations were exceedingly difficult to parse. Babies born to families in lower socioeconomic brackets were more likely to be low birth weight, premature, and have younger mothers, all of which were strongly correlated with SIDS.[27] Furthermore, the inverse relationship between socioeconomic status and SIDS incidence was not unique—it held true across infant mortality generally.[28]

Parental correlations presented sources of speculation, and gendered, racial, and class-based associations cultivated unfavorable appraisals of women, minorities, and low-income families. Studies searching for discernable associations of SIDS with parental demographics, medical histories, or habits hovered

uncomfortably close to implicating parents. For all their benevolent intentions, home visits presented further occasion to critique parents. When health
professionals traveled to families' homes—even with the intent of offering
assistance—they inquired about nearly every facet of SIDS episodes. Although
nurses were trained specifically not to interrogate parents, the mere act of soliciting information about SIDS deaths could ignite feelings of liability. As one group
of parents in Nebraska explained it, "Questioning [itself] creates doubt, anxiety,
and guilt."[29]

In considering familial circumstances as potentially hazardous, specialists
were liable to perceive disadvantaged families themselves as unhealthy. Mothers became conspicuous subjects of speculation. Epidemiologists and visiting
nurses typically asked SIDS mothers about their personal or caretaking habits
(such as eating patterns, weight gain during pregnancy, or how and when they
took their babies outside).[30] Investigators and home visitors also recorded
women's marital and employment status, assessed the quality of their homes and
their sorrow for their child's passing, as well as adjudged their mental capacities.

These appraisals dated back to the 1960s, when pathologists started reg-
istering families' home environments. In Theodore Curphey's project in Los
Angeles, home visitors noted whether homes appeared disordered, unhygienic,
or unkempt. One typical remark documented that the "household conditions
are not the best—untidy." Another noted that the family resided in "a small
but adequate 2 bedroom home which appeared clear and well-kept."[31] A separate summary described a grieving parent as an "unmarried 18yr. old mother,
who seemed genuinely fond of baby, [and] was at work when death occurred."
This report treated the mother's marital status and "fondness" for her child as
legitimate, pertinent notes. Additional turns of phrase also suggested doubts
about mothers' believability: qualifiers such as "mother denies . . ." or "mother
claims . . ." betray some uncertainty on the part of interviewers. Other language was more direct. One report mentioned that "there were no suspicious
actions on the part of the parents and they appeared to be genuinely upset."[32]
Another described a mother who displayed "no more emotion than usual
when discussing infant's death but appears to be a conscientious mother possibly above average intelligence."[33] Even when commentators defended parents,
they divulged underlying reservations about parents' innocence. A pathologist in New York, for example, attested to one couple's innocence by explaining
that their residence—"nicely furnished and immaculately clean"—was "obviously the home of a responsible married couple who could be expected to take
good care of their offspring."[34] Other descriptions further reiterate that overlaying, suffocation, and parental blame had real staying power because of circumstantial uncertainties. Many death scenes involved children found wedged
between bed surfaces, crib slats, or walls; others involved parental alcohol

consumption.[35] In some cases, parents themselves worried their child had suffocated. One mother who blamed herself said she "wished she knew what she had done."[36] Despite their best intentions, home visitors were, at least on some level, appraising parents' care for their babies.

Margaret Pomeroy, one of earliest nurses to become involved in SIDS research and visitation protocol, as well as a strong advocate for SIDS parents, betrayed larger cultural prejudices in her defense of the single SIDS mother. She noted that "one might suppose that the unmarried mother would not be as deeply affected and might even feel a certain amount of relief when [SIDS] occurs. But this is most decidedly not the case. After all, she chose to keep her baby and to raise him alone, which is not easy. She arranged her life around this decision, and suddenly the need is no longer there. She is left desolate, and often does not have the family support that others do at a time like this."[37] While making the case that unwed mothers might have been especially in need of support services, Margaret Pomeroy intimated that unwed mothers, because of the cultural perceptions of their "situation," were targets of suspicion if SIDS occurred. Other work implicated that some SIDS mothers were deficient. A 1972 study of 226 infant deaths (47 of which were officially SIDS) assessed mothers' intelligence levels. Researchers determined that the group of SIDS cases had "an excess of mothers whose intelligence and domestic efficiency were below average."[38]

Similar pronouncements impugned families in need. In 1974, at an International Symposium on SIDS held in Canada, a California physician reasoned that SIDS incidence rates varied by class because "those people with a better background take better care of their children, and they take them seriously and give them better care." His colleagues wondered whether locational declines in SIDS "might be indeed a reflection of care and fussing enough." Others further speculated that some decreases, especially in inner-city areas, might be "due merely to 'the pill' and relaxation of abortion laws, so that every child is a wanted child and carefully nurtured."[39] A local newspaper piece in 1981 connoted that medicine was learning that where SIDS occurred, "the 'home standard' was lower . . . and that included a lower standard of infant care."[40] A study published in the *New England Journal of Medicine* in 1986, based on death scene investigations in Brooklyn, New York, determined that "poor judgment by the caretaker of the infant . . . [was] an important contributing factor in almost all of the deaths" studied.[41] These appraisals bore resemblance to those of nineteenth-century mothers whose "ignorance and vice" led to their babies' deaths by overlaying.

In the second half of the 1900s, defenders of disadvantaged groups pointed out that SIDS also occurred in more privileged populations.[42] But lower-class and minority families were distinctly disadvantaged and mistreated in the aftermath of SIDS. Across the United States, upper-class families routinely benefited from more information and clear communication. They were more likely to be asked permission to conduct an autopsy, to be provided information, and to be offered counseling.[43] White families were much more likely to receive any explanation at all for their child's death. While 41 percent of white families learned their baby's autopsy results within one week, only 28 percent of black families heard as quickly. On the opposite end of the spectrum, just 5 percent of white parents never heard any results from their child's autopsy but 23 percent of black families never heard back.[44] Poor families were also less likely to have private family physicians with whom they could consult, and parent groups (predominantly white middle-class organizations) struggled to connect with inner-city and minority SIDS families.[45] While 75 percent of upper-class families victimized by SIDS in 1973 reported that they had heard of SIDS before, only 48 percent of lower-class families were familiar with the condition.[46] Disadvantaged Americans were simply not well or promptly informed of the SIDS diagnosis.

Even more disturbing, similar deaths in white families were almost two times as likely to be explained as SIDS compared to those in black families, which were nearly four times as likely to be explained as "suffocation."[47] In Abraham Bergman's 1972 national survey, 57 percent of white families were offered SIDS as an explanation for their child's death compared to only 27 percent of black families. And, while only 3 percent of white parents were told their baby had suffocated, 11 percent of black families were told as such.[48] When asked about his death-coding procedures, one Alabama coroner replied that suffocation—not SIDS—was the real culprit, since "blacks do not know how to care for their children properly."[49] As Bruce Beckwith summarized, "Far too often an infant [death] in a 'nice' family is SIDS, but in other families an identical kind of death is interpreted as suffocation, neglect, or deliberate infanticide. It is unfortunately not rare for parents of SIDS victims to be treated as suspected criminals in many communities."[50]

Formal indictments were anomalous, but those few SIDS parents who did face formal criminal charges or jail time were indeed lower class, minorities, or both. Despite their being atypical, Abraham Bergman described these outlying cases as "illustrative of the suspicious attitude that is prevalent throughout the country."[51] They certainly exemplify how disadvantaged families were criminalized after SIDS.

After John and Pat Smiley lost their daughter Genya to SIDS, they were jailed for involuntary manslaughter. At their home in southern California, John and Pat Smiley discovered Genya one afternoon after sleeping in late. They were unable to afford a crib, so Genya slept in a drawer, a fact the prosecution employed as evidence of neglect. The day of Genya's death, the sherriff's office helped respond to the couple's call for an ambulance. Enforcement asked both parents about their drug and alcohol use, separated them, and had them take drug tests before placing them both in jail. Ovidio Penalver, a medical student at the University of Southern California who had worked the previous year on the SIDS management survey, read about the Smileys in the newspaper. He immediately contacted Abraham Bergman and got in touch with the couple to reassure them. SIDS parent activists, outraged, took up the Smileys' case, which was ultimately thrown out.[52]

Roy and Evelyn Williams, a black couple from the Bronx, were similarly tried for criminal neglect in the death of their son. Police questioned the couple separately and incarcerated them with a $1,000 bail. At the time of her baby's death, Evelyn had been undergoing treatment for postpartum depression, a detail that increased suspicion. Roy and Evelyn remained in prison for five and six months, respectively, before they could meet bail. Abraham Bergman testified on the Williams' behalf at their court hearing in New York, but he was never even called to bear witness. After hearing the details, the judge threw out the case. As Bergman snidely described, the Williams were "free—free to live with their memories of spending half a year inside a New York City jail mourning for their dead baby."[53] After fielding criticism for the city's handling of the case, the renowned New York medical examiner Milton Helpern reflected that "the Williams baby occupied a crib with an older sibling infant and was found dead by the father, who initially told the police that the child had not been fed for several days." "The conclusions of the Medical Examiner in a death due to neglect," he continued, "are not arrived at by caprice."[54] Helpern further explained that the Williams case followed standard investigatory protocol. Elsewhere, Helpern passionately defended his department's handling of sudden infant mortality, protesting that critics who insinuated his office presumed infant deaths were criminal acts were not only wrong but were "interfering with the research program we are carrying out."[55]

John and Billy Mae Price, a young, poor couple in South Carolina, also had to pass through the legal system. Their case also reflects how challenging it could be to differentiate SIDS and child abuse. When the Prices arrived at the hospital, the emergency room doctor who received them noticed a bruise on their baby's head and then became aware that the couple's first child had died similarly when she was four months old. He considered the possibility of child abuse and called the police. John Price was imprisoned and prevented from attending his son's funeral before being released. When asked about his experience, he told a reporter, "I don't think they treated us right at all."[56]

UNEASY THOUGHTS

Accounts detailing possible criminality in SIDS episodes did not help in exonerating parents. Neither did media translations of medical research, which dutifully covered the theory of the month club. Even though journalists reported that sudden unexplained infant deaths were caused by "real disease" and were not the fault of parents, their pieces painted a confusing picture.[57] Papers and magazines printed articles on SIDS correlations and constantly suggested that medicine was just on the cusp of resolving SIDS. Headlines such as "'Crib Deaths' Answer Seen Imminent" and "Sudden Infant Death Causes Uncovered" mingled with titles relaying various theories, like "Biochemist Links Crib Death to Low Level of Sugar in Blood," "Antibodies Found in Lungs of SIDS Victims," and "California Researchers Report They Have Identified a Bacterium Linked to Crib Deaths."[58] Furthermore, periodic coverage of infanticide, abuse, and other accidents confused for SIDS sustained ideas about smothering and suffocation.[59] Indeed, one disconcerting facet of the history of SIDS is that so many case reports either strayed from the definition or else accentuate how convoluted it was. Numerous children in the 1970s and 1980s, for example, were said to die from SIDS when they were well over one year of age.[60]

Medical investigations, for all their diversity, shared an important commonality: they endeavored to deconstruct the theory of suffocation. Indeed, many investigators considered it their personal project to dispel the association between SIDS and smothering. But doctors working to disprove smothering found it a difficult notion to discard. Regardless of physicians' protestations, parents remained caught in the grips of the suffocation premise. Joyce Hanlon died from SIDS when she was a little over four months; her mother found her in her crib with a blanket wrapped around her head, speculating that Joyce had suffocated.[61] Circumstances like this led many parents to assume that not only had their child suffocated, but it had also suffered. Consider the following description of a typical case: "the death scene is often one of disarray. The infant is frequently found wedged into the corner of the bed, far from where he was put down to sleep. Blankets are often heaped up, and sometimes cover the infant's head, giving rise to the invidious thought of possible suffocation."[62] When pressed, even doctors adamant that SIDS was not synonymous with overlaying or smothering had to concede that both were literal, if rare, possibilities.[63] As late as 1990, pathologist Richard Naeye permitted that "accidental smothering by a parent . . . remains a possible cause of SIDS."[64] Even more, it was often difficult, if not impossible, to distinguish between SIDS and intentional suffocation by homicide based on an autopsy.[65] As Marie Valdes-Dapena admitted, "Autopsy findings in cases of suffocation with a soft object are usually the same as those in a typical crib death."[66] Comments like these hearkened back to descriptions of overlaying from previous centuries.

The admission that known suffocation and SIDS cases presented similarly raised forthright concerns about discerning between SIDS and infanticide. In a 1968 article published in the *Mount Sinai Journal of Medicine*, psychiatrist Stewart Asch stated that a majority of crib deaths were in fact episodes of maternal infanticide instigated by postpartum depression (PPD). Asch based his conjecture on his professional observations and experience with PPD and a single study in England from 1927 suggesting that over 40 percent of female admissions to the State Criminal Lunatic Asylum were due to infanticide. By his explanation, new mothers suffering from PPD often experienced suicidal ideations. Their babies could be endangered if they experienced a sort of "confusion and alternation of identities" between themselves and their babies, a mix-up that could lead the mother to transpose her suicidal aims onto her baby. Asch also thought the epidemiological correlations were suspicious: SIDS cases co-occurred with the PPD time frame, appeared similar at autopsy to suffocation (the most common mechanism of infanticide), and tended to happen during early morning hours (the "period of greatest agitation in depressed individuals") and winter months (when adult suicide rates also peaked). According to Asch, a "large proportion" of sudden infant deaths were probably "covert infanticides" that resulted from "confusion in identities between mother and fetus/baby . . . [whereby] infanticide may occur in place of suicide."[67]

Asch's proposition provoked both criticism and approval. In 1977, using vital statistics from 1950 through the early 1970s, two epidemiologists denounced Asch's hypothesis as "untenable." They did locate an increase in infant homicide rates, but found that no decrease in infant homicide rates occurred after SIDS became an official death certificate coding.[68] That same year, in a chapter on intentional accidents, the sixteenth edition of the textbook *Pediatrics* wondered whether "a significant proportion of *crib deaths* may actually be the result of parental assault." Physicians ought to be suspicious, the piece stipulated, "whenever there is a long delay between the time the child was last seen alive and the discovery of death." This alarmed physicians studying SIDS, who knew that often SIDS parents did not discover their child for hours. The chapter's author, a professor of pediatrics at Albert Einstein Medical College in New York, went as far as to indicate that many SIDS deaths "most likely . . . represent instances of deliberate injury inflicted on children by parents or caretakers and are made to simulate accidents."[69]

A decade later, pathologist Alan W. Cashell defended Asch's supposition in the *American Journal of Forensic Medicine and Pathology*. Cashell described two cases, one of murder and the other of attempted murder, as "evidence that homicide should be considered as a cause of sudden, unexpected death in infants even when autopsy reveals no specific findings." Cashell argued that a sizable number of annual SIDS deaths were "actually murders," and urged his colleagues to conduct scrupulous postmortem exams.[70] Asch and his supporters were responding to a somewhat new cognizance, but their observations were redolent of SIDS' historical ties to overlaying.

While parents and doctors were still groping for its legitimacy, SIDS became all the more delicate given the nation's heightened consciousness of child abuse. In the 1960s, interest in child abuse exploded in the medical and public sectors. Attention had been slowly mounting since the mid-1940s, when a pediatric radiologist named John Caffey published an article describing X-rays from six children with subdural hematomas. Together, they also had twenty-three fractures and four contusions. None of their injuries were explained.[71] Caffey offered abuse as one possible explanation. He thought it was conceivable that parents might miss a head bump that caused a hematoma, since sometimes even a small accident could do so, and often the symptoms were delayed from the time of injury. But that explanation did not hold up with the bone fractures. Parents would have observed those injuries, and they exhibited visible symptoms almost immediately. Whatever events caused his six patients' fractures, Caffey reflected, "were either not observed or were denied when observed."[72] In other words, either those parents missed something significant, or they were lying. The implication sparked what scholar John E. B. Myers called "a small but steady stream" of interest in child abuse.[73] Almost two decades later, in 1962, when Henry Kempe and a group of colleagues published "The Battered-Child Syndrome" in *JAMA*, as Myers writes, what had been "a trickle of writing" on abuse evolved into "a torrent."[74]

Kempe's article was a watershed in child protection, but it is easy to see how it muddied the waters with regards to the SIDS diagnosis. Kempe and his co-authors identified the battered-child syndrome as a "clinical condition in young children who have received serious physical abuse." They cited it as a "frequent cause of permanent injury or death." Kempe advised that the syndrome be considered in a number of different situations, ranging from the presentation of highly visible symptoms such as bone fractures or a subdural hematoma to more subtle expressions such as "failure to thrive." One of the indications was "any child who dies suddenly." Battered-child syndrome victims, "as a general rule," were usually under three years old, and "most, in fact are infants."[75] Abusive parents were not necessarily clinically psychopathic or visibly disturbed; cases occurred "among people with good education and stable financial and social background." To anyone working on SIDS, these circumstances sounded strikingly familiar. Kempe's recommendation, indeed his entreaty, was in essence that the battered-child syndrome be on the differential diagnosis list for a SIDS case. "A physician needs to have a high initial level of suspicion of the diagnosis of the battered-child syndrome . . . in any child who dies suddenly."[76]

Stories on child abuse multiplied in major national media outlets. The magnified awareness precipitated a new era of protective services for children.[77] It also had the effect of heightening suspicion surrounding sudden infant death. As Abraham Bergman observed in 1973, "increasing publicity being given to another neglected problem, child abuse, has tended to direct more suspicion to families of SIDS victims."[78] Doctors and others heard simultaneous, conflicting messages. On the one hand, they were instructed to be attentive and perceptive to possible child abuse cases, in which sudden infant death was a major red flag.[79] From another corner, they learned to dispel any inclination towards accusation in the exact same situation. While pamphlets and informative literature tried to distill the distinctions between child abuse or neglect and SIDS, the reality looked much murkier.[80]

Beyond its presentation, the battered-child syndrome posed a problem for diagnosing SIDS because it appeared quite prevalent. In the mid-1960s in Los Angeles, for example, pathologist Theodore Curphey estimated that around 2 percent of infant deaths were the result of abuse.[81] A 1980 analysis the Department of Justice produced exclaimed that "some observers believe that child abuse has 'reached epidemic proportions.'" Before more formal surveys, it was impossible to nail down actual incidence rates, but reported cases had escalated rapidly following Kempe's 1962 article, and virtually all professionals agreed that the real extent of abuse was just starting to come into focus. One researcher called child abuse the "major killer" of American children, suggesting that it might cause up to fifty thousand deaths per year. Two alternative estimates placed the number of children who died annually directly because of abuse at between a few thousand and more than sixteen thousand.[82] The government funded the first major systematic study around 1980. That year, it documented over 625,000 cases in which abuse or neglect led to visible harm; by 1986, that number had increased to over 930,000.[83] The notion that child abuse, and abuse-related mortality, were relatively regular occurrences, and that researchers could only discern "the tip of the iceberg," did not take any pressure off SIDS families.[84]

The literature suggested that child abuse was so under-recognized in part because physicians were blind to such horrific parental wrongdoing—that they were literally incapable of believing parents had the capacity to be abusive. This disbelief inhibited physicians from noticing signs of abuse or asking parents about the subject.[85] This behavior flew in the face of prevailing claims of SIDS researchers and affected parents who indicated medical professionals often assumed abuse. Regardless, rising attention to child abuse, especially given its associations with poverty, did deepen SIDS' controversial character.[86]

Smothering was a resilient feature in SIDS research, if for no other reason than the notion constantly needed to be negated.

SIDS AND FAMILIAL BEHAVIOR

The notion of abnormality and the risk factor framework for SIDS also facilitated understated ties to suffocation and parents. Alternative investigations into SIDS extended beyond the confines of biomedicine and hospital walls, and they touched on the thorny issue of familial misconduct. Lewis Lipsitt, a leading psychologist at Brown University who directed the school's Child Study Center and founded the journal *Infant Behavior and Development*, began working on SIDS just as medical scientists were becoming wed to the notion that SIDS resulted from a complex, convoluted combination of various errors. Lipsitt's perspective held that infancy was a pivotal phase of learning and adaptation, and the discrete timing of SIDS was paramount. His hypothesis was behavioral, though he suggested that physiological irregularities were also crucial—these could compromise infants' learning and make them susceptible to SIDS.[87] He called the human infant a "reciprocating organism." Babies, he said, were highly responsive, and their primary task was to learn. Infancy was "practice for the future."[88] Lipsitt theorized that some kind of learning disability instigated SIDS. Constitutional abnormalities might blend with environmental factors to produce what Lipsitt called a "reflex response failure," and he was particularly concerned with failures related to breathing. When an infant experienced respiratory blockage, Lipsitt explained, its natural response was to take "defensive action." Lipsitt thought SIDS infants might have never learned to correctly clear their airways, thus failing to take the appropriate "defensive action" when something threatened their ability to breathe.[89]

Lipsitt contended that physical weaknesses could become "activated" by environmental conditions. Underlying anatomical shortcomings might inhibit learning by suppressing a baby's natural reflex responses or impairing its ability to learn vital responsive behaviors, such as clearing an airway. These factors could "combine and interact to constitute a 'learning-disabled' infant who may succumb to SIDS if presented fortuitously with a life-threatening situation."[90] Susceptible babies raised in environments that, for whatever reason, failed to "teach" them adequate respiratory responses, might in turn fail to respond to oxygen deficits, and die.[91]

Lipsitt's learning disability theory involved three composite shortcomings: the infant's anatomical deficiencies, the mother's qualities or background, and the interactive relationship between both parties. He was earnest in his insistence that researchers refrain from "value judgments concerning how 'good the mother is with her infant,'" but still at the base considered both SIDS mothers and infants to be "deficient in some unknown number and type of dimensions that might otherwise lead to a smoothly interacting, reciprocal relationship."[92] Mindful of his work's suggestive nature, Lipsitt implored medicine to broaden its perspective:

> Sometimes the presentation of findings which suggest that style of living may be implicated in the deaths of infants causes consternation. Few of us would like to believe that the behavior of parents or the milieu in which infants are raised, which the parents may not be able to alter, can be legitimately tagged as contributors to death. However, we must look beyond the accusatory paranoia which so frequently accompanies the SIDS phenomenon and try to find the fortuitous and seemingly benign conditions in the lives of families and infants which appear to be implicated as SIDS precursors. Smoking behavior is one such condition.[93]

The general concept that a learning disability gave rise to SIDS gelled with medical scientists' prevailing belief in multiple causality. Furthermore, it left room for variation while still accounting for the specific age frame for SIDS, and also merged the physical with the mental. In other words, Lipsitt's idea—that SIDS could occur when underlying "subtle perinatal hazards and constitutional insufficiencies" were "compounded by the failure of experience to prepare the infant for later threats to survival"—heeded the dominant science across the social and technical disciplines.[94] Work such as Lipsitt's demonstrates how scholarship began to treat SIDS as part of a highly complex nexus of infant, parent, familial, and environmental constitutions and interactions.

Psychoanalyst Arno Gruen trained at New York University and worked as a psychology professor at Rutgers University for seventeen years. Remembered predominantly for a book on the "autonomous self," Gruen published a little-known but fascinating piece on SIDS in 1987. His idea was based on "arousability." As Gruen explained, a baby's ability to either be aroused or to arouse itself from sleep was directly related to its environmental circumstances. Specifically, a baby's arousal abilities depended on its "experience with intensity of stimulation particularly during early development." Arousability was "determined by the interplay of stimuli and responses between the infant and its mother."[95] At first glance these notions appear subtle deviations from Lipsitt's work, and Gruen was not alone in his contentions about arousal. Research contending that SIDS babies had problems with arousal response mechanisms even fit well with ongoing sleep medicine research.[96] Yet Gruen used these notions to further a psychiatric theory for SIDS that was brimming with sexism. Gruen's hypothesis conveyed that mothers were at least partly to blame for SIDS. He argued that a baby's ability to become aroused was decided by its early exposure to stimulation and interplay, both of which were the exclusive charge of its mother.

Gruen suggested that mothers, by interacting with their babies with "tenderness and love," created a "life-supporting mesh of stimuli" for their children. When the mesh weakened, he cautioned, "structural maturation and maintenance [of the baby] become seriously impaired."[97] With these ideas in mind, Gruen studied the interactive patterns of parents who had lost children to SIDS.

Between 1981 and 1985 Gruen conducted interviews with fourteen sets of parents who had lost a child to SIDS in the previous decade. He assessed the "unconscious feelings of resentment and aggression in interpersonal relations as revealed through mother-father interaction, contradictions in statements, omissions in accounts, [and] phantasies and dreams."[98] Gruen's adverse appraisals of the women he interviewed were conspicuous. Consider the following representative excerpts: Mrs. A "gave the impression of a person with insufficient energies for building a self of her own" and seemed to have grieved "only for herself," rather than her child. Mrs. B, a "lonely, alienated feeling woman" had a "dissociative quality" and a "minimal capacity for empathic relatedness." Mrs. C. "seemed capable yet at the same time childlike." Mrs. E was a "woman who appears unable to extend love to anyone," and her "'guilt' feelings do not seem so much to be based on empathy for what [her] little boy suffered, but worry about what others would say about her image as a mother." Mrs. G's "insistence on the appearance of happiness, her persistence on smiling while speaking of sad and upsetting things, suggest . . . a great deal of dissociated hatred and hostility."[99]

Gruen concluded that the mothers he interviewed "appeared in need of mothering" and depended entirely upon their husbands for confidence.[100] SIDS mothers, he observed, adopted "dependent" roles in their families; their literal status as "dependents" in their own homes, he said, opposed their own conceptions of themselves as wives and mothers. That distance, Gruen continued—between the observed reality that his mother subjects were dependent and their own ideas of themselves as caretakers—cultivated unconscious resentment. Their resentment led mothers to reject "their child's *aliveness, independence or uniqueness.*"[101] In contrast, Gruen described that the fathers in his study group "demonstrated an exceptional degree of mothering" and were "clearly highly solicitous and prone to caretaking."[102] This interpretation of fathers' propensity for "mothering" was not complimentary. Gruen regarded the fathers in his study as more capable than their spouses yet still participatory in a harmful episode of role reversal. Not leaving any doubt as to his interpretation, Gruen conveyed that the behavior of SIDS mothers "'confirms,' despite cultural denial, the 'dependency' and essential 'weakness' or 'inferiority' of women."[103] Babies deprived of sufficient tactile stimulation—a function "determined by the quality of the mother's lovingness"—could suffer inhibited arousal capabilities.[104] A mother's "rejecting attitude toward her infant . . . is not being proposed as a cause of SID[S]," Gruen clarified, but "it is proposed as being a factor in the pre-disposition for SID[S] if the rejection is unconscious."[105]

Gruen said his findings could offer practical applications. If mothers' disassociations could be rectified, their children might be saved. Gruen referred to research on scoring systems to identify high-risk babies, recounting conclusions from Sheffield that health counselor visitations decreased the SIDS "expectancy rates." Gruen thought this evidence bore out his hypothesis, and that his idea helped explain the study's results. As he described, "being an object of concern and interest to another person [the health visitation counselor] reduced the mother's narcissistic resentment towards her child as well as her conflicts about dependency on her husband."[106] The researchers who implemented the visitation system in Sheffield had argued that it conferred some advantage for infants that reduced their vulnerability to SIDS; Gruen thought it conferred some advantage to mothers that enabled them to function more satisfactorily as caretakers.

Gruen's work was unsound in a number of ways. His methodologies were distorted. Gruen conducted interviews years after parents had suffered the loss of a child and thus was retroactively evaluating parents' psychological states at the time of the SIDS event. By the mid-1980s, scholarship substantiated that the death of a child exerted powerful and lasting physical and mental impacts on parents. Gruen's interpretations were subjective, but even if one were to accept them, it is reasonable to assume that the SIDS parents he interviewed experienced long-term personality and emotional adjustments as a result of their loss. Gruen's protocol would have been better suited to evaluate the effects of SIDS on individuals, marriages, and families, instead of the circumstances preceding SIDS. Lastly, Gruen's descriptions speak for themselves; they vilify mothers.

Gruen's mother-blaming was not new or unusual. Indeed, scholars have shown that mother-blaming has existed in many forms throughout history. Molly Ladd-Taylor and Lauri Umanski distinguish three categories of women most vulnerable to charges that they are "bad" mothers: those in nontraditional family situations or minority mothers, those who "would not or could not protect their children from harm," and those whose children "went wrong." Historically, when children die, Ladd-Taylor and Umanski elaborate, "mother-blaming abounds." Especially after it was understood under the umbrella of "risk factors" and "risk groups" that spliced with parental behaviors, SIDS was ripe for mother-blaming.[107] Furthermore, in the decades following World War II, psychiatry and related fields ascribed to a particular strand of "antimaternalism" that manifested in a "narrow, psychologically focused form of mother-blaming." The ideal mother was a perfect blend of the right psychology with the right biology.[108] Many psychiatrists stressed the issues of "separation and individuation" of a child from its mother, and the approach lent to blame. In her survey of mental-health journals published in the 1970s and 1980s, scholar Paula Caplan found that professionals "were overwhelmingly indulging in mother-blaming."[109] Arno Gruen's hypothesis is a prime example of this scenario.

Gruen published his work in the fledgling journal of the Association for Pre-natal and Perinatal Psychology in 1987. The piece does not appear to be widely known or cited. His more extensive unpublished research, however, circulated among the "SIDS Behavioral Network," a research group consisting of forty-eight international professionals across academic disciplines that Lewis Lipsitt specifically convened to draw attention to possible behavioral and psychological factors related to SIDS.[110] In soliciting feedback on it, Lipsitt exposed Gruen's research to an invested readership. Writing to his colleagues, Lipsitt described that Gruen's thesis would be "undoubtedly controversial in a world that tends to deny that any psychological factors or behavior have anything to do with SIDS."[111] That Lipsitt considered Gruen's work suitable for circulation is telling, and Gruen's ideas did gain some approval. Prominent anthropologist Ashley Montagu supported Gruen's conclusions in an unpublished letter to the *New England Journal of Medicine*. Montagu contended that "inadequate maternal care" and a failure to adapt to postnatal breathing errors were factors in SIDS. He specifically referenced Gruen's study as a compelling demonstration of how "the failure of mothering is the principle factor in producing the conditions which lead to SID[S]."[112]

Implicating apnea, a pair of researchers had proposed an idea similar to Gruen's in 1975. Psychiatrist Steven Friedlander and long-time SIDS researcher Edward Shaw contended that apneic episodes were not the result of a biologi-cal process gone awry but instead "were invoked by the SIDS infant when ten-sions in his environment (and particularly the tensions of parentally-induced anxiety) become too severe for the infant's 'normal' coping mechanisms to atten-uate." Apnea was not a physical pathology but a "psycho-social dysfunctional-ism."[113] Endeavoring to veer away from a strictly medical framework for SIDS, proponents of such psycho-social theories saw SIDS as the cumulative result of social epidemiological factors, rather than anatomic epidemiological factors. The social governed the physical. For Friedlander and Shaw, apnea was "the end-point of a continuing process of tension-induced psycho-physiologic regression, in which the infant is able, finally, to effect an 'escape' from a situation that is no longer tenable."[114] SIDS was the result of an evolutionary defense mechanism; babies reflexively tried to "escape" from unfavorable living conditions in which they had unmet psychological (emotional) and physical needs. "We believe that the epidemiology of SIDS," they said, "paints a convincing picture of a psycho-socially dysfunctional environment. It is dysfunctional because it causes the death of the infant." Given this conclusion, their additional specifi-cation that this "in no way implicates the parents in any 'blameworthy' sense" hardly mattered.[115] These attempts to step outside the proverbial box and consider the importance of social factors in alleviating SIDS—an admirable aspiration—ultimately did point fingers at parents.

CONCLUSION

For American families, risk factors offered little peace of mind. Media reporters informed parents that their only "refuge" from SIDS was in statistics.[116] The chance was about one in 350. Most parents probably found no solace in those odds, and SIDS parents certainly did not. For them, SIDS was not the output of a risk-assessment equation or an unfortunate statistical possibility. Lynnda Reed lost her son Kenny in 1976. Reed was helping her daughter get ready for a Valentine's Day party when she "had an awful premonition" and went to check on Kenny. In an instant, she became a "SIDS parent." Five years later in an interview, Reed recoiled at questions about "high-risk" categories. For all the risk profiles doctors produced, as far as Reed was concerned, "CHANCE . . . [was] the only 'known' factor in causing SIDS." "Most SIDS parents really don't like statistics," Reed said, "because people read those statistics and then categorize or stereotype us."[117]

Reed's observations were poignant. The theory of the week club and the risk factor framework were meant to help solve the problem of SIDS. But in time they weakened the precept that SIDS was totally unpreventable and unpredictable. SIDS correlations with certain groups of people (such as lower-class Americans) and certain behaviors (such as smoking) contributed to colloquial assumptions that SIDS was associated with lower "home standards . . . and . . . a lower standard of infant care."[118] Establishing risk correlations ultimately made it all too easy, Bruce Beckwith warned, "to be judgmental to the parent who is suboptimal in the view of society, who falls short of our concept of ideal."[119] Furthermore, the risk factor framework laid the foundation for diverse new hypotheses that called parents, as well as SIDS itself, into question.

Bruce Beckwith's observation that "the diagnosis of SIDS places the pathologist in the position of being judge and jury" foreshadowed an attempt to refine the SIDS diagnosis.[120] In 1989, the SIDS definition was amended to require death scene investigations. SIDS became "the sudden death of an infant under one year of age which remains unexplained after complete postmortem examination, including an investigation of the death scene and a review of the case history."[121] Every home and family struck by SIDS became subject to professional review—it is not hard to imagine that families asked to reenact SIDS death scenes using dolls, as is done in criminal cases, felt like they were suspects.[122] Despite the impetus to reorient sudden infant mortality and vindicate families, the construction of SIDS under the risk factor framework still left families vulnerable to accusations. Because of its own ambiguities, the SIDS diagnosis confused just as much as enlightened, and villainized just as much as it humanized sudden infant death. In other words, the medicalization of SIDS both exculpated and incriminated families. In the 1960s and beyond, no one felt this pressure more fully than parents themselves. Parents struggled just as much as professionals to sort out SIDS' strains, and while they did not necessarily take comfort in risk factors, in research hints, in statistical odds, or in population associations, they did find support in one another.

5 · MOBILIZATION
SIDS Activism

By the middle of 1968, Americans could see death all around them. After the Tet Offensive and the My Lai Massacre, the United States descended into the depths of its involvement in Vietnam. The death toll was climbing quickly into the tens of thousands. The Civil Rights Movement had been shaken to the ground by the assassination of Martin Luther King Jr. in April; his death touched off upheaval across the country, including major riots in Chicago, Baltimore, and Washington, DC. Dozens of Americans died in the turmoil. Barely two months later, Bobby Kennedy was assassinated. In July, more race riots broke out in Cleveland, Ohio, and Gary, Indiana. Nationwide, crime and homicide rates were escalating to new heights; over the decade, serious crime rates rose by 62 percent. In 1968 alone 13,650 Americans were murdered.[1] All of the year's horrific deaths were hammered into the public's consciousness—it was practically impossible to escape from them. Juxtaposed to these very public losses, thousands more deaths, of young babies, were endured in private homes and lives. Losses to "crib death" were still brimming under the surface of the nation's schizophrenic attention. Parents and families affected were out of sight, and they coped in isolation.

In July of that year, before the turbulence in her own city at the Democratic National Convention, before women's liberation groups hosted the famous protest of the Miss America Beauty Pageant in Atlantic City, and before the Tlateloco Square student massacre at the Summer Olympics in Mexico City, Carolyn Szybist was home in her tiny second-floor apartment near Chicago's North Side, flipping through *Redbook* magazine, when a piece on crib death caught her eye. Szybist, a passionate and creative emergency room nurse with a determination one colleague initially dubbed "pushy," had encountered crib death before. In the ER where she worked, babies brought in dead on arrival without any clear reason were quietly known as "those babies." One of the first cases of "those babies" Szybist witnessed had ended with her performing a posthaste baptism to help solace the child's hysterical mother. That was almost a decade earlier, but Szybist remembered it vividly; three months after the baby girl died, her parents had read Szybist's engagement announcement in the paper and sent her a crystal rose vase.

Szybist consoled other parents and read other articles, but the *Redbook* piece spoke to her. Across the country, Szybist read, "for 50 or 60 mothers each morning—more than that on winter mornings, fewer in the summer—the moment of return [to their child's crib] is a tragedy they could never forget." She knew this. She was one of those mothers. On a comfortably cool Saturday morning exactly three years prior, Szybist had returned from working a night shift to find her son, Larry, dead in his crib. Now, after three years of grieving and despondency, Szybist was ready. She copied down the address for the National Foundation for SIDS (later renamed the National SIDS Foundation, NSIDSF) and wrote that she wanted to get involved.[2]

Szybist became hooked. She made some calls and started up an NSIDSF chapter in Chicago. Its first parents' meeting was cathartic. "Our stories were different. Our feelings were the same," Szybist recalled, "and I cannot describe the joy that happened in finding each other." By coincidence, the American Academy of Pediatrics (AAP) was meeting in Chicago that fall, and Szybist asked Abraham Bergman to speak to local parents. He agreed and left Szybist with media and professional contacts that "flung [her] into the fray." Szybist's involvement deepened as she fielded interview requests and met with physicians and coroners. The Chicago NSIDSF chapter sprung up so quickly and with such participation that less than one year later, in the spring of 1969, the NSIDSF offered Szybist a board position and put her in charge of chapter development.[3] Szybist chaired major projects for the NSIDSF, including orchestrating the first National Parent/Medical Conference on SIDS and planning nursing education. She consulted with burgeoning local and hospital programs seeking to address SIDS, and became vice president of the NSIDSF in 1972. In 1976, Szybist was appointed executive director.[4]

Szybist's immersion in the NSIDSF stands out because Szybist had a medical background and occupied leadership roles, but other parents matched her personal commitment. Across the country, parents' activism and ensuing policy changes brought the NSIDSF into the purview of hundreds of other affected families, who saw in the organization the promise of fellowship and an outlet for frustration and sadness. SIDS organizations like the one to which Carolyn Szybist devoted herself extended to parents through informal group therapy, political activism, and channeled organizational ambitions. They offered the hand of optimism, and many parents (almost exclusively middle class and white) accepted it.

Although the NSIDSF eventually succumbed to financial deficits and internal disputation, parents' efforts forced SIDS into the nation's consciousness. SIDS parents and their allies assembled a small but meaningful national activist organization. The NSIDSF was categorically devoted to "fixing" the manifold problems associated with SIDS. It highlighted the ways in which America mismanaged SIDS and then helped inspire legislation, funding, and attention, all of which compelled federally operated sudden infant death organizational centers. Parents brought SIDS out of the shadows; with professional allies, they made the private loss of SIDS a public matter. Most importantly, in forming the NSIDSF, parents like Carolyn Szybist came together, and their fellowship and activism eased their pain.

PARENTS COME TOGETHER

The genesis of SIDS organizations was inspired by the successful legacies of mass-based associations like the National Tuberculosis Association and the National Foundation for Infantile Paralysis. Both groups intended to overcome particular conditions (tuberculosis and polio); they taught that the combined, focused efforts of motivated professionals and laypeople could overcome the nation's most feared diseases. Founded in the 1960s in the shadows of such behemoth examples, SIDS organizations worked to mirror their forerunners' successful strategies. Compared to their predecessors, SIDS groups were much smaller—at their peak, even combined, they had a mere fraction of the membership and funding of older models. The initial mobilization of parents affected by sudden infant death highlighted both the numbers of sudden unexplained infant mortality and the long-term suffering it induced. In less than two years in the early 1960s, three major organizations flowered on the coasts: the Mark Addison Roe Foundation in New York, the Washington Association for Sudden Infant Death Study in Seattle, and the Guild for Infant Survival in Baltimore. In all three cases, parents who felt alone and confused compelled action.

In 1958, Jed and Louise Roe, a middle-class couple living in Greenwich, Connecticut, took their son Mark to see his pediatrician, Dr. J. Frederick Lee, for a well-baby exam. Lee pronounced Mark a healthy six-month-old. Just two weeks later, in October, the Roes found Mark dead in his crib. Almost as fazed as Mark's parents, Lee pushed for an autopsy. The results indicated Mark had died from acute bronchial pneumonia. This baffled the Roes. Distraught and confused, they struggled to come to terms with the sudden loss of their son. Despite receiving autopsy findings, they felt tormented by the inexplicability of Mark's death. Jed Roe became obsessed with finding out what had happened to his son. He met with physicians all over New York and poured through medical literature, to no avail. When the Roes failed to locate any foundation devoted to babies like Mark and their families, they started one of their own.

In August 1962, the Roes founded the first lay organization devoted to the problem of sudden infant death. The Mark Addison Roe Foundation began with hardly any funding, a small board of trustees, and a handful of medical advisers. The Foundation's mission was to heighten awareness of sudden death in infancy as a recognizable syndrome, and it pledged to "promote, stimulate, and support research in the diagnosis, treatment, and cure of sudden, unexpected death in infants."[5] From its origins in a basement office, the Foundation set up national headquarters in New York City and rebranded itself as the National Foundation for SIDS in 1967.[6] In 1976 it moved again, to Chicago, and became the National SIDS Foundation.[7] (That name is used throughout to prevent confusion.) Its nucleus was parent volunteers. They staffed the office, responded to phone calls and mail inquiries, and distributed self-produced educational literature on sudden death in infancy. Each year the NSIDSF sent out tens of thousands of SIDS brochures, maintained a membership of a few thousand, and coordinated with local professionals to advance the organization's goals.[8]

A similar story unfolded on the West Coast. In September 1961, Fred and Mary Dore discovered their three-month-old daughter Christine deceased in her crib. Christine's autopsy declared that "acute pneumonitis" had caused her death. As coroner Leo Sowers explained to the Dores, this explanation was in reality a "catch-all phrase to include the sudden and unexpected deaths of previously healthy infants." Like the Roes, the Dores were bewildered and overcome with grief. When she learned that Seattle typically experienced somewhere between thirty and fifty similar cases each year, Mary Dore began collecting newspaper articles on "crib death" and scanned obituaries to connect with other families who had lost babies. By one description, she became "a one-person support group for the parents of 'crib death' victims."[9]

Mary and her husband, a state senator in Washington, continued to seek answers. When they came up short, the Dores compelled the Washington State Medical Association to establish a committee to study cases like Christine's. The committee was unable to locate any organized research collaboration on sudden death in infancy, and advised its governing organization to allocate $20,000 for an inaugural study on the topic. Meanwhile, the Dores continued coordinating with other parents and medical allies to lobby for state legislation. Senator Dore introduced a bill mandating that all sudden unexpected deaths statewide in children younger than three years old be reported and studied at the same central location, the University of Washington Hospital, at no cost to parents. The bill passed in March 1963.[10] Shortly thereafter, the National Institute of Child Health and Human Development (NICHD) agreed to host a conference on the issue, and awarded two University of Washington physicians, Bruce Beckwith and Abraham Bergman, funding to conduct a study on sudden death in infants.[11]

In 1965, the University of Washington, in collaboration with the Dores, formed the Washington Association for Sudden Infant Death Study. The group had a three-tiered mission—to support Washington families, to foster community understanding and awareness of sudden infant deaths, and to promote research—with the ultimate goal that sudden infant death gain formal recognition as a disease.[12] The Washington Association, run by a board of officers and volunteers, asked members to contribute just one dollar annually. The Association was overwhelmingly committed to assisting parents whose babies had died inexplicably. In 1969, in lieu of a standard description of its activities and purpose, the Association pointed to "one of hundreds" of letters of appreciation it had received to describe its work:

> How can we ever thank you enough . . . for the literature, and for all the moral support given so generously! . . . We realize most families who lose children in this way are not given this most needed assurance . . . and people can say the cruelest things, even friends . . . for no one seems to understand! . . . and they ask such terrible questions. How do all those families who do NOT receive information (such as we), ever return to carrying on a normal existence? . . . I feel life would seem absolutely hopeless, had we not by chance been given your address.[13]

A third similar situation transpired in December 1963 in the Baltimore area, when Saul and Sylvia Goldberg lost their daughter Suzanne. The Goldbergs aspired to establish a branch of the Roes' foundation, but chose instead to form their own organization, the Guild for Infant Survival (it became the International Guild for Infant Survival in 1968). The Guild considered itself "humanitarian" above all else; its foremost objective was to counsel and aid grieving parents. The Guild did concern itself with medical research, but even this was intended as a "source of understanding and comfort for those who experience this tragedy, in order to dispel their strong feelings of guilt and inadequacy." It treated medicine as an important source of solace for parents, and hoped its own work would inspire research, but did not strictly participate in medical projects. Alongside professional allies, members networked to offer personal consolation and guidance to parents victimized by sudden infant death. This outreach, in conjunction with public relations efforts, was meant to bring the "seriousness, scope, and nature of this major public health problem to full public attention, in order that aroused concern will stimulate increased medical interest, activities, and facilities toward the solution of these needless deaths."[14]

For the most part, the NSIDSF overshadowed other SIDS associations. By its tenth anniversary in 1972, the NSIDSF had expanded significantly. Drawing momentum from grieving but persevering parents like Carolyn Szybist who found consolation through activism, the organization grew haphazardly. Starting in the late 1960s, the NSIDSF expanded through subsidiary chapters in Denver, Detroit, Chicago, Minneapolis, Connecticut, and Long Island; others were forming in Massachusetts, California, Miami, Florida, and upstate New York. By 1974, the NSIDSF consisted of more than thirty-seven chapters. By 1980, it had fifty-seven.[15] In different locales, NSIDSF chapters ranged in formality from "kitchen table operations" to "sophisticated computerized models."[16] The Foundation expected each chapter to adopt its larger mission but encouraged chapters to give precedence to local parents' needs and practical realities. NSIDSF chapters worked closely with professionals in various sectors of the community, developing ties with hospitals, clinics, funeral homes, churches, schools, and local government.[17]

The NSIDSF propagated three central, intertwined messages. First, it strove to raise awareness that SIDS existed. (In 1980, one Wisconsin NSIDSF chapter's newsletter wished the national office's new public relations director luck by saying, "May you make SIDS as well known as the Kenner products from 'Star Wars' and 'The Empire Strikes Back'!"[18]) The NSIDSF also defended SIDS as a "real disease" equivalent in severity to many well-known childhood maladies. Lastly, it upheld the message that SIDS was entirely unpredictable and unpreventable. The NSIDSF made use of "all facets of communication" to raise awareness and propagate these lessons. Its members eagerly met for interviews with print, radio, and television media sources, spoke at local events, mailed out literature on SIDS, and even put together a one-minute public service announcement that reached a national audience in 1977.[19]

When it was founded, the NSIDSF upheld research as central to its work. Starting in the late 1970s, the NSIDSF began offering modest research fellowships to medical students or health professionals. Each award consisted of a grant for $1,000 (later increased to $5,000) for the successful applicant to pursue a SIDS research project over the course of an eight- to twelve-week period under the supervision of an approved advisor. The NSIDSF created the award expressly to "expose and cultivate interest in students to pursue SIDS research" more than for any anticipation that recipients' work might generate a solution.[20] It also contributed funding to major research projects nationwide. Its offerings were impressive for such a small organization—it gave $100,000 in 1984 alone—but they were paltry.[21] With severe financial limitations and parent volunteers who wanted to become personally involved in the Foundation's work, education and family counseling presented realistic objectives. The NSIDSF was dedicated to parents and families above all else, and it accentuated support and advocacy.

SIDS families knew better than anyone that the devastation of infant death was permanent; some parents had waited decades for the chance at information and support that the NSIDSF offered. One parent from Missouri wrote to the NSIDSF's national office asking how to join a local chapter. Her son had died twenty-four years earlier. "How can I help?" she asked. "I would do anything to help relieve some tortured parents from going through what I have for 24 years and probably [will] the rest of my life."[22] In 1979, Ana Maris Luker similarly asked about getting involved with parent support networking. Her son had died from "crib death" in 1953. Even after such a long time (during which she raised seven children), Luker continued to read everything she could about SIDS and wanted to help other families who suffered her ordeal. "Even though our son would be twenty six years old," she explained, "we still hurt and will miss him and suffer his loss all our lives."[23] The same year, *Pediatrics* published a SIDS mother's poem (anonymously at the time) commemorating the fourteenth anniversary of her child's death. The poem's author was Carolyn Szybist. Recalling the piece's origins, Szybist remembered sitting in her office at the National SIDS Foundation late in the evening. Coming to terms with the date, she broke down, and turned to her typewriter. The piece, she described, just "came out of my fingers. Complete, never edited. Almost channeled."[24] Entitled *The Tenth of July*, Szybist's poem expressively conveyed that the loss of SIDS was a never-ending tragedy parents carried with them throughout their entire lives:

It was so many years ago
When you left us.

Why you died
No longer matters.
But the when remains
And serves, one more time, as a memorial
To remembering.

Today is very like that day long past
Clear and cool and out of reason
For the midst of Summer.
It stirs the memory so carefully submerged
Until today.

And it matters.
Because you were.

My mind does not mourn yesterday.
It mourns today.
The images that pass before my eyes

Do not recall the infant son
But see you running through my house
A teenage child in search of food and gym shoes and maybe me.

I do not mourn you for what you were,
But for what can't be
The unfinished life we didn't share.
The very briefness of that life
Has reached this day and makes me pause and know
I miss you.[25]

It was precisely because SIDS affected parents so lastingly and profoundly that the National SIDS Foundation's primary investment was in families. The NSIDSF was structured as a parent-to-parent community network to provide families with information, compassion, and support. Initially, it involved only SIDS families, but as SIDS itself morphed in the public and medical spheres, that changed. By 1980, the group had expanded to attend to apnea monitoring families.[26] It promoted an extended-family feel. Chapter newsletters recounted national, regional, and state news relevant to SIDS, as well as event and research updates such as future conferences or television appearances, but they were invested in local parents and communities. Mailings documented birth announcements and expressed congratulations when member families welcomed new life into their homes or celebrated birthdays and anniversaries.[27] They concluded with memorial sections, ranging in prototype from simple statements to poetry or lyrics, to commemorate losses suffered.[28]

Newsletters also included informative inserts and announced dates, times, and locations for parent support meetings. They called on readers to partake in fundraising activities, politics, and small-scale community events.[29] Members orchestrated charm and T-shirt sales, designated local "SIDS Weeks," and hosted magic shows, craft fairs, raffle giveaways, bike-a-thons, dances, picnics, dinner theaters, fashion shows, and bowling nights.[30] Organizers intended that these events would bring families together, raise money, and draw attention to their cause.

TAKING SIDS TO CONGRESS

Parents had been lobbying the federal government to become involved in sudden infant mortality since the 1960s. So far, they had been at least partly successful, winning some sponsorship for conferences, research, and the SIDS national management survey. But by the early 1970s, parents and their allies were clamoring for money and attention. They were tired of what they interpreted as lip service from the government pledging its commitment to SIDS. As the Guild for

Infant Survival explained, the NICHD had tried to mollify parents by repeatedly assuring them that SIDS was a "high priority for attention and action" while it allowed SIDS research to languish.[31] In early 1972, parents helped effect a Congressional hearing with the Subcommittee on Children and Youth (a subset of Senator Walter Mondale's Committee on Labor and Public Welfare). It led to a joint resolution that the government ramp up its attention and funding for SIDS. In 1973, attendants at another session disputed exactly how the government should do so.

In 1972, Mondale, a Democratic senator from Minnesota, commenced the caucuses with an emotive description of SIDS that matched almost verbatim the words Carolyn Szybist had encountered in *Redbook* in 1968: "Every night several million American mothers feed their babies, put them in their cribs, and say goodnight. The next morning they return, greet their children and begin another day of care. Yet, every morning, anywhere from 30 to 60 mothers return to find their babies lying dead in their cribs." Mondale asked why, if SIDS was the number one killer of American babies, the nation's effort against it appeared so stagnant. He was flummoxed: "I just can't understand how we can all agree that this is the largest killer of infants in this country, and everybody agrees that this statistic is unarguable, yet we have no notion other than the vaguest idea what is causing it, to the point that we do not even want to warn parents because if they should ask questions, we can't answer them. How can we be in this predicament?"[32]

At the time, SIDS still lacked a code in the *International Classification of Disease*. Research projects had done very little to resolve any of the scientific or humanistic issues associated with SIDS. Funding had increased but was still minimal. Interest was only nominally higher. In 1972, the NICHD received just thirteen applications for research projects specific to SIDS, and numerous proposals were rejected due to "poor scientific merit."[33] Jay Arena, president of the AAP, explained that most physicians never saw SIDS. The people who actually confronted SIDS cases were *not* physicians, medical students, or scientists—they were coroners, police officers, firemen, and funeral home directors. They were families, friends, and neighbors. SIDS parents still felt isolated in their suffering.[34]

The Congressional hearings threw light on parents' grievances. Professionals' responses to SIDS and SIDS families ranged from very careful and thoughtful to destructive. Parents reported being asked accusing questions: How many times did you hit the baby? Did your other child hurt the baby? Did you allow your dog to bite the baby? Did you squeeze your baby? Did you have an accident you were afraid to tell anyone about? Didn't you check your child during the night?[35] A SIDS mother from Seattle shared that when she was leaving the hospital with her subsequent newborn baby, a nurse told her, "'I heard you suffocated

your last baby. I hope you take better care of this one.'"[36] Even well-meaning professionals could deepen parents' suffering. Some physicians' intent to alleviate
parents' self-blame likely contributed, unintentionally, to errors in SIDS management. By one medical examiner's explanation, parents tended to blame themselves "until someone knowledgeable tells them differently."[37] Physicians lacking
an intimate understanding of SIDS may have felt emotionally compelled to offer
parents alternative causes of death intended to reduce their suffering, but this
inadvertently compounded confusion and impeded comprehensive SIDS management and analysis.

Indeed, most parents were exasperated over jumbled investigations and
autopsy protocols. NSIDSF president Judith Choate explained that it was "the
rule, rather than the exception, that families must wait months to hear the results
of an autopsy."[38] Even when they were performed, autopsies, especially without interpretation, confused many parents. Some parents learned that their
child had died from alternative causes, ranging from pneumonia to suffocation to bronchitis, and sometimes formal postmortem reports conflicted with
what families had learned from their doctors.[39] Most parents agreed that more
transparency surrounding autopsy and death certification would have been healing: "a great amount of unnecessary suffering could have been eliminated," one
couple explained, "by three little words, Sudden Infant Death, written on a piece
of paper called a death certificate."[40]

The myriad diagnoses and information they received, in combination with
suspicion on the part of others, cultivated in SIDS families a deep desire to
know something—anything—about what had happened to their child. The
construction of the SIDS diagnosis did not change the fact that these families
felt starved for information. In the mid-sixties, before SIDS was coined, one desperate mother whose baby had died three years earlier heard about Theodore
Curphey's work in California and wrote to him requesting information. After
explaining the litany of explanations offered to her by various medical personnel ("Can you see my confusion?" she entreated him), Nancy Barton appealed,
"if anyone has anything, any kind of information that could enlighten me it
would be really appreciated." She even provided a self-addressed, stamped enve-
lope to facilitate a response. (Curphey was not able to even read Barton's letter
until six weeks after she penned it. He responded after another four. His reply
probably offered Barton little peace of mind, and in fact presumably deepened
her confusion by continuing to hedge around several labels.)[41] Another determined grandparent wrote to Curphey asking, "1. What else is known about this
terrible thing? 2. Can it be prevented? 3. What research, if any, is being done
in this field and where? 4. Any other facts you can give me." She mailed copies of
the dispatch to multiple of Curphey's colleagues, various health agencies in Los
Angeles, the Children's Hospital in Washington, DC, the National Institute for

Child Health, and even the Academy of Medical Sciences Institute of Pediatrics in Moscow, from which she received a very thoughtful (and timely) response.[42]

In the 1960s and beyond, heartbroken parents wrote to the NSIDSF detailing their stories, searching for guidance and reassurance. "I mainly want to know if you think I killed my baby or did she really die from 'crib death'?" a young mother from Oregon wrote. "And what is 'crib death'[?]" she continued, "Please help me as soon as possible. I don't want to kill my new baby." Another mother, from New York, wrote, "I need your help I am going to end up in a mental hospital if I don't get some help from someone soon. I am so lonely."[43] Countless parents praised the NSIDSF as the only source that truly helped them overcome the loss of their babies. As one parent explained, "For some strange reason the knowledge that someone else shared that same factor gave me a feeling that I wasn't alone."[44]

This shortfall broached the broader topic of "SIDS publicity," and attendees at the Congressional hearing voiced philosophically different ideas about the values and risks of public awareness. SIDS activists understood that the media could help acquaint the public with SIDS. At the same time, inaccurate or sensationalized pieces had the propensity to spawn confusion or sustain suspicions about parental culpability. Not everyone agreed that publicizing SIDS was appropriate or necessary. The NICHD strongly opposed widely disseminating information on SIDS. Especially in the pages of publications like *Infant Care*, specifically developed for new and expecting parents, it would be futile to dwell on a problem as dark as SIDS, it said. Beyond "being of no help," advising parents about SIDS "would rather be harmful by raising anxiety and fears and not providing ways of confronting them." Pediatrician Jay Arena concurred that publicizing SIDS broadly was a "questionable strategy" that could "create such a family disturbance that it would be unlivable." Arena warned that "a greater harm would be done by over-publicizing this condition [SIDS] until we know a great deal more about it." The AAP backed the Children's Bureau's decision to refrain from printing SIDS information in its advice publications for parents. As far as it was concerned, telling new parents about SIDS would do little else besides "raise apprehension and fear."[45]

SIDS parents disagreed. For them, information was the linchpin in recovery. Judy Choate conceded that awareness might initially stir fear but argued that fear would subside quickly. Another mother thought SIDS would never be overcome and eradicated without more awareness. "We may be saving young parents from worrying about SID[S]," she explained, "but we are not saving their babies. Let this disease be known . . . and let it be conquered."[46] Allowing that there were more and less appropriate times and places to conduct information campaigns (SIDS literature "shouldn't be reading room matter in gynecologists' offices," one father said), parents did not think medical uncertainty justified silence.[47] In a brief but scathing exposition on the extent and reality of "crib death" in America in 1975, affected father Richard Raring declared that SIDS was not receiving the public outcry and attention it deserved. Raring was outraged over medical and lay ignorance of crib death. Most medical schools did not teach about the phenomenon, he said, and pediatricians were unfamiliar with it because they dealt exclusively with living patients.[48] Raring insisted on heightened awareness and rejected as illegitimate the notion that knowledge about crib death would unduly frighten new parents. The "added increment of worry," he said, "falls far short of being justification for ignorance."[49] Another father, Arthur Siegal, offered a flawed analogy that accentuated how the paradoxes ingrained in SIDS were not limited to its medical definition. Siegal compared knowing about SIDS to knowing that cigarettes cause cancer, saying that he thought "everybody should have the knowledge that such a disease does exist, so that if confronted with it a person might be better able to maintain his sanity."[50] However, information about the cigarette-cancer connection empowered Americans to act, if they wanted, to prevent disease progression: stop smoking. Information about SIDS offered no parallel preventative options. As Bruce Beckwith explained, "The needs for providing public information on current research . . . impose a cruel hoax upon the parents of past and future SIDS victims."[51]

The government levied no direct opinion on publicity, but after the 1972 hearings, the Senate passed (by a vote of seventy-seven to zero) a resolution to make SIDS a research priority and extend counseling services to affected families.[52] Mondale introduced legislation to enact those measures. His bill charged the NICHD with conducting SIDS research. It mandated that the NICHD enact professional and public educational programs, bestow grants to approved researchers, provide information and counseling to families affected by SIDS, and periodically evaluate and document the status of SIDS knowledge.[53] It also made stipulations for implementing SIDS "information and counseling projects." At its core, the bill was aimed to amplify research dollars for SIDS and to build "regional infant death centers" to choreograph SIDS management.

Before Mondale's bill passed as the Sudden Infant Death Syndrome Law of 1974, two Congressional hearings debating the proposal revealed significant disagreements about how the government should intervene on SIDS. Government representatives testified against the bill, opposing it on the grounds that the legislation was "duplicative and unnecessary." From their perspective, the bill would not confer new advantages. Their offices had contributed financial support for research projects, coordinated efforts to ensure SIDS was coded in the International Classification of Diseases, and hosted multiple research conferences. Far from disagreeing that SIDS was a significant ordeal, witnesses on behalf of government organizations contended that they were already responding appropriately and sufficiently to it.[54]

Much to parents' frustration, the NICHD habitually quoted its more-favorable funding allocations for *affiliated* research—research that pertained to SIDS but was not necessarily directly intended to study SIDS. As the Institute explained, related research was crucial to "the development and clarification of our knowledge of SIDS and represents the best investment of our research funds at this time."[55] Supporters of the SIDS bill broke the NICHD's numbers down into their constituent parts, showing that funding for SIDS alone was minis-cule compared to the swelled numbers implied by the NICHD's affiliated fund-ing estimates. No one did this more evocatively than Saul Goldberg, the head of the International Guild for Infant Survival, who calculated that the NICHD had committed a mere $4.50 per lost child.[56] Rejecting the claim that funding for related research would further the fight against SIDS, Goldberg and other parents demanded research specific to SIDS. "The stories of Pasteur and rabies, Salk and polio, Ehrlich and syphilis—and many others—" Richard Raring wrote to the subcommittee members, "are stories with the same plot and same ending. None were doing research that would be called just 'pertinent' or 'relevant.' In every case they were single-mindedly searching for the cause and cure of a single, specific disease, with nothing else to divert their full attention."[57] Raring's per-spective, shared by others in attendance at the hearing, was understandable. He was a SIDS father incensed by the absurd and persistent vacuity of SIDS knowl-edge. But his take was equally flawed. Research indicated that SIDS was probably not a single disease pathway. And, for each of Raring's examples, an alternative story of accidental discovery and triumph existed. Medical revelations like peni-cillin, pap smears, and X-ray diagnostics were all realized haphazardly. From a logical perspective, the NICHD was correct that related research projects—in areas such as infant and prenatal development or immunology—just might pro-duce an unanticipated breakthrough in SIDS. It was entirely possible that tan-gential research would turn out to be the keystone in solving SIDS.

Parents like Richard Raring, along with their Congressional allies, blended critical observations with personal experience and high emotions. They faulted the NICHD for failing to promote interest in SIDS among young researchers and falling short of its responsibility to fund research, and charged that the orga-nization was contributing to SIDS ignorance. In the end, SIDS parents made a lasting impression. The bill passed.

For SIDS activist organizations, the 1974 SIDS Law was a major landmark. Parents could anticipate help and funding. From 1974 to 1976, the NICHD received almost four times the number of SIDS research proposals, and funded six times as many, as during the seven years from 1964 to 1971.[58] In 1975, the Department of Health, Education, and Welfare distributed twenty-four grants to establish SIDS "community information and counseling projects." Each proj-ect was expected to promote, help fund, and synchronize four basic aims: obtain autopsies, notify parents of autopsy results, correctly use the SIDS label on death certificates, and provide information and counseling for affected families.[59] The legislation intended to amend the variable and inconsistent practices then in existence, and parents were excited at the prospect of competent, capable management programs. But the year after the SIDS Law passed, one legal scholar's analysis summarized that "the statutory bases underlying SIDS management by official agencies leads to the conclusion that the majority of death investigation systems, as presently constituted, are either fundamentally insensitive to the need for implementing SIDS management programs or are unable to do so for lack of funds, know-how, or legal authority."[60]

Despite implied simplicity, each state was responsible for implementing its own SIDS project. As happened after the famous *Brown v. Board of Education* case that mandated school desegregation twenty years prior, states adopted different approaches and different timelines. A handful of states already had essentially identical laws on their books before 1974, and in those areas the SIDS Law resulted in few changes. In other places, the NSIDSF had highly functional chapters up and running that were already working towards the same goals as the newly implemented centers. In these locations, the boundary lines between NSIDSF chapters and state-run SIDS information and counseling centers were ambiguous. Given that both the government SIDS projects and the NSIDSF aspired to vast objectives with little personnel and no clear division of labor, it is not surprising that both groups experienced moments of success and failure, friendship and frustration.

SIDS INFORMATION AND COUNSELING CENTERS

In July 1975, the federal government launched the first SIDS information and counseling centers.[61] These state programs endeavored to assume responsibility for implementing and standardizing the same measures as the major epidemiological studies in the 1960s, but they also partook in more concerted and extensive efforts to achieve widespread social and medical understanding. Much like the NSIDSF, SIDS centers sought to become involved in any activity related to SIDS.[62] Most received barely enough money to retain a sufficient staff.

Even with little funding, a patchwork of SIDS programs sprang up across the country. By 1980, thirty-seven SIDS information and counseling centers across thirty states were up and running.[63] Each center operated individually yet shared the overarching goal of adherence to the "Four Point Program." The most essential broad objectives for SIDS programs nationwide were to provide families with humane, compassionate counseling and information and to teach professionals who encountered SIDS and victimized families about how to respond to the diagnosis.[64] SIDS centers struggled to perfect the organizational aspects of tracking SIDS, although they were more effective in altering social responses. Professionals and lay volunteers at SIDS centers were deeply invested in the humanitarian aspects of SIDS; they relentlessly stressed that SIDS was "real" and focused their attention predominantly on the task of treating parent survivors.

States building new information and counseling centers looked to existing programs for guidance. Oregon was an obvious choice. Its SIDS protocol (initiated in 1971) had served as the model for the national legislation, and it came out glowing after Abraham Bergman's 1972 management survey. Bergman had called it the "best organized statewide system" for handling SIDS anywhere in the country.[65]

Larry Lewman, Oregon's deputy chief medical examiner, described his state's general death investigation system as "the secret" to effective SIDS management. He promoted Oregon's conventional procedures (for all deaths, not just for SIDS) as the antidote to the nation's problems with handling SIDS cases, a situation so dire he referred to it as "a horrible national scandal." Oregon had supplanted its "outdated" coroner program in 1959 with a medical examiner system. (In contrast to the position of coroner, which was an elected post with no mandatory professional scientific or medical prerequisites, medical examiners were appointed, licensed physicians.) Lewman specified that medically trained pathologists were the most critical assets underlying any functional death examination program, and even cited the coroner system itself as the country's "greatest obstacle in attempting to humanize and standardize the handling of SIDS." Investigations, Lewman asserted, "should be left to medical professionals and must not be entrusted to lay coroners and police."[66]

Oregon's approach mirrored that from research in Cleveland and Washington: a central location received case referrals, performed autopsies, orchestrated parent interviews, and distributed information. Lewman's office hired a nurse coordinator who specialized in SIDS and traveled to every county to instruct professionals. Thus, in each county there was at least one public health nurse designated to conduct SIDS work and visit affected families. To foster professional awareness, SIDS cases were presented in "case of the month" conferences, medical education lectures, and police agency presentations.[67] The Oregon NSIDSF operated separately from the state's medical examiner offices, but both groups coordinated to refer one another cases.

When she advised local professionals how to start building successful SIDS projects, NICHD director Geraldine Norris stressed that establishing a "reliable system for identifying SIDS cases" was the "keystone for a successful information and counseling project" and recommended that organizers focus on those plans first.[68] Indeed, the practical aspects of coordinating informational exchanges with parents and disseminating information about SIDS were at the

heart of SIDS projects' daily existence. The Four Point Program of SIDS management (originally conceived as the "Bill of Rights for Families of SIDS Victims")
was every center's foundation; it incorporated the principal time-sensitive tasks
of (1) obtaining autopsies, (2) promoting the correct use of SIDS on death certificates, (3) notifying families of the cause of death promptly, and (4) following
up with families to offer counseling and information.[69]

Every SIDS center was geared towards improving community handling
through professional education. According to one estimate, between 200 and
250 people could be involved in any given SIDS episode, and the hope was to
reach all of those individuals to ensure each one was a positive source of support
for SIDS families.[70] The idea was that "every personal contact a SIDS family has
during the course of its crisis has either a positive or a negative influence on the
resolution of its grief and period of bereavement." The two most crucial initiatives
dealt with enhancing knowledge of SIDS and improving families' initial treatment. The educational protocols were hardly profound; the centers preached
basic learning points and simple directives. "The MOST IMPORTANT role" for
hospital personnel, for example, was "just to be there. Be available to listen and
answer questions."[71] Factual and informative literature developed together by
the NSIDSF and SIDS centers conveyed the "basic facts" of SIDS, summarized
research updates, and dispelled certain "myths": the diagnosis was not rare, did
not involve suffering, and was not related to suffocation, contagion, or heredity.
No one was at fault in SIDS deaths, and no known prevention existed.[72] Literature emphasized that "SIDS is a REAL DISEASE, just as cancer, heart disease,
and multiple sclerosis are real diseases."[73] If "confusion and ignorance about the
disease" often exacerbated SIDS families' suffering, simple cognizance—lifting
the "veil of ignorance surrounding crib death"—was treated as the antidote.[74]

Curricula designed for first responders stressed SIDS identification and initial treatment of parents.[75] Even if first responders lacked detailed information
on SIDS, they could help by reassuring traumatized parents and offering sensitive care. First responders like police officers, emergency medical technicians,
and firefighters were coached how to sensitively handle sudden infant deaths.
Lessons emphasized that SIDS families must "be treated with the same degree
of compassion and sympathy as any other family who has lost a loved one."[76]
Although without an autopsy first responders could "only *suspect* SIDS as the
cause of death," they were schooled to "always give the parents the benefit of
the doubt and assume SIDS until an autopsy proves otherwise."[77] Instructive
guidelines recommended attempting CPR regardless so that parents felt something was being done to help.[78] Police officers were encouraged to complete
investigatory duties sensitively and obtain information using an interview or dialogue style rather than interrogating families. Reflecting the approach that SIDS

was a crisis event, officers learned not to "pressure the parents for answers," since they "may really not remember details."[79] Training for nurses, who might play a long-term counseling role, often entailed even more comprehensive materials.

SIDS centers made notable gains. Heading into the 1980 fiscal year, they existed in thirty-seven states and served about half of the national population.[80] From 1973 to 1978, the number of SIDS cases confirmed by autopsy rose from 70 to 80 percent. SIDS centers boasted a higher infant autopsy rate than the national mean (they averaged a rate of 52 percent, while the national average fluctuated in the mid-fortieth percentile).[81] SIDS programs conducted an estimated two thousand professional education training sessions annually, and the national SIDS program office prepared and distributed over 400,000 copies of SIDS educational materials.[82] Anecdotal evidence from grant application reference letters also shows that SIDS centers experienced qualitative successes.[83] Health professionals pointed to SIDS educational sessions as "excellent learning experience[s],"[84] and many parents were deeply touched by the attention SIDS centers paid them in a time of need.[85]

Still, the extent to which SIDS centers benefited all Americans who experienced SIDS is not entirely clear. Intermittently, leadership enacted measures to reach less-privileged groups. In Chicago, for example, a nurse hosted parent coffees for urban families and teenage parents. The gatherings were expressly intended to bring the benefits of parent-to-parent support from middle-class suburbia to the inner city. The same location also worked to transcribe literature into other languages and locate translators to improve its services to minority and non-English-speaking families.[86] The SIDS center in Springfield, Illinois, took up similar initiatives, acknowledging how grossly underrepresented and underserved minority families were within SIDS parent groups as well as its own activities. Staff there commented that their own literature—representative of that used nationally—was predominantly directed towards middle- and upper-middle-class, two-parent, educated families. In attempt to remedy this apparent problem, they recommended that information sheets use "simpler words" and avoid "complex sentence structure," while still refraining from being "either condescending or insulting." They also proposed that literature be developed for non-traditional families such as working mothers or single parents.[87] There are no remaining records of whether or to what extent these types of simple initiatives met success. One reporter's assessment that such inequalities were periodically "discussed, but not resolved" appears to have been quite accurate.[88]

Beyond this gulf, SIDS centers also came up against personnel and organizational challenges. The distinctions between government-mandated SIDS information and counseling centers and NSIDSF chapters were frustratingly blurry. SIDS centers commonly requested help and advice from nearby NSIDSF chapters, often even borrowing NSIDSF literature verbatim. SIDS centers and the NSIDSF shared the same interests and objectives and, for the most part, joined together in community outreach and education projects.[89] But this meant that SIDS centers always leaned heavily on the small subset of the population to which they were accountable—SIDS parents. To a certain extent, some parents felt taken advantage of. Two scholars described that NSIDSF parents felt like they were "working as ancillaries" to SIDS centers and had unexpectedly "lost some of their autonomy and much of their morale and momentum."[90] The NSIDSF had initially reveled in its success compelling the government to fund SIDS centers, but for some that outcome turned out to be bittersweet. The NSIDSF, Carolyn Szybist gauged in 1980, had "found itself in the unique position of having created most, if not all, of its external competition."[91] Within just a few years, many parents began to question the utility of the centers and in some places even opposed their continued existence.[92]

The federal mandate that states operate SIDS information and counseling centers lapsed in the early 1980s. After the Maternal and Child Health Block Grant of 1981, money previously allocated for SIDS centers was relayed to individual states. States gained some freedom in allocating money and implementing programs, but they lost a lot of dollars. Beginning in October 1982, SIDS was lumped in with other maternal and child health programs (such as such as adolescent health, genetic diseases, disabilities, and hemophilia) under the "health service" sector of states' grants. Since each state was responsible for coordinating and distributing its own block grant funds (some of which opted to channel money directly to county health departments), SIDS centers after 1982 followed separate trajectories by state. Many of them scaled down or else suspended their SIDS centers.[93]

At another Congressional hearing on SIDS in 1985, parents berated the government for drastic cuts to SIDS funding. Not only had the government dropped categorical funding for SIDS programs in the states, it also slashed investments in SIDS research. After peaking at around $3.3 million in 1981, SIDS-specific research money fell to about $600,000 in 1985.[94]

THE NSIDSF'S RETIREMENT

The NSIDSF barely outlived the centers it helped establish. While it was working alongside SIDS centers, the NSIDSF was simultaneously laboring to overcome long-standing defects. In the first place, the group was beset by the same homogeneity that characterized SIDS centers: its ranks were filled with mostly white, middle-class families. In 1971, Joel Alpert, chief of pediatrics at Boston City Hospital, described that "effectiveness of the parent groups seems to be largely limited to middle-class parents . . . the poor, who are at highest risk, are not being reached."[95] Abraham Bergman similarly lamented that the NSIDSF was predominantly composed of white middle-class Americans. Neither the NSIDSF nor the Guild for Infant Survival, he assessed, had successfully extended support to lower-class or minority families. Whereas 10 percent of middle- or upper-class families identified parents from activist groups as the most helpful person or organization after SIDS occurred, none of lower-class families surveyed mentioned any member of a parent group as their most helpful resource. Bergman's remark that "such families do not tend to be joiners" is uninstructive in attempting to explain these disparities.[96]

By 1980, Carolyn Szybist described the NSIDSF as deep in the throes of a "'basic survival' crisis."[97] It suffered most from two serious administrative stumbling blocks: financial setbacks and organizational obscurity. The NSIDSF was in an almost constant state of financial insecurity. In the late 1970s things were dire, and although the organization remained afloat, fundraising bedeviled it through the remainder of its existence.[98] With growing expanse and shrinking resources, the NSIDSF's indefinite organizational structure became increasingly problematic. Multiple individuals said that a "lack of planning" and a "lack of strategy" were major defects.[99] One member explained that "anyone who has been involved with the NSIDSF for very long knows that it has lacked a real plan since its onset."[100] Its constituents were frustrated at the overarching shortfall of integration and cooperation among branches. The disconnect between NSIDSF chapters and the national office—described by Szybist as a "limited partnership"—plagued the group through its most trying years.[101] Many chapter representatives felt left "in the dark" and unaware of what was happening with the organization at the national level.[102]

The NSIDSF's pairing of disorganized bureaucracy with crippling funding shortages was hardly a recipe for success. Beyond threatening the organization's survival, both issues also had the unwanted effect of distracting attention from the NSIDSF's real purpose, its mission to aid families.[103] In the 1980s, the flowering of multiple groups invested in the same issues created a more competitive environment that proved too much for the NSIDSF's own weaknesses. In that decade, groups that concerned themselves with SIDS splintered and also grew in number, resulting in a complex array of organizations that made for a tangled network. Some NSIDSF chapters seceded to form independent groups. Some states retained their own SIDS information and counseling projects. And new associations popped up. Alongside the NSIDSF and SIDS centers stood other associations offering similar services to parents who had lost children, such as the Compassionate Friends, Aiding Mothers and Fathers Experiencing Neonatal Death (AMEND), and Share Pregnancy and Infant Loss (Share).[104] By the early 1980s, the NSIDSF had eighty chapters and was starting to crumble from within. In 1987, it merged with a handful of SIDS groups scattered across the country into the SIDS Alliance. In 2002, the SIDS Alliance expanded its scope beyond SIDS to focus on stillborn losses and all sudden, unexpected infant deaths, changing its name to First Candle.[105]

CONCLUSION

Evidence suggests that the SIDS Law and SIDS centers were more an outcome of revisions underway—instigated by parent and physician activists—than they were creators of change. Surely SIDS centers contributed to improvements in the ways SIDS cases and families were treated; evaluations and feedback from hundreds of medical professionals and from numerous parents indicate especially that professional educational training initiatives SIDS centers orchestrated had real results.[106] Yet the influence of federal SIDS programs emanated from shifts in cultural awareness, curiosity, and reactions to SIDS that were gaining traction beforehand. The onset of federal funding and formal government involvement in SIDS management was a product, not a root cause, of a heightened consciousness of SIDS.

The NSIDSF also never met its "ultimate objective" of eliminating SIDS.[107] In the 1970s and early 1980s, it fell victim to some of the same problems plaguing medicine and research: constant funding shortages, discrepancies among beneficiaries, a lack of public attention, and a constantly veering long-term direction. The stalled success in the medical arena no doubt contributed to the NSIDSF's difficulties; medicine's inability to furnish explanations meant that parents were unable to provide newly affected families with answers. The obstacles to drawing out medical solutions to SIDS made it increasingly challenging to successfully run a condition-based organization.[108]

Even while the NSIDSF failed to persevere as an independent association and to eradicate SIDS, it did have mixed success with its other purposes, especially those of helping parents and educating Americans.[109] Even though one SIDS center reflected in 1979 that "SIDS still has a social stigma . . . probably due to an uninformed public regarding SIDS as a disease," it is undeniable that the NSIDSF helped move SIDS "out of the closet" and into the realm of "becoming a household word."[110] The Foundation's work raised the national consciousness of SIDS and supported thousands of parents and families who suffered a loss. It also instigated some improvements in SIDS management, both through its own endeavors and through effecting the SIDS information and counseling centers. SIDS centers, in turn, furthered the NSIDSF's objectives to promote professional awareness of SIDS and enhance families' treatment through their professional education programs.

More than any measurable successes or failures, though, the real significance of the NSIDSF escapes quantification. Perhaps no one was as dedicated to the mission of supporting SIDS families as the parents who became involved in SIDS organizations—armed with a special faith in the therapeutic powers of peer-networking, they were unfailingly devoted to helping other victimized parents. The Foundation offered them a venue for connections and support they desperately needed, and it positively relieved their suffering. Parents formed close, lasting bonds, and the relationships they built through the NSIDSF were restorative. Reflecting on her experience getting involved with the Foundation, Carolyn Szybist reminisced, "I was healing. I wasn't alone. There were so many of us."[111] When parents met one another, they "had the wonderful feeling that someone understood and cared," and that they were "no longer fighting . . . grief alone."[112] "When I began to talk to mothers who had lost children," said Sandi Boshak, "I learned that my feelings of loss and emptiness and guilt were not unique. Because I was able to share the experience with them, I was able to pull through."[113] In 1972, Abraham Bergman admitted that he hoped the NSIDSF would no longer exist in another five years because Americans would be so much more aware and understanding of SIDS; "'that's when we will have achieved our goal,' he said, 'when a family feels no more guilty about losing a child to crib death than they would if the child died of pneumonia, meningitis, or leukemia.'"[114] If parents' sentiments are any indication, the NSIDSF may not have exactly realized Bergman's wish, but it certainly helped.

The NSIDSF and SIDS centers prioritized the psychological and emotional aspects of SIDS. They focused above all else on attending to parents' need for "disease credibility assurance."[115] Both groups believed in the adage that "in knowledge there is power": "for SIDS parents, knowledge about the syndrome, about the grief process, and about the impact of such a death . . . helps them to cope with the immediate impact of the death and, in the long term, helps them to accept the loss and get on with their lives."[116] But given the awful situations in which they found themselves, knowledge could only carry these parents so far. In one talk explaining "what to say" and "what not to say" to SIDS parents, nurses learned that most parents felt like "SIDS" was not sufficient to explain their predicament. "In this age when medical science has discovered so much, has made such tremendous advances, the fact that this elusive killer is still undiscovered is difficult to understand," the presenter stated. "Had the baby died of some well-known disease or disorder, there would be no need to further explain, no need for further questioning."[117]

In other words, to a certain extent, these groups were fighting an unwinnable battle. Even their best and most heartfelt efforts could not change the fact that the SIDS diagnosis—and its counterpart prevailing paradigm of inexplicability and unpredictability—left victims wanting. Even parents provided ample and accurate information about SIDS suffered profoundly from guilt and self-reproach; the most steadfast professional reassurances were "not enough to stop their [SIDS parents'] pain." SIDS offered them *some* explanation, but it was so far from definitive that parents continued to "develop their own 'theories' which incorporate[d] blame or self-doubt."[118] And as much as the NSIDSF and SIDS centers asserted that SIDS was a "real disease" in the same way as cancer, the reality is that SIDS was distinguished among other culprits in childhood death for its uncertainty and its suddenness. As one parent put it, every SIDS story ended with questions.[119] The SIDS label—the main tool on which the NSIDSF and government SIDS centers relied—might have been mitigating, but it was still incomprehensible. In this way, SIDS itself fell short of fully reassuring and relieving parents. The history of the NSIDSF and the state SIDS information and counseling centers confirm this; indeed, this exact flaw in the diagnosis made the NSIDSF and SIDS centers' emotional, informational, and personal support emphases that much more coveted and influential.

6 · CAUSE FOR ALARM

Warren Guntheroth had been in the SIDS game for his entire career. He grew up in Oklahoma during the Great Depression, and moved north to Boston for school as a young adult. Harvard granted him a full scholarship for undergraduate and medical school. In the 1950s, Guntheroth joined the faculty at the University of Washington, where he founded the institution's pediatric cardiology department. His colleagues remembered Guntheroth as a passionate and a confident practitioner—when he suffered a heart attack that eventually led to his death in 2012, he walked himself from his office to the emergency room and started directing the residents treating him. Guntheroth had attended the 1960s conferences on sudden death in infancy, kept up with the "theory of the month club," and published on the topic. At the 1963 conference, he had speculated about the idea of a "near-miss" SIDS baby—an infant who seemed to somehow evade death. Implicit in his idea was the notion that sudden infant death was preventable, and that did not sit well with his peers. In 1969, Guntheroth returned to the submission, presciently suggesting that sudden infant death babies might have "instability" regulating their breathing during sleep. He wondered whether it might be possible to locate "triggers" for babies who struggled to breathe, adding that "a portable monitor would be very inexpensive, and a patient who is at risk and who had a respiratory infection, for example, could have a small monitor." "This may cause a great many neuroses," Guntheroth said, "but at least it *is* a possibility of doing something in terms of prevention."[1] In 1972 Alfred Steinschneider provided the key link for Guntheroth's supposition: apnea. In his published work, Steinschneider asserted that apnea was the potential trigger, monitors the potential solution. Before investigations revealed them as erroneous, those ideas exerted powerful influence over SIDS research ideologies and investigations.

In 1973, Warren Guntheroth began prescribing breathing monitors that could be used at home to fearful couples who came to see him after their babies had stopped breathing and almost died. Terrified of repeat episodes, parents were taking turns staying up all night to watch their babies. Guntheroth thought home monitors could help. Small portable devices with wires that attached to babies and measured vital signs, monitors sounded an alarm if they detected a breathing stoppage or slow heart rate. Most models sounded at around seventy decibels (approximately the same sound level as an average vacuum cleaner). This was the exact scenario Guntheroth had envisioned in 1969, and his sleep-deprived patients welcomed the help. Guntheroth recommended monitoring "based less on a conviction that home monitoring would prevent SIDS than as a way of reducing the anxiety of parents."[2]

Across the country, other American families were turning to similar cardio-respiratory monitors for the same reasons: they were desperate for anything that might protect their children from sudden infant death. In Wisconsin, in 1978, Cathi Hoven-Sparks lost her daughter Nicole to SIDS. Nicole's high-tech monitor—akin to the one Guntheroth recommended—did not save her life. Before she died, Nicole's older brother Shane also had a home monitor, pre-scribed for apnea. Shane lived. In 1980, when Cathi had another child, Jacob, doctors told her and her husband that Jacob fell into two ostensible "high-risk" categories: he had an older sibling who had died from SIDS and he presented with breathing abnormalities. His doctors diagnosed Jacob with "near-miss" SIDS, eponymously conveying that he had come close to succumbing to SIDS. They recommended monitor treatment—the same prescription that had seem-ingly saved Shane and failed Nicole. Cathi and her husband dutifully operated the monitor and tracked Jacob's condition in their home. When journalists, medical professionals, or peers called monitors' legitimacy and effectiveness into question, Cathi vehemently defended Jacob's near-miss SIDS diagnosis and his monitoring treatment. Cathi spoke openly about her family's trying experi-ences with SIDS and near-miss SIDS, and eventually launched a support group specifically for families with monitors.[3]

The experiences of physicians like Warren Guntheroth and families like that of Cathi Hoven-Sparks capture some of the most loaded questions surrounding SIDS and apnea in the 1970s and '80s. Their decisions personify doctors' and families' fraught efforts to prevent SIDS. Based on the theory that apnea could result in SIDS, thousands of parents across the nation outfitted their nurseries with electronic monitors. In the hopes of preventing SIDS, these families reset their lives to accommodate monitors. Grounded in the research suggesting that infants suffering from sleep apnea may be at risk for SIDS, home monitors offered an intriguing, if imperfect, preventative treatment.

The development and proliferation of home infant apnea monitors was a cru-cial part of the story of SIDS. Monitors arose as the product of a timely series of collisions between a few overlapping intellectual and physical developments in medicine and society. Their applications had real consequences for families as well as SIDS research. Monitors emerged in hospitals, moved to private homes, and spawned additional SIDS-related diagnoses and complications. Around monitors coalesced fascinating contemporary debates regarding medical technology, patient autonomy, home health care, and investigatory clinical treatments. Monitors embodied the risks SIDS posed to a child and its family, and fueled the conflation of ideas about vulnerability, prevention, and safety with hopes for infant health and familial security. Medicine introduced monitors as an exciting possible remedy for SIDS, yet it never produced any clear evidence that monitoring had any ability to measurably reduce or prevent sudden infant death. The devices re-circuited the very issues they sought to overcome. Monitors obscured rather than clarified SIDS' causes, reshaped rather than removed sources of guilt, and displaced rather than dissolved anxieties about SIDS.

MONITORS AND MEDICINE

Apnea monitors and SIDS research crossed paths during a window of historical opportunity. Infant apnea monitors moved to the center of SIDS management in the 1970s and 1980s due to related circumstances in organized medicine. Technological monitors proliferated in critical care medicine, neonatal intensive care arose as a distinct province within the hospital, and infant sleep science emerged as a prominent medical interest. The contemporaneous advents of technological monitoring, newborn intensive care, and sleep medicine all cultivated a context both favorable and receptive to the pairing of apnea monitors with SIDS.

In the decades after World War II, a vast array of technological equipment and treatment modalities flowed into and out of hospitals. Ranging from defibrillators to contraceptives, dialysis machines to surgical techniques, and screening instruments to respirators, in the postwar era technology increasingly became a component in medical practice. Monitors were one form of new medical gadgetry. Electronic monitoring of patients became especially popular in such high-profile arenas as organ transplantation, burn units, and fetal heart monitoring; it also gained a reputation as an advanced form of medical practice via placement in nascent hospital critical care centers.[4]

Monitoring patients' vital signs was part and parcel of the modern intensive care unit (ICU). While monitor technology came of age, a growing number of hospitals began designating separate ICUs for the most critically ill or postoperative patients. In the mid-1950s, the Children's Hospital of Philadelphia introduced the first postoperative care space specifically for infants. It had an around-the-clock nursing staff, and by 1962 had expanded to become the first infant ICU. In the next decade, newborn infants claimed their own ICU spaces in hospitals across the country. Neonatal intensive care units (NICUs) offered protected spaces and specialized, comprehensive medical attention for the most vulnerable, complex, or demanding patients. Monitoring was fundamental in the NICU. Any number of basic physical measurements—blood pressure, heart rate, breathing rate, or temperature—could prove crucial in determining a baby's course of care.[5]

It was here that infant respiratory monitors made their debut. Typically, nurses shouldered most of the responsibility for tracking infants' vital signs, and newborns susceptible to breathing problems commanded vigilant observation.[6] Monitors were initially touted as a help to overstretched nurses and a way to ease the burden of constant surveillance in the NICU. Breathing monitors could supplement (or possibly even in the future replace) nurses, releasing them from consuming observational duties and enabling them to care for more patients. In 1960, the developers of one breathing monitor described that their "efficient and reliable" device, "wherever it has been in use," was "welcomed most enthusiastically by the nursing staff, who, liberated from the necessity of watching the baby every few minutes, are able to confidently get on with their routine duties." Monitors also brought the possibility of improved care, since they might remove the potential of human mistakes in patient monitoring.[7] Even in high-functioning critical care units, promoters warned, potentially fatal breathing pauses could "escape the attention of the nursing staff for several minutes."[8] A breathing monitor could offer hospitals and NICU staffers peace of mind by alerting professionals and acting as a sort of insurance policy against the flaws of human observation.[9]

Throughout the decade, infant breathing monitors were sold as an essential component in any respectable NICU. By many descriptions, the NICU was predicated on the possession of "sophisticated" or flashy electronic equipment for around-the-clock physiological monitoring; to a certain extent, medical technology and the NICU were contingent.[10] Infant respiratory monitors fit directly into this mindset, coexisting with nurses as allies in the most innovative newborn infant hospital care centers.

While monitors and NICUs matured through the 1960s, the science of infant sleep had been expanding. In the 1960s, documenting infants' sleep behaviors, operating ICUs, and monitoring vital signs electronically all converged in the hospital. In 1972 Alfred Steinschneider roped these developments into the SIDS arena. His timing could not have been better. SIDS researchers, including Warren Guntheroth, had previously raised the prospect of sleep apnea as a cause for sudden infant death. An article published in 1965 in the *American Journal of Diseases of Children* described a small case study of four sudden infant death babies. Lead author L. H. Stevens argued that the cause might have been severe apneic episodes. "Part of the large island of infant mortality that is called sudden unexplained death," he posited, "may represent no more than those hapless individuals who experience these [apneic] episodes in their severest and most intolerable form and perish."[11]

The apnea explanation itself was not new when it prospered. Rather, the circumstances in the 1970s constituted a favorable environment for the apnea explanation, making it appear newly appealing. The apnea theory and apnea monitors thrived beginning in the 1970s because they met a ready audience. Researchers were eager to locate a framework for SIDS that discredited the lingering concepts of overlaying and suffocation, and they now accepted the notion of abnormality. Sleep apnea also accommodated SIDS epidemiology—it accounted for SIDS correlations with sleep and night hours, and jibed with the long-standing belief that breathing was somehow implicated. Most of all, it was practicable. As one pediatrician at the Johns Hopkins Hospital exclaimed, Steinschneider's article had raised "the possibility of identifying infants at risk from SIDS before the final event."[12]

After Steinschneider asserted that "prolonged apnea . . . is part of the pathophysiologic process resulting in SIDS," SIDS and apnea became so entangled that the distinctions between them became distorted.[13] In the Medline database, from 1966 through 1972, just one article referenced SIDS and sleep apnea in conjunction. In the six years after Steinschneider's piece, from 1973 through 1979, 99 articles referenced SIDS and apnea together; in the next three years, from 1980 to 1982, 335 articles referenced them jointly.[14] The profusion was exponential. In the opening sentences of a review article taking stock of the entire SIDS field in 1980, Marie Valdes-Dapena reported that the sleep apnea theory was "pre-eminent; it supersedes all others." "So prominent is it, in fact," she continued, "that in the minds of both our lay and scientific communities, an unfortunate tendency has arisen—whereby pathologic apnea is equated with the sudden infant death syndrome, as though the two were one."[15]

"ALARMING BABIES"[16]

A number of academic research centers designed studies to examine SIDS, sleep apnea, and monitoring. They sought to evaluate and assess the potential role of monitors in medical treatment for apnea. The prestigious Massachusetts General Hospital (MGH) in Boston conducted the most influential trials. MGH was not the only hospital to commence home monitoring studies—others were quickly underway at Columbia University, Stanford University, and before long at the SIDS Institute in Baltimore (a research organization that opened in 1980 with Steinschneider at the helm), for example. But MGH's program and outcomes significantly shaped the ideas, methods, and direction of home monitoring in the 1970s and 1980s. It acted as a guidepost for virtually every subsequent program nationwide, and played a pivotal role in entwining home monitors with SIDS.

Lead investigators in Boston, Daniel Shannon and Dorothy Kelly, coordinated a home monitor study in 1973 to "evaluate the effectiveness of home management of life-threatening apnea in infants with near-miss sudden infant death syndrome."[17] Typically, near-miss SIDS involved prolonged apnea, cyanosis, or any apparently life-threatening event that required resuscitation. By incorporating near-miss SIDS into their study, MGH researchers bestowed no small measure of legitimacy upon the concept. The initial MGH patient group consisted of eighty-four near-miss infants who suffered from prolonged sleep apnea, defined as twenty seconds or longer. (This was longer than Steinschneider's original measurement of fifteen seconds or longer; twenty seconds henceforth became the standard measure for a prolonged apneic episode.) Shannon and Kelly combined diagnostic testing with meticulous observation to ascertain apnea, and treated patients with monitors. Their conclusions supported the sleep apnea hypothesis, sanctioned the use of home monitors, and established a template to ascertain at-risk babies.

Some of the criteria were modified over time, but the most important factors for ascertaining at-risk babies were whether an infant was the sibling of a SIDS victim, whether he presented with prolonged apnea, and whether he had any history of near-miss SIDS. Parents of at-risk babies underwent specialized preparation at the hospital. Staff taught them how to attach electrodes and operate monitors, which were set to alarm after twenty seconds of inactive breathing. In the event of an alarm, parents were instructed to observe first: watch for signs of breathing and color change. If their baby's skin changed color, parents should stimulate immediately; if not, they should wait thirty seconds before taking any action to reactivate breathing. If necessary, interventions were to progress from least to most aggressive. Parents began with "gentle stimulation" (minimal shaking), for example, before engaging in "vigorous stimulation" (prolonged or repetitive shaking). Their last resorts were CPR and bag-and-mask resuscitation. Mothers and fathers were also trained to maintain comprehensive records documenting the details of every alarm occurrence.[18]

Parents monitored their babies at home for an average of seven months. Twenty-seven infants required resuscitation at least once, and four died. In three of the deaths, parents had not heard their monitors alarm and were prevented from reviving their child. In response, MGH amplified the alarm volume and began working to incorporate an alternative device that would itself stimulate a baby after thirty seconds. In the fourth case of death, one of the child's parents previously "had a frustrating experience with home monitoring" and "refused" monitoring.[19]

Shannon and Kelly concluded that there existed "a significant risk of severe life-threatening apnea in infants who have experienced near-miss SIDS." They recommended carefully supervised home monitoring for any baby that had ever needed resuscitation, and explained that parents needed twenty-four-hour access to professional medical, technical, and psychological counsel. (When they wrote that monitoring ought to be "carefully supervised," Shannon and Kelly meant that it needed to be prescribed and overseen by a doctor.) The MGH team's conclusions, that (1) "infants who have experienced near-miss SIDS are at great risk of recurrent apnea, hypoxia, and sudden death" and that (2) "most deaths can be prevented by supervised home monitoring of respirations and appropriate intervention by parents trained in resuscitation," was tantamount to a ringing endorsement of Steinschneider's apnea theory of SIDS causation and a mandate to pediatricians, researchers, and hospitals to invest in and commit to home monitoring regimens.[20]

By 1980, the infant apnea monitoring protocols at MGH were functioning as a yardstick for emerging programs wherever they existed.[21] For eligible families, in-hospital training lasted twenty-four hours, incorporated informational videos, and entailed a comprehensive educational regimen taught by nurses and physicians. There are no data recording the extent to which parents in the MGH program used it, but they were provided around-the-clock access to professional help should they want or need assistance.[22] Families returned to the hospital every month for follow-up pneumograms—recordings of overnight vital signs during sleep. Using standardized event sheets, parents detailed the exact circumstances of "real" alarm events (as compared to mechanical malfunctions), including the number of times the alarm sounded, whether the child was awake or asleep, whether the child was breathing, his skin color, and their own exact responses. In addition, parents kept meticulous daily journals—medical professionals wanted to know about a child's medications, activities, eating schedules, sleeping habits, as well as "anything else unusual."[23]

WHAT DOES THE DOCTOR SAY?

Physicians were disinclined to directly challenge the apnea theory of SIDS causation, but the pages of medical journals expose an icy divide over its applications. Many physicians were extremely apprehensive, if not outraged, over the widespread use of monitors. They had a number of specific disputes. Perhaps the most important and vocal points of criticism dealt with efficacy—first regarding the links between apnea and SIDS and second of monitoring itself. While monitors grew in popularity, infant sleep apnea was still obscure. The exact nature of the relationship between SIDS and apnea was definitively unknown.

Apnea and SIDS were so jumbled together in the 1970s and 1980s that most laypeople, and even many professionals, had difficulty separating the two. Clinicians described that "the public and health care providers are not well-informed about the distinctions between SIDS and infant apnea."[24] In 1974, researchers surveyed a randomly selected group of pediatricians about the treatment of apneic babies. The 379 responses they received make plain that there was overwhelming uncertainty, even among specialists, about SIDS and apnea. "The striking differences in opinion regarding the relationship of SIDS and apnea revealed by this study suggest that widespread public confusion about this relationship is mirrored in pediatric opinion," they said, and "the academic pediatricians and practitioners appeared to be equally uncertain."[25] The connection was further muddled since so many babies exhibited signs of apnea. Steinschneider himself reported that sleep apnea was a "virtually universal occurrence" in babies and even noted that most affected babies resumed breathing on their own.[26]

Critics declared that there was no conclusive proof home monitoring could effectively prevent SIDS. In one contribution to The Lancet, a skeptical physician observed that no studies demonstrated monitors "had any effect on morbidity, mortality, or infant survival." The same physician went on to query: "If specially trained nurses on eight-hour shifts miss nearly 40% of apneic spells in an intensive care setting, isn't it reasonable to expect that parents on 24-hour shifts, seven days a week, for several months will not do as well?"[27] Many doctors and parents justified home monitoring on the grounds that it was "our only defense" or "the only (available) wheel in town," but in the words of one practitioner, it was "a rather bent wheel."[28] Physicians calling attention to the lack of evidence regarding monitors' efficacy derided the practice as little more than a manifestation of the "classic clinical pressure to 'do something, anything!'"[29] Another physician thought the evidence in support of monitoring was so scant as to profess that "physicians and the public have been brainwashed."[30]

Opponents took issue with monitors' operative demands and safety. For them, monitors were faulty at best and hazardous at worst. The technology was far from perfected, especially for home use; most devices were unreliable and expensive. Some lacked the ability to detect certain kinds of apneas, and parents reported high false-alarm rates and finicky mechanics.[31] Even newer models were seriously limited in their capacity to reliably detect apneas, alarm accurately, and prevent SIDS. As one observer summarized, "all monitors have limitations."[32] Some parents even reported that their babies learned that the alarm beckoned their mothers, and figured out how to set it off on their own, either by interfering with the device or holding their breath.[33] Beyond questionable accuracy, Bruce Beckwith warned that monitors, particularly in "inexperienced hands" (and by this he meant parents), could be "downright dangerous": "electrodes and wires always raise the possibility of electroshock or strangulation."[34] Indeed, in the mid-1980s, the FDA started receiving reports documenting hazards, injuries, and even one fatality associated with infant apnea monitors.[35] In 1988, a frustrated pair of researchers also referenced two deaths that appeared to be a result of electrocution from monitoring.[36] No longitudinal studies existed to guarantee the protracted safety of monitoring.

Lastly, skeptics harangued monitors for their deleterious psychosomatic effects in the home. Monitors were deeply disruptive and stressful; their adverse effects on parents and families were no secret. Opponents argued that the unproven treatment did not warrant the harmful home environment they engendered. And they were especially angry over the "crass commercialism" of inventors and sensationalized media reports that indicated otherwise. Beckwith charged advertisers with jumping the gun on home monitors and "inducing hysteria for purely economic motivations."[37] Such concerns were not ungrounded; advertisers did falsely market various devices as capable of preventing SIDS.[38]

These types of apprehensions did not deter physicians who saw monitors as the most promising direction in SIDS prevention. In fact, proponents of monitors were more than willing to concede most of their critics' points. Professionals agreed that monitors were technologically deficient and needed all kinds of improvements. They concurred that monitoring should be carefully confined to medical prescription and professional oversight—parents should not be monitoring babies at home unless a physician authorized them to do so. Steinschneider worried that without professional supervision, the country risked unnecessarily placing "oodles and oodles of babies" on monitors.[39] He also admitted that monitors caused parents "tremendous anxiety."[40] Dorothy Kelly at MGH explained that monitor therapy had the potential to become a "major disruption" to families and that "the whole endeavor can seriously threaten family stability unless accompanied by an elaborate support system."[41]

Despite the fact that physicians backing monitors essentially assented on some level to nearly every criticism they met, they fundamentally interpreted the circumstances differently. Rather than discontinue monitoring because it was unproven, they issued edicts for expanded research and development to accumulate evidence and improve the technology. Steinschneider rightly pointed out that "it is axiomatic in medicine that no proposed therapy become a standard of practice until its efficacy has been demonstrated."[42] He and his supporters rejoined parents' struggles by refining channels of psychological, technical, and medical support for monitor families. They touted home monitoring as an improvement over hospital monitoring, which was equally, if not more, expensive, exhausting, worrisome, and disruptive to family life.[43]

Finally, advocates had a powerful weapon in their arsenal: affirmations from parents that monitors had been a welcome help. Supporters argued that monitors offered parents some measure of security and a "certain amount of control over [a] child's well-being."[44] "Faced with a tangible risk of a severe or potentially fatal episode," Steinschneider explained, "parents did cope effectively with the imperfect mode of treatment offered and were overwhelmingly grateful for the availability of an instrument that made it possible for them to care for their infants at home."[45] Shannon and Kelly at MGH similarly relayed that 75 percent of the parents with whom they worked said monitoring reduced their anxiety.[46] Furthermore, physicians in favor of home monitoring argued that opponents were "totally unjustified to blame . . . anxiety on the monitor."[47] Parents' anxiety, they said, was a product of the fearful situation in which they found themselves—it would have existed regardless of any monitor.

Interestingly, proponents and detractors were tuning in to their patients' concerns. Parent operators of apnea monitors, trained to manage complex medical equipment in their own homes, were tapping into practices unlikely to have been delegated outside the medical establishment in previous decades. In a way, monitoring transformed lay parents into medical caretakers. Physicians who prescribed monitors were inviting parents to engage in medical care with them, widening the tightly constricted circle of practitioners. Doctors who rejected monitors, on the other hand, were broadening their prescriptive worldviews to account for patients' mental and emotional well-being. Both camps were responding to their patients' individual interests.

"AT HOME WITH A MONITOR": PARENTS WITH APNEA MONITORS

To consult the medical literature on apnea monitors is to confront the uncomfortable reality that their effectiveness was very much unresolved. Reviewing parents' accounts of their experiences with monitors—as related in the media, didactic materials, and filtered through medical papers—is an entirely different exercise in unease. One instructive booklet for families with monitor babies informed parents that the "first alarm that happens at home is one you will probably never forget!"[48] Its cheery tone was dismally ironic. Parents who returned home from the hospital with a monitor literally saw their lives transform overnight. These devices were complex and imperfect; they were originally designed for hospital NICUs. They did not translate easily to home life: they heightened anxiety and tension, were often precursors to manifold mental health problems, disrupted family life, and impacted relationships.[49] The National SIDS Foundation was exactly right in its assessment that "the intensive care unit of the pediatric ward, we could say, moves . . . into the home."[50]

Monitors restricted parents' daily lives. Most families used a monitor for more than six months, and felt confined or tethered during that time. One mother said the device was so constricting that she felt "'like a prisoner' and 'strangled.'"[51] Working mothers found it difficult to maintain employment.[52] A majority of families used their monitors all the time, rather than as recommended, only during periods of sleep.[53] Parents learned to avoid noisy activities ("don't take chances!"), including routine things like running the dishwasher, vacuuming, or showering, and to remain within ten seconds' distance of their child at all times.[54] Monitors alarmed often during the day and the night, ranging from ten to over thirty per day.[55] In one extreme case, a child's alarm sometimes went off up to fifty times during the night.[56] Parents that had been staying awake all night to watch their children breathe now recounted staying awake at night to watch their monitors.[57] An interesting "informal survey" of Canadian parents tapped into the pervasiveness of the stress monitors sowed, indicating that babies picked up on their parents' anxiety. "The baby knows something is going on," Pamyla Haines explained.[58]

Husbands and wives also experienced strains. In one study, 10 percent of couples felt distant. They reported marital discord from differing attitudes about the "need and importance of the device."[59] Anne Barr, an NSIDSF parent who authored an advice booklet for monitor families, confided that "sex, or lack of it, can also be a problem." "Obviously," she said, "the tense atmosphere created by life with the monitor is not conducive to good sexual relations."[60] Although mothers and fathers both were trained and involved in monitoring care, mothers disproportionately shouldered the responsibility. One study found that mothers were the primary operators of monitors twenty-two hours daily, and concluded that "the mother was the family member whose life was most affected."[61]

Financial costs burdened many families, although a few avenues materialized to temper the charges. Some families obtained partial insurance coverage. More often over time, parents acquired hand-me-down donated equipment or rented used apparatuses. Otherwise, device costs approximated $1,500. Additive charges to account for parent training, home visits, and twenty-four-hour access to medical and technical respondents could bring totals up to as high as $4,000.[62] An MGH follow-up analysis found the average family incurred more than $2,500 in medical bills and remained in debt from monitor-related costs for between one and three years.[63] In one newsworthy instance, an equipment company in Florida took a family to court for failing to pay its monitor bills (it had mistakenly believed that insurance was covering the $210 monthly fees for the device). Kathleen Brady spoke about her dilemma on a radio show: "If they take it away, she dies," Kathleen said of her daughter Ashley's monitor. "I can't believe everybody's putting money before a baby's life." A listener who happened to deal in monitors contacted Kathleen to offer a replacement.[64]

Stimulation protocols could make parents further anxious. Professionals' directives to "gently stimulate" a baby involved anything ranging from a touch to a slap to light shaking. "Vigorous stimulation" entailed a harsher touch or aggressive shaking. Some parents were taken aback by these instructions.[65] One couple admitted, "we feel almost ashamed of ourselves to be rough or to cause [our daughter] pain, but that is what the doctors have recommended."[66] Without offering details, an anecdotal report in 1985 described that there were "cases in which overenthusiastic resuscitation by parents in response to an alarm has led to serious damage to the infant."[67]

These concerns are interesting given that, during the same decade, shaken baby syndrome became its own item of medical and social distress. In 1974, John Caffey, the same physician whose 1946 article had stimulated professional medical attention to child abuse, described "the whiplash shaken infant syndrome": a condition whereby "manual shaking of infants by the extremities or shoulders" brought on "whiplash-induced intracranial and intraocular bleeding, but with no external signs of head trauma." At the time, Caffey recommended that a broad public education campaign be coordinated to teach parents about the dangers of shaking babies.[68]

As monitoring grew more common, parents increasingly formed support networks to help each other cope with its tribulations. In Boston, parents met monthly and parent "graduates" of the monitoring program were incorporated into training schedules. MGH also issued a newsletter, "Parent Cable," for monitor families.[69] These activities inspired parents in other parts of the country, like Cathi Hoven-Sparks, to actuate similar channels of support. Some groups even offered qualified babysitting personnel during meetings.[70] The emergence of monitor-specific support groups implicitly speaks to parents' difficulties with monitors while still indicating parents' underlying dedication to monitoring.

Perhaps what is most striking about parents' accounts, though, is their overall *satisfaction* with monitoring. Parents did report misery at first. They acknowledged that monitors caused intense anxiety and isolation, and often precipitated depression or mental health problems. Mostly, however, parents reported being grateful to have monitors. They said their anxieties with a monitor, however heightened, would have been worse without it. They adjusted; frustrations and fearfulness gave way to a familiar, manageable routine. Anne Barr informed parents that they would likely experience three distinct phases with their monitor: an initial or "breaking-in" phase, an adjustment phase, and a "time afterward when the monitor has become part of the family."[71] Barr reassured parents they would eventually see the monitor as a "trusted friend in the house."[72] And indeed, many parents agreed that overall, monitors reduced, rather than cultivated, anxiety; some described their devices as "well worth the trouble," a "blessing," or even, "an Angel of God watching over your child."[73]

Numbers further testify to parents' faith. By the middle of the 1980s, MGH had recommended monitoring for almost 1,500 babies. More than 750 babies were involved in an ongoing trial in Baltimore, and more than 650 had been prescribed home monitors at the Children's Hospital of Philadelphia.[74] In California, professionals prescribed more than 1,800 home monitors.[75] This was just the tip of the iceberg. Hundreds of other babies were enrolled in home monitor programs nationwide, stretching from Massachusetts to the Midwest, the South to the Northwest, and to the noncontiguous states. At the Kapiolani Women's and Children's Medical Center in Honolulu, Hawaii, physicians estimated in 1985 that about 70 percent of infant patients were using monitors "at any given time."[76] A pair of practitioners in West Virginia in 1983 described home apnea monitoring as "quite common" in their state, "as well as in the rest of the eastern United States."[77] In the rural mountainous regions of the West, home apnea monitor use skyrocketed by 450 percent in just five years.[78] In 1983, nurse Kit Bakke identified fifty operational apnea programs throughout the U.S. and Canada, twenty-eight of which complied with her survey request. The respondents (which represented less than half of the existing apnea programs on the continent) had supervised 1,570 monitoring cases just in the previous twelve months.[79] All of this evidence only delineates physician-managed cases. Four years later, accounting for cases with *and* without formal medical oversight, the Congressional Office of Technology reported an estimate that 40,000 to 45,000 home infant apnea alarms were in use across the nation.[80] Already by 1981 there were about thirty home infant apnea monitor models on the market.[81] One manufacturer, Healthdyne, Inc., was a home health equipment company founded by a SIDS father who left his job as an aerospace engineer after his son died. By 1986, it had sold around 70,000 home apnea monitors and was worth an estimated $134 million.[82]

These thousands of parents were willing to take the bad with the good—as Barr explained, "for monitor parents, the old saying 'better safe than sorry' takes on special meaning."[83] For them, the possibility that a monitor could save their child far outweighed whatever problems the device may have introduced. As far as they were concerned, if their child was still breathing, the apnea monitor had worked. They perceived that every time they responded to an alarm, they were saving their child's life.[84]

RECHARGING THE ISSUES

In 1972, apnea monitoring presented a potential resolution for SIDS. It offered a targeted area for research, the ability to discern at-risk babies, and protection. Its possibilities reignited hopes of lifting the shroud of mystery from SIDS and clarifying its unknown facets. Yet home apnea monitors produced new language for talking about familiar concerns—they may have reshaped the questions, but they did not change the conversation. Monitors failed to overcome parental guilt and did not improve conceptual coherence of the SIDS diagnosis; they rewired rather than resolved the central dilemmas surrounding SIDS.

Instead of alleviating guilt—a universal facet of SIDS—monitors exposed parents to alternative sources of guilt. The devices offered concerned parents a measure of solace, but it was sharply qualified. Hesitant parents felt they had little option but to accept monitors' drawbacks. One mother explained that she would "throw that machine out the window" if she could obtain her doctor's permission.[85] Many parents saw their monitors as a "necessary evil."[86] Because monitors insinuated that SIDS might be prevented, they posed the "additional psychological risk" of subjecting parents to even more direct accusations. In the event that a child on a monitor died, his parents were vulnerable to accusations (both internal and external) that they were implicated in their child's death.[87] Monitors may have come across as a technology that could assume responsibility for a child's well-being, but they required human operators. If a monitor did not fulfill its life-saving purpose, parents were not necessarily absolved. Some medical articles even explicitly cited parental "noncompliance" and "nonuse" of home monitors as explanations for infant deaths. These charges were directed at parents specifically noted for their low socioeconomic status, minority racial identities, and lack of medical insurance, and a high proportion were unwed mothers.[88] The implications refashioned the guilt and blame related to SIDS to accord with the apnea-induced version of the diagnosis.

The ambiguous notion of near-miss SIDS similarly encapsulates how apnea monitoring accommodated the existing discourse. The concept of near-miss gained real traction under the apnea rubric. It is not surprising that near-miss was a disputed term (one sardonic article title published in Australia asked: "'near-miss' or 'near-myth'?"), and criticisms spanned from technical to abstract.[89] Some researchers thought near-miss or "aborted crib death" incidents "rarely turned out to be crib deaths in the end."[90] Writing in 1976, Bruce Beckwith estimated that only about 5 percent of SIDS cases were preceded by any kind of near-miss event.[91] Some physicians worried that near-miss was not related to SIDS at all.[92] Others took issue with the term's virtually total reliance on the subjective testimony of parents.[93] Even professionals who accepted near-miss as a legitimate and useful moniker were perturbed by the lack of any uniform definition or standardized criteria with which to measure it.[94] Furthermore, near-miss was a fluid item of medical grammar, employed as a symptomatic adjective to describe both infants and events as well as used as a diagnosis itself. A baby, for example, might be described as *suffering* a near-miss SIDS or as actually *having* near-miss SIDS. The distinction was hazy.

Despite its limitations, many prominent physicians defended near-miss. They suggested that near-miss babies *were* different, somehow, from controls.[95] The prevalence of the term near-miss in both professional and colloquial literature—it was frequently embedded in the titles, abstracts, and contents of medical and media articles—attests to its perceived utility. Near-miss not only constituted a risk factor for SIDS, but also shaped the profile of another discrete patient population: near-miss babies. The result was a sort of "diagnostic sprawl"; by way of the apnea theory and apnea monitoring, "near-miss" grew from being a risk factor for SIDS into a treatable condition on its own.[96] Exemplifying this trend, two neurologists at the University of Virginia were even working on developing a monitor device that could "help parents determine whether their infant suffers from symptoms that indicate the need for further medical care." They envisioned that it could be a "universal . . . screening device" for SIDS, akin to a smoke detector, since "every infant is at some risk."[97]

In 1983, Alfred Steinschneider and Marie Valdes-Dapena published an article on SIDS, near-miss, and apnea. In favor of maintaining the near-miss concept, they suggested doing away with the particular expression and replacing it with a new label: an "apparently life-threatening event."[98] This terminology—an *apparently* life-threatening event—was implicitly ambiguous. In 1986, the National Institutes of Health formally recommended discarding the term near-miss SIDS in favor of the alternative nomenclature: "apparent life-threatening event syndrome," or ALTE (pronounced *all-tee*). The official definition was based on caregivers' perceptions: "an episode that is frightening to the observer and that is characterized by some combination of apnea . . . color change . . . marked change in muscle tone . . . choking, or gagging."[99] By name and definition, supposition was built into the concepts of near-miss and ALTE. Apnea and monitors played a key part in spawning near-miss and then ALTE, both of which dispersed parental guilt and siphoned the uncertainty of SIDS into diagnostic offshoots. In spawning both designations, apnea monitoring distributed the problems ingrained in SIDS instead of resolving them.

THE PARTIAL DEMISE OF APNEA

The apnea theory was never totally stamped out. Like the previous hypotheses of status thymicolymphaticus and accidental mechanical suffocation earlier in the twentieth century, the apnea theory suffered a series of blows that gradually revealed the full extent of its flaws, but monitoring was never fully outmoded. One reason the theory only partially fell from grace is that parents upheld it. Another is that it was practically impossible to conduct controlled clinical trials on home monitoring as a prevention tool for SIDS.[100] Initial problems with the apnea theory for SIDS sprang from doubts about its foundations. Babies' breathing patterns, particularly while they slept, were evidently erratic. Pediatricians had yet to decipher the boundary between "normal" and "abnormal" breathing, especially among newborns. Medical consensus held that slightly abnormal breathing was expected in infancy, at least to a certain extent.[101]

Following from the question of when infant apnea might be ordinary, prolonged apneic episodes resemble a strange pediatric phenomenon known as "breath-holding spells." Babies or toddlers (two months to two years) simply stop breathing, sometimes for as long as a minute. Often, they lose consciousness and pass out. The spells are reflex responses and completely involuntary— children have no control over them. Frequently, they "occur when a young child is angry, frustrated, in pain, or afraid."[102] One physician who proposed apnea as a cause for SIDS a full seven years before Steinschneider's article noted that an apneic episode severe enough to induce cyanosis in an infant appeared "identical to that observed in older children experiencing breathholding spells."[103] Based on its absence in the scholarship (this confusing overlap was scarcely mentioned in medical literature), breath-holding did not pose a major challenge to the apnea theory nor contribute to its demise, but it did underscore that practitioners were operating with very incomplete knowledge of "normal" pediatric breathing and "abnormal" infant apnea.

Researchers consistently failed to reach decisive conclusions about the connection between apnea and SIDS. One team surveyed eleven apnea programs in California and found that infants who had monitoring recommended suffered comparable SIDS rates to infants who were not prescribed monitors. Both groups "were at equal risk of dying of SIDS."[104] A research team headed by Joan Hodgman, a leading neonatologist in southern California who helped establish one of the nation's first NICUs in 1961 in Los Angeles, and Toke Hoppenbrouwers, a Ph.D. in neuroscience and clinical psychology, opined that "a growing number of studies" (including their own) were not documenting any differences between apneic and control infants. Although they were sensitive to the fears of parents, Hodgman and Hoppenbrouwers warned their colleagues that "we should not lose sight of the fact that the effectiveness of home monitoring has not been established." "In a climate in which the indications for treatment are unknown," they continued, "we should be cautious."[105]

Research across the Atlantic was most damaging (which is remarkable given that monitoring was regarded as a uniquely American convention). British practitioners were more universally suspicious of apnea monitoring. They pointed out that near-miss babies had "an excellent survival rate with or without monitoring."[106] In December 1982, David Southall hammered the first major crack in the apnea hypothesis. Southall examined over 1,000 infants, five of whom died from SIDS. He measured no prolonged apneas in any of the babies who died. Based on his study, prolonged apnea was not predictive of SIDS.[107] In a repeat study in 1983 consisting of more than 9,000 babies and twenty-nine SIDS deaths, Southall again found *no* differences between SIDS babies and controls in electrocardiac functioning or pneumogram readings. The twenty-nine SIDS infants showed no signs of apnea prior to their deaths. If anything, the children who exhibited abnormal pneumogram readings were more likely to live. Southall again concluded that apnea was not predictive of SIDS.[108] Not surprisingly, he was an outspoken critic of monitors. "Experience in the use of home monitors has been disappointing," Southall reflected, arguing that little reasoned evidence existed to justify home monitoring as an approach to SIDS. When other large-scale projects started reviewing cases, they showed that very few SIDS babies had ever experienced apneic episodes. Collectively, in fact, they demonstrated that there was "no difference in breathing patterns between infants who subsequently died of SIDS and controls."[109]

Through the 1970s and 1980s, the American Academy of Pediatrics (AAP) condoned home monitoring among its professional constituents. The organization never advocated or endorsed monitoring, but it also never specifically advised against its professional use. In 1975, the AAP issued a formal statement expressing concern about monitors "sold over-the-counter and advertised to prevent SIDS," discouraging their sale. It recommended continued research trials to amass further evidence.[110] Three years later, a Task Force on Prolonged Apnea updated the society's stance. The AAP declared that intensive observation ("24-hour surveillance") was crucial in managing prolonged apnea and allowed that electronic monitors, either in the hospital or in the home, may "be useful adjuncts to 24-hour surveillance." Task force members noted the psychological challenges of monitoring and again called for more research, "because a definitive causal relation between prolonged apnea and SIDS has not been established."[111] In 1985, the Academy reaffirmed that the relationship between SIDS and apnea was unknown.[112] It advised pediatricians to "evaluate and treat each case individually. Those who believe there is a relationship between prolonged apnea and SIDS and/or home monitoring may be helpful should prescribe monitoring; those who do not are not obligated to prescribe monitoring and should not feel pressured to do so. All should recognize and communicate that monitoring cannot guarantee against SIDS."[113] Monitors were "physician's choice." The AAP's responses to the professional controversy over apnea monitoring before the late 1980s were noncommittal.

Other investigations sowed more grim doubts about SIDS and near-miss. In 1977, British pediatrician Roy Meadow published the first paper explicating Munchausen syndrome by proxy (MSbP). Meadow described a pair of cases in which mothers lied about their children's health histories and symptomology. Their behaviors, Meadow explained, were "reminiscent" of Munchausen syndrome itself, a condition Richard Aster first described in *The Lancet* in 1951 to categorize patients that "consistently produce false stories and who fabricate evidence so causing themselves needless medical investigations, operations, and treatments."[114] The mother Meadow directly identified as a "first example of 'Munchausen syndrome by proxy'" was tampering with her six-year-old daughter's urine samples.[115] Five years later, Meadow published an article reporting on nineteen cases of children "with clear evidence of massive and persistent fabrication by a parent of both the history and the signs." With a greater case pool, Meadow more explicitly discussed the features of MSbP. He described the "impressive" medical detail of mothers' fabrications—their methods "combined cunning, dexterity, and, quite often, medical knowledge."[116] Meadow thought pediatricians still "should teach" that "mothers are always right," but his testimony implored caution. His findings taught that doctors should harbor at least some skepticism.[117]

Most of Meadow's cases involved epilepsy (a seizure disorder), but subsequent investigators linked his observations to apnea and monitoring.[118] A study in 1986 directly connected MSbP to recurrent infant apnea; the authors reviewed a series of monitoring cases and documented a subset of babies whose parents' behaviors were "compatible with the entity described as Munchausen syndrome by proxy." They relied on Meadow's descriptions and further identified MSbP as "a form of child abuse." For babies presenting with apnea, they specified, MSbP could present with any number of the following features: "(1) history of multiple resuscitations (especially in the hospital setting), (2) no recognizable cardiorespiratory abnormalities between episodes, (3) resuscitations begun only in the parent's presence, (4) need for resuscitation documented by others; and (5) a sibling with a similar illness or death."[119]

The next year, David Southall, the pediatrician who provided evidence seriously disputing the apnea theory, published a case study that followed two babies with bizarre histories of apnea. He thought their presentations matched descriptions of MSbP. Suspicious of foul play, Southall sought help from authorities and set up covert video surveillance. What he and his colleagues observed was appalling; they watched both babies struggle violently against their mothers, who were suffocating them using bedding or clothing items. Surveillance teams interrupted within seconds of both events.[120] Prompted by this experience, Southall began a similar, larger project. Between 1986 and 1991, he treated fourteen babies whom he suspected were victims of abuse. Just as before, Southall and his colleagues employed covert video surveillance, and just as before, the tapes revealed disturbing results—caretakers suffocating children. Southall, no doubt deeply distressed by his findings, counseled physicians to contemplate the possibility of abuse "under certain circumstances."[121] In the middle of Southall's study, Roy Meadow made overt connections between SIDS and MSbP. "Careful clinical and pathologic investigation, combined with laborious psychosocial studies of families, has disclosed," Meadow stated, "that a significant proportion of children previously labeled as having died of SIDS are likely to have been killed by their parents."[122]

The ties between abuse, MSbP, apnea, monitoring, and SIDS suggested that death investigation protocols needed to be altered—"the acceptance that death by suffocation sometimes masquerades as SIDS should lead to reevaluation of the use of the term and of the most appropriate investigations for infants who die suddenly and unexpectedly," Meadow explained.[123] In the middle of 1989, the National Institute of Child Health and Human Development organized an expert panel to assess the state of SIDS knowledge and research twenty years after the diagnosis was constructed. The team recommended amending the 1969 SIDS definition to incorporate new details. To account for the notion of abnormality, it removed the "unexpected by history" phrasing from 1969. It incorporated an age limit of one year, since over 90 percent of cases occurred in babies less than six months old. The panel also concurred that diagnosing SIDS required a death scene investigation. The experts reemphasized the importance of autopsies but added that unless a thorough scene investigation was also performed, SIDS could not be diagnosed. The new definition in full read: "The sudden death of an infant under one year of age which remains unexplained after a thorough case investigation, including performance of a complete autopsy, examination of the death scene, and a review of the clinical history."[124]

Amid this development, several highly publicized murder cases—originally misdiagnosed as SIDS—also increased suspicion.[125] One was particularly arresting. In March 1994, New York police went to speak with a quiet, forty-eight-year-old woman. Waneta Hoyt suffered from osteoporosis, high blood pressure, and diabetes. With thinning hair and the physical sadness of five of her children's deaths weighing her down, Waneta looked much older than her age. Raised in upstate New York, Waneta had dropped out of high school to marry Timothy Hoyt in January 1964. They welcomed their first son, Erik, in October of that year. Erik was a healthy baby, but he died when he was just three months old. No autopsy was conducted, but Erik's death was understood as a crib death case. Waneta and Timothy had a second son, James, shortly thereafter, and a daughter, Julie. One Thursday morning in September 1968, when James was just over two years old and Julie was not yet two months, Julie died. Exactly two weeks later, so did James. Waneta told medical authorities Julie had choked on rice cereal; James had suddenly collapsed after he finished his breakfast.

Before SIDS even had a name, Timothy and Waneta Hoyt were parent victims of sudden infant death. When they had a fourth child, Molly, in the spring of 1970, the couple took extra precaution. Timothy and Waneta brought Molly to the hospital after just a week because she was turning blue. Unable to locate abnormalities, physicians discharged Molly after two weeks. When Alfred

Steinschneider came across Molly's case, he had her admitted for care at his own Upstate Medical Center in Syracuse. Molly was hospitalized and monitored for fifty-two days. During her stay, she never experienced a prolonged apnea episode and her exams were all normal. Two days after Molly went home, Waneta grew fearful for her life and brought Molly back to Upstate. Eleven days later, Molly went home with an apnea monitor. The next morning, she died.

Noah Hoyt, Waneta and Timothy's fifth child, was born one year later. In light of their family's medical history, Noah's parents returned to Steinschneider. Noah spent a little more than a month in the hospital with no problems. They day after they left, Waneta returned to the hospital with Noah, frightened that he was turning blue. They spent another month in residence, went home, and came back again the next day. After six additional days in the hospital, Noah and Waneta returned home for the third time. Noah died the following day. Waneta visited the graves of her five children every year. To her neighbors, she was a tragic local figure, almost a myth. She lived with her husband and their adopted son, Jay, quietly for another two decades.[126]

Despite the fact that only Noah received an autopsy, each of the Hoyt children's deaths was recorded as an episode of sudden infant death. The Hoyt babies were atypical for more than sheer numbers—they were anonymously inscribed into pediatric medicine. Molly and Noah Hoyt, M.H. and N.H., were the two infants whose deaths led Alfred Steinschneider to conclude in his 1972 article that apnea was implicated in SIDS. When New York police went to speak with Waneta Hoyt in 1994, they started the process of unraveling Steinschneider's entire argument, which had been rooted in the "H. family." Years after police authorities first grew suspicious about the multiple deaths in the "H. family," they were able to identify the Hoyts and subpoena Noah's medical records. Separate external expert reviewers thought the case was a homicide.[127]

Within hours of bringing Waneta Hoyt in for questioning, police had her confession in hand. It was chilling. "I caused the death of all of my five children," she said. Of Erik, Waneta explained: "I held a pillow . . . over his face while I was sitting on the couch. I don't remember if he struggled or not, but he did bleed from the mouth and nose." Waneta admitted pressing Julie's face into her own torso until Julie stopped struggling. The morning James died, Waneta "wanted him to stop crying . . . [and] used a bath towel to smother him." When Molly came home from the hospital, Waneta "used a pillow that was in the crib to smother her." Recalling Noah's death, Waneta said: "I held a baby pillow over his face until he was dead." "I could not stand the crying," Waneta continued; "it was the thing that caused me to kill them all, because I didn't know what to do for them."[128]

Waneta Hoyt was tried for murder on all five counts. She rescinded her initial confession, alleging that it had been coerced. During her trial, four nurses

from Steinschneider's team testified that Waneta Hoyt had "showed little interest" in her babies while she was in the hospital. Nurse Thelma Schneider said
she and her peers had approached Steinschneider and "expressed our fears—we
had a gut feeling that something was going on," she said. "Either [Steinschnei-
der] was in total denial or not being very objective." An ambulance worker who
responded to the Hoyts' emergency calls, Robert Vanek, felt skeptical after James
died. "Three in a row? It bothered me," Vanek remembered. In September 1995,
Waneta Hoyt was convicted and sentenced to seventy-years to life in prison.
The judge stated that her penalty was for "depraved indifference to human life."
She died in jail in 1998 from pancreatic cancer, still proclaiming her innocence.[129]

The Hoyt case, sensational in its own right, was even more incredible for the
fact that the family had formed the foundation for Alfred Steinschneider's landmark 1972 article linking SIDS to apnea. The misinterpretation is as telling as
it was crippling. Steinschneider's report suffered from multiple methodological
weaknesses. In a letter published in *Pediatrics* in 1973, physician John Hick challenged Steinschneider's interpretations. In acerbic tone, Hick pointed out that
the "prolonged apnea recordings" Steinschneider discussed were hardly severe
enough to warrant concern. He was also suspicious that no one except the
mother ever witnessed any problems whatsoever with the "H. family" babies.
Hick even wrote that the "circumstantial evidence" indicated "a critical role for
the mother in the death of her children."[130] But even the editors of *Pediatrics*
seemingly sided with Steinschneider, printing his retaliation and expressing how
"particularly impressed" they were with his statements that "*failure to define the
cause* of a sudden death can never be used as a support for the diagnosis of child
abuse" and that "no such evidence was available" in the given "H. family."[131]

Steinschneider's conclusions, beset as they were with problems, flourished
in the mid-1970s in part because physicians working on SIDS were so deeply
invested in discounting the notion of smothering and in differentiating SIDS
from infanticide. SIDS researchers—even with dissimilar notions—were
actively trying to create *distance* between SIDS and homicide, not contend with
their similitude. Even though Abraham Bergman disagreed with Steinschneider's endorsement of home monitoring, for example, his perspective on the
relationship between child abuse and SIDS sheds light on how Steinschneider's
theory was able to survive at all. When asked about the possibility of mistaking
child abuse for SIDS, Bergman told a reporter that he would "rather let one go
free than accuse 99 wrongly of having been responsible for their child's death."[132]
Waneta Hoyt's conviction in the 1990s brought these concerns—largely mar-
ginalized in the 1970s—into new light. The Hoyt case should have been the final
nail in coffin for the apnea theory, but it more so reintroduced prickly questions
about SIDS.[133]

CONCLUSION

By the end of the 1980s, SIDS researchers were still at a loss to explain things to parents. As Dr. Mark Pearlman, director of an apnea center in New Jersey, remarked in 1988, "we have more information than we have ever had . . . but it has only created more questions."[134] The apnea theory added confusion to SIDS, and the monitoring of tens of thousands of babies did not demonstrably reduce SIDS. The apnea hypothesis introduced technological monitoring in American homes and blurred understandings about whether medicine and parents could prevent SIDS. The actual physical process of alarming babies constitutes a vivid historical symbol of parents' and doctors' shared struggles to manage confusing research and distressing messages about SIDS. Monitors may have offered parents the façade of safety, but they were a highly problematic intervention. Indeed, the science discounting apnea as a cause for SIDS also ended up revolving back around to suffocation, infanticide, and abuse. Monitoring instruments embodied both fears of SIDS *and* hopes of preventing it; they relocated medical care from the hospital to the home and scattered the problems surrounding SIDS far more than they solved any.

No medical studies ever documented evidence monitoring worked. But parents' stories speak for themselves; they explain why and how thousands of families did not care that scientific medicine only equivocally confirmed monitors' efficacy. Beverly Whitney lost her son Todd to SIDS, and her daughter Debbie was on a monitor after his death. She hated the monitor—"it was a nightmare," she said. But one night Beverly ran to respond to an alarm and found her daughter "sweaty and ice-cold," just like she had found Todd. Screaming, Beverly started shaking her daughter, then tried to resuscitate her. Her husband joined in, and somewhere between "all the flopping and shaking," Debbie resumed breathing. The next day, the Whitneys put a microphone next to Debbie's alarm.[135] Thousands of other parents like the Whitneys perceived monitors as a life-saving trade-off. It was "easier to adjust" to monitoring than to losing a child, they said; every time they heard an alarm, it was the chance to rescue their baby's life.[136]

7 · SLEEP LIKE A BABY

In one of the first professional infant care books, published in 1911, pediatrician J. P. Crozer Griffith observed that there was "sometimes a great deal of needless anxiety among mothers" about how their babies slept.[1] More than a century later, in light of new questions, schismatic professional recommendations, and SIDS, the simple act of laying a baby to sleep became an even more uneasy ritual for many American parents.

Sudden unexpected infant deaths have always been connected to sleep, but in the later years of the twentieth century two threads in pediatric sleep medicine became especially closely related to SIDS. One dealt with babies' actual physical body positioning and placement for sleep—specifically, whether a baby laid on its stomach (prone), back (supine), or side. The second piece more broadly involved the circumstances of a baby's sleep environment—its bed, bed placement, and bed company.

Despite the fact that researchers always considered sleep a central feature of SIDS, they were mostly uncritical of prevailing sleep advice until the mid-late 1980s. Such elementary matters as sleep positioning or location were mentioned but not critically assessed for the first two decades of concerted research. Certainly, SIDS researchers were interested in babies' sleep, but they were most attentive to aspects of sleep that corresponded with or stemmed from the apnea theory. Rather than scrutinizing such plain issues as body placement or bedding characteristics, researchers studied complex, measurable neurological and anatomical components of sleep. In other words, those facets of babies' sleep that came to be most intimately—and controversially—tied to SIDS at the dawn of the twenty-first century remained on the outskirts of SIDS research for most of the twentieth century.

The details surrounding how and where babies slept were never far from the minds of SIDS researchers and worried parents, but the lack of science undergirding widespread customs and ideas about how babies should sleep is telling. As two physicians remarked in 1990, "although doctors have changed their opinions about the best sleeping position for babies from time to time and place to place, it is curious that the actual benefits and disadvantages have received so little 'critical scrutiny.'"[2] Before the 1990s, most American mothers laid their babies to sleep on their stomachs. This convention originated with American caregivers. Organized medicine, which considered prone sleeping a harmless preference until research indicated otherwise, espoused it. In contrast, the practice of "co-sleeping" (when family members—in this case, parents and babies—sleep together) has a long history of stigmatization.

Although investigators documented a correlation between prone sleeping and sudden infant death, it was decades before they interpreted it as problematic. In the U.S., epidemiological researchers inquired about sleep positioning but did not deem it a legitimate area of causation. In the U.K., likewise, evidence of the correlation between stomach sleeping and sudden infant death surfaced as early as the 1960s; by the 1970s, the association was statistically significant.[3] Yet, because of contemporary customs, in neither location did physicians fret. Thus, despite available evidence, the medical establishment was slow to assess infant sleep position as a contributing factor in SIDS.

The wavering history of pediatric sleep science demonstrates that convictions about what constituted "safe" for sleeping babies changed drastically over time. Where this history dovetails with SIDS, two things become apparent. First, SIDS researchers were blinded to those aspects of sleep that they eventually recognized as most relevant. This was the case for a number of reasons: investigators were committed to discounting anything that tied SIDS to suffocation, they were initially wedded to a framework that did not consider conditional risk factors, and they were led astray by the apnea theory. Secondly, SIDS research outcomes benefitted profoundly from international scholarship. When SIDS researchers collaborated and exchanged data across international borders in the 1980s, they were able to ascertain simple bedtime measures that effected what countless theoretical proposals, decades of research, and tens of thousands of apnea monitors had all failed to do: demonstrably reduce SIDS rates.

BEDTIME: AN EXERCISE IN STOICISM

Over the course of the twentieth century, Americans increasingly regarded where, how, and with whom babies slept as crucial parenting decisions. For the greater part of the nineteenth century, parental advice literature did not discuss sleeping. In the late 1800s, however (especially after the advent of germ theory), manuals began to address children's sleep with regularity.[4] By the early 1900s, children's sleeping patterns and habits were regarded as important to survival and development; by the 1920s, the subject had been thoroughly "problematized" and constituted a "consistent new level of concern" for parents.[5]

In the last decade of the nineteenth century, physicians and child development professionals began advising mothers to approach bedtime with unwavering uniformity and measured emotional and physical distance. Contributors to popular periodicals such as the Ladies' Home Journal, for example, condemned the apparently widespread practice of cradle rocking. They castigated cradle rocking for accustoming infants to undue attention at bedtime and warned mothers that the practice "should be early abandoned, and even when essential, used in most careful moderation."[6] Amateur and professional directives against cradle rocking were part and parcel of a broader perspective on infant sleep that taught that mothers who coddled their babies around bedtime would suffer manifold consequences. Infants needed to be put to bed at stable times, professionals said, without any fanfare—no cooing, cradling, or rocking.[7] Making bedtime a ritual in stoicism would "teach" babies how to sleep. Regimented sleeping was considered an important component in parental discipline, advantageous for both a baby and its mother. A baby accustomed to poor sleeping protocol, characterized by irregularity and excessive maternal attention, could develop unwanted attributes later in childhood, such as clinginess or dependency. Mothers who pampered their babies at bedtime or maintained lackadaisical sleep regimens were also needlessly subjecting themselves to exhaustion.[8] Pandering to a baby around its bedtime would "make a slave of the mother," warned one leading pediatrician.[9]

Along with observing regular sleep schedules and avoiding pampering activities such as cradle rocking, solitude became another staple in properly training an infant to sleep well. Prior to the late 1800s, Americans were generally accepting of close-knit sleeping arrangements, in both their own homes and in public establishments such as hotels. Babies often slept in the presence of adults, and young children frequently slept together; the collective arrangements were practical and seen as conducive to sleeping. Beginning in the late nineteenth century, that consensus shifted. Professionals taught that children should sleep by themselves; company became incompatible with sleeping and was increasingly perceived as unhygienic.[10]

For the same reasons that babies needed to be "trained" to adhere to strict sleeping schedules without excess attention from their mothers or nurses, they needed to learn to sleep alone—promptly. The sooner a baby was sleeping in solitude, the better. "In every way," one mother advised in 1890, "it is best for a child to sleep by himself."[11] Another reflected that "putting children to sleep in the same bed with old or feeble people [was] a course always detrimental to the health of the young."[12] Experts touted added benefits of solitary sleeping for married couples: privacy, improved sexual relations, and fewer disturbances. (In turn, they also thought witnessing sexual activity could exert deleterious effects on a young child through its entire life course.) Isolating sleeping children would benefit a family's health twofold: it would produce better sleep and promote children's healthy moral development. In comparison to the shared family sleeping arrangements more prevalent through most of the nineteenth century, the onset in the late 1800s of the strict "rule" that babies sleep separately amounted to a "revolution in traditional arrangements for children."[13]

This advice became increasingly insistent in light of overlaying. Most American medical professionals agreed that "an infant, of course, should never sleep in the same bed with its mother"; a separate room was best.[14] Although in the twenty-first century separate sleeping has been framed as a choice, at the turn of the twentieth century it was a definite class issue—having a separate sleeping surface (much less a separate room) for a baby was a costly luxury. In his influential book *The Diseases of Infancy and Childhood*, leading pediatrician L. Emmett Holt asserted that babies needed separate beds "in order to prevent the danger of overlying by the mother, which among the lower classes is a frequent cause of death."[15] In a separate work, *Save the Babies*, Holt listed "sleeping in bed with the mother" as one of various stipulations "which are bad for all babies."[16] In the first editions of *Infant Care*, the widely read booklet prepared by the U.S. Children's Bureau, mothers read that their babies should always sleep in beds alone and preferably in rooms alone, especially because "not a few young babies are smothered while lying in bed with an older person."[17] Physician Norman E. Ditman's manual *Home Hygiene and Prevention of Disease*, published in 1912, argued that separate sleeping was an easy intervention for preventing exhausted working mothers who "sleep like logs" from inadvertently killing their babies: "we want to teach parents," he said, "that the life of an infant under one year of age is never safe in bed with a mother."[18] With this danger, professional warnings against shared sleeping shifted in tone, from a stern suggestion against an "ill-advised" situation to a rigid directive against a "downright dangerous" decision.[19]

Physicians in the early 1900s approached sleep positioning in infancy (how a baby's body was positioned while it slept) as "a matter of not the slightest consequence," as Dr. J. P. Crozer Griffith articulated in his guidebook on infant care.[20] Reflecting this sentiment, he specified that a sleeping baby was welcome to "assume any position most comfortable to it."[21] Griffith's commentary stood mostly alone—infant positioning was infrequently mentioned in advice books. The topic did not appear in *Infant Care* until the 1955 edition, which offered some frank remarks on the matter. It stressed that both back and stomach sleeping were perfectly alright, although it advised that babies who spit up frequently (as many babies do) would likely be "better off" sleeping on their stomachs. Interestingly, the booklet noted that mothers sometimes worried about babies who preferred to sleep on their stomachs, "for fear their babies won't get enough air to breathe this way." To such worriers, the text offered relief: "it is perfectly safe for a baby to lie on his stomach on a firm, flat mattress, on which he can move his head from side to side easily." Continuing on, *Infant Care* conveyed that babies who were "said to smother usually die not from lack of air to breathe but from some rapid, overwhelming infection. Many doctors feel it is safer for babies to sleep on their stomach than on the back."[22] Furthermore, babies who slept on their stomachs were perfectly capable of turning their heads to the side for air "when on a firm, flat surface without a pillow." The pamphlet also explained that parents could "do one another a service by spreading knowledge about this, and by urging, in their communities, that careful diagnosis be made of such sudden deaths." The 1962 edition of *Infant Care* noted that spreading the word about the safety of stomach sleeping and the fallacy of accidental mechanical suffocation reports in newspapers "would help to prevent the feelings of guilt that now crush those parents who would not otherwise understand that the loss of their baby was due to no fault of their own."[23] All of these sentiments directly reflect the ongoing medical discourse at the time that castigated the accidental mechanical suffocation (AMS) framework and favored a respiratory infection explanation.

Stomach sleeping was never specifically promoted over back sleeping for scientific reasons. Instead, it was gradually and slightly acknowledged as "probably the better position in which to place the baby."[24] As one pediatrician reflected in the 1990s, "I am not sure why we have placed infants on their stomachs. It just sort of evolved."[25] In the first half of the twentieth century, American pediatric literature developed a subdued proclivity for stomach sleeping, based mostly on parents' preferences and pragmatic thinking. Babies seemed to sleep more soundly on their stomachs, and parents feared that a baby sleeping on its back might choke to death if it spat up. Their partiality for stomach sleeping appeared both entirely sensible and harmless. No scientific studies evaluated the pros and cons of different positions; as the American Academy of Pediatrics (AAP) Task Force on Infant Positioning and SIDS noted in 1992, medical professionals in the United States "have tended to offer advice [on babies' sleep positioning] that seems most logical and to be guided by general custom."[26] In 1950, Katherine Bain, with the Children's Bureau, epitomized this trend when she clarified that a baby who slept on his stomach was "in no more danger of smothering than if he were sleeping on his back."[27] Given the relative medical indifference and the parental partiality for prone sleeping in the twentieth century in the United States, it was "common practice" for parents to lay their babies to bed on their stomachs.[28]

Midcentury parenting advice also maintained that separate sleeping was best for mother and baby. Professionals may have been slightly more understanding of a mother's desire to place her infant's crib near her own bed, but they still were wary that doing so would precipitate undue maternal anxiety. With her baby so close, a mother was prone to "lie awake listening to his breathing, and worrying about his every sniffle or hiccup." Given that "at first, a baby's breathing is somewhat irregular," new parents were likely to be alarmed by all kinds of harmless noises. The best way to minimize those needless fears was simply "not to have the baby's bed too near at hand."[29] In a 1963 edition of *Infant Care*, the Children's Bureau further observed that "babies are noisy roommates" and pointed to separate rooms as a simple measure that could help mothers sleep better and help married couples maintain privacy.[30]

The clear penchant in the postwar era that babies sleep alone in separate rooms maintained the early twentieth-century concerns about overlaying under the "new" guise of AMS even while often dismissing AMS as an illogical maternal fear. In midcentury editions of *Infant Care*, a separate subheading in the chapter on "things you may have misgivings about" was reserved for smothering. "Many parents worry needlessly for fear their baby will smother," writers said, "either from sleeping on his face or getting his head covered with bedclothes." The authors blamed excessive concerns over smothering on misguided newspaper coverage of AMS. The texts clarified that infection, the signs of which could be "so slight" as to go unnoticed even at autopsy, was the typical culprit—not suffocation.[31] But in a concession akin to one later SIDS researchers had to make, *Infant Care* acknowledged the risk of accidental suffocation by parents. It specifically advised readers not to give in to the temptation to share a bed with a baby, saying, "There is some danger that an infant can be smothered in the bedclothing or pillows or hurt by an adult rolling over." Lest there be any confusion, *Infant Care* put the advice candidly: "let the baby sleep alone."[32] By the postwar era, psychologist Willard Caldwell reflected, the "myth" that it was dangerous for parents and babies to sleep together was "well established."[33]

LAID TO REST: REVISITING INFANTS' SLEEP

Given the syndrome's almost universal occurrence during sleep, SIDS researchers were obviously concerned with sleeping. After 1972, the apnea theory compelled all kinds of research into sleeping, but for the most part it was specialized. One prevalent arena of investigation, for example, was sleep cycles. Modern sleep research in the 1960s differentiated between active sleep—characterized by irregular breathing and heart rate, tiny muscle and body movements, and bursts of movement in the eyes—and quiet sleep—a more consistent, controlled, still bodily state with regular breathing and heart rates. Science labeled active sleep "rapid eye movement sleep," or REM sleep, and quiet sleep simply "non-REM sleep."[34] For most adults, one complete cycle through restive and active sleep took about ninety minutes. Infants completed one cycle in just fifty minutes. At term, babies spent about equal time in active and restive sleep, but as they grew spent more time in quiet sleep. By the time they were eight months, babies spent twice as much time in quiet as active sleep.[35] When scientists started to document significantly more episodes of apnea during active sleep, learning more about babies' sleep cycle development became a pressing mission.[36] With apnea as the leading contending cause of SIDS, and the note that apnea occurred much more frequently during REM sleep, every extra minute a baby spent in REM sleep could matter. Increasingly, it looked as though babies who had some abnormality or developmental delay in their sleep-state organization might be at risk.[37] More studies inquired into REM cycles, sleep stages, neurological patterns, and the subtle fluctuations in vital signs during sleep.

Such research exemplifies how SIDS sleep research in the U.S. was specialized and highly sophisticated in nature. Few SIDS researchers devoted concerted attention to the specific conditions and location where babies slept as potential causes. Topics such as body placement or bedding appeared strikingly elementary in comparison to detailed medical investigations into particular aspects of sleep. Doctors continued to agree that parents could lay their babies to sleep however they preferred. Separate sleeping was perceived as so customary that it hardly warranted comment. Basic facets of sleep thus bring out the continued problems and paradoxes of SIDS. The context of SIDS—and specifically its purpose of negating the impression of suffocation—obscured pertinent details and clouded medical reasoning. The two issues of sleep position and sleep location failed to garner critical attention during the peak years of SIDS research. Some Americans, however, paid cursory but persistent attention to how an infant's body was placed to sleep, and their low-level interest indicates some underlying suspicion, or at least confusion, regarding the issue.

Harold Abramson was a rare physician who saw bedding, position, and location as all important. In 1944, when he analyzed 139 cases of AMS, Abramson offered nearly identical prescriptions for safe sleeping as those decreed by the AAP more than fifty years later. He contended that babies should never sleep with pillows and that crib mattresses should be flat. He urged that "unnecessary articles" (such as pillows, blankets, or toys) be removed. "No practice should be more emphatically condemned," Abramson added, than laying a baby together with its mother in her bed after feeding, because "overlaying may be caused by the mother who falls asleep." Lastly, Abramson was struck that 68 percent of the babies in his study had been discovered on their stomachs, lying facedown in the prone position. In comparison, just 17 percent of bodies were found lying on their backs.[38]

Given his findings, Abramson questioned the safety of placing babies facedown for sleep. In retrospect, Abramson's word of caution about prone sleeping, which failed to compel the most attentive medical researchers for another half-century, stands out: "attention should again be called to the preponderance of infants under 5 months of age who were found in the 'face-down' posture on death from smothering." He even contended that the prone posture could be causative in AMS, as opposed to merely correlative. Infants still gaining head and neck mobility might struggle, Abramson postulated, to adjust their positioning or find open airways among heavy bedding materials. "It seems reasonable," he concluded, "to recommend that the routine nursing practice of placing infants in the prone position be avoided except during such times as the babies are constantly attended. The practice should, furthermore, be entirely done away with at night."[39]

For the most part, Abramson's contemporaries set his ideas aside. Because they were invested in repudiating AMS, interested professionals were trying to upset Abramson's overarching suggestion that suffocation was the primary mechanism acting in sudden infant death. Pathologists Irene Garrow and Jacob Werne, for example, wryly noted that if Abramson was correct about AMS being an appropriate way to describe most sudden infant deaths, then certainly mothers should follow his advice. But they thought Abramson's interpretation was fallacious and that sudden infant mortality had nothing to do with mechanical suffocation. From their perspective, AMS was not an appropriate description and Abramson's advice was absurd. Contending instead that an infection was at play, Werne and Garrow suggested that if anything, stomach sleeping might *reduce* a baby's chances of sudden death by minimizing its chances of contracting pneumonia (by promoting "postural drainage of infected secretions").[40] Keith Bowden, a physician in Australia, agreed with Werne and Garrow and concluded, "There should be no departure from . . . the usual ritual observed in putting a baby to bed."[41]

Although the next wave of investigators—who participated in categorizing SIDS—documented a correlation between prone sleeping and sudden infant death, it took decades before researchers determined that the association mattered. Epidemiological studies inquired about sleep positioning but did not deem it a legitimate area of causation. Lester Adelson and Eleanor Kinney's project in Cleveland in the 1950s documented infants' sleeping positions; notably more babies in their study died on their stomachs.[42] Theodore Curphey's study in Los Angeles County also recorded observations about sleeping position, and his team's qualitative case report descriptions noted babies' typical sleeping positions. In one series of 189 cases, 108 babies (57 percent) were found on their stomachs. Contemporary visiting nurses' data sheets inquired about a child's position in the bed, clothing, and typical sleeping arrangements (whether it normally slept with anyone).[43] In the U.K., likewise, medical evidence of the correlation between stomach sleeping and sudden infant death began to emerge as early as the 1960s. The relationship cropped up at both international conferences on sudden infant death in the 1960s, and by the 1970s, available evidence indicated that the association was statistically significant.[44]

Why did researchers brush aside these data? At the time, the finding that most babies died on their stomachs carried little weight precisely because most American children slept on their stomachs; researchers thought the statistic offered "no sound basis for any type of rational solutions to the problem." "Certainly, most children who are found dead under these circumstances are observed to be lying on their abdomens," Lester Adelson allowed in 1963, but he was unconcerned—in light of prevailing customs, the correlation hardly seemed significant.[45] Researchers at the University of Washington discounted similar findings. Their study in the mid-1960s revealed that most babies were found on their abdomens; some were on their sides, and only 4 percent were on their backs. Yet because this distribution appeared to align with general sleeping practices, the authors clarified that "no conclusions can be drawn about the effects of sleeping position."[46] Afterwards, they conducted a side project to "find out how normal babies sleep." Investigators surveyed 214 parents and over 90 percent reported that their children slept on their stomachs.[47] The assessment that most "normal" babies slept on their stomachs muted the possibility that prone positioning was relevant to SIDS. The finding that most SIDS babies were discovered on their stomachs, rather than appearing noteworthy, was seen as a foil, a confounding factor.

Yet it is intriguing that even while Americans portrayed that they were convinced that sleep positioning was not germane to SIDS, they were unwilling to jettison the idea altogether. Americans discussed the possible relationship between stomach sleeping and SIDS recurrently, in manifold venues, for most of the twentieth century. In hindsight, the extent to which the association was well-documented, debated, and then dismissed is striking. Physicians, SIDS centers, and the NSIDSF asked parents about sleep positioning in studies and home visits; many parents, in turn, were openly suspect. These decisions and questions betray suspicions adamantly denied in words.[48]

Parents voiced concerns about whether stomach sleeping had a hand in SIDS from the 1940s through the 1980s. In 1948, one father, convinced his son had died as a result of sleeping on his stomach with his face down, as advised by the child's pediatrician, went as far as to commission a private research firm to collect information on children in the Los Angeles area who had died from suffocation. The firm's report apparently indicated that almost all of the infants were indeed lying facedown.[49] The same year, an anonymous parent editorialized in the *Woman's Home Companion* that her child had died because its doctor had instructed that the child be placed on its stomach for sleeping.[50] From the 1960s until the 1980s, public health nurses who visited SIDS families were schooled in how to respond to one of parents' most frequent questions: "Are all infants found on their tummies?"[51]

Observers were similarly skeptical. At the Congressional hearings before the House Subcommittee on Public Health and Environment in August of 1973, Tim Lee Carter, representative from Kentucky, asked Gerald LaVeck, director of the NICHD, about the typical position in which SIDS babies were found. LaVeck directed Carter to the study from King County, recalling its findings that around 90 percent of infants were discovered on their stomachs. LaVeck noted, just as others had before him, that most babies were put to sleep on their abdomens. Carter repeated the statistic, musing that it was "rather unusual." He seemed taken aback but abruptly commenced a separate line of questioning about whether SIDS babies could be predicted in any way. A few minutes later, he asked the audience for a show of hands "who suffered this disaster, have had youngsters . . . die from SIDS," and returned to the positioning issue. Carter proceeded to ask each parent in attendance to identify herself and share the position in which she had found her baby's body. One by one, they answered. Mrs. Hawkins—on his stomach. Mrs. Goldberg—on his stomach. Mrs. Giffin—on her stomach. Mrs. Harold—stomach. Once Carter had heard from all the parents present, he simply stopped, passing the baton back to the chairman running the show, and a new representative stepped in with a fresh battery of inquiries.[52] Reading the record, one can almost see Carter scratching his head.

The next year, in 1974, pediatrician Beverley Bayes matched Carter's hesitations in a letter she wrote to the *New England Journal of Medicine*. Bayes linked stomach sleeping to the increasingly prominent premise that SIDS resulted from apnea and hypoxia. "Could it be that our culturally determined habit of placing infants in the prone position to 'prevent aspiration,'" she asked, "actually causes decreased pulmonary ventilation in sleep?" Bayes was especially concerned about satiated infants with full stomachs, who might experience added pressure against their diaphragms and struggle to breathe effectively. She suggested that a respiratory expert put together a project to study whether "the mechanical compression of the prone position maintained for several hours can, in fact, alter ventilation and lead to hypoxia." Even though Bayes knew prone sleeping alone was unlikely the only causative agent, she thought it could be a trigger that might fatally impact babies with any number of other potential risk factors.[53]

Despite available data, the medical establishment was slow in assessing sleep position as a contributing factor in SIDS. Medical researchers did not seriously consider the proposition that prone sleeping might be implicated in SIDS until the mid-late 1980s. Of course, it would be unfair to expect historical actors to notice or interpret data in modern ways. But given that professionals so persistently asserted that sleep position was not a causative factor in sudden infant mortality, why did they bother to continue to inquire about it at all? And what took them so long to take notice? Their actions did not line up with their words.[54]

Before the late 1980s, sleep positioning as a cause for SIDS was incongruent with researchers' convictions. By the later 1980s, however, the risk factor framework had been firmly established; with the apnea theory falling out of favor, the risk factor framework was more accepting of the proposition that sleep positioning could be a component. Furthermore, the inclusion of international data on SIDS epidemiology forced American medicine to contend with the issue of sleep positioning.

Certainly, the history of SIDS research is punctuated by (mostly western) international scholarship, predominantly by virtue of academic conferences, but in the latter half of the 1980s transnational informational exchanges escalated. Compared to the global collaborations and discourse that blossomed in the late 1980s, SIDS medicine had been isolationist. Before the mid-1970s, most experts asserted that SIDS rates were stable across international borders. But stark disparities within the U.S. compelled more scrupulous reviews. It turned out that SIDS rates were as inconsistent globally as within America. In the U.S., average incidence rates ranged between two and three cases per thousand live births. In Israel, rates were as low as 0.31 per thousand. Finland and Sweden also had low rates, of approximately 0.4 and 0.5 per thousand, respectively. SIDS incidence in Japan was 1.2 per thousand. Tasmania and certain parts of New Zealand, on the other hand, had exceptionally high rates, ranging from 4.4 to 8 deaths per thousand live births.[55]

In 1985, a British pediatrician practicing in Hong Kong planted a seed in *The Lancet*. In the first four years of the 1980s, David P. Davies reported, Chinese pathologists documented only fifteen cases of SIDS (a rate of 0.036 per thousand live births). At first, Davies doubted that such an exceedingly low incidence was "real." Instead, he thought SIDS was probably underreported in China or was "masquerading as other causes of death." But after he learned about the rigorous postmortem standards employed by the Chinese and spoke with several leading pathologists, Davies became convinced that China's low SIDS rates were not an error of diagnosis. Any baby found deceased in a home was taken to one of just two sites, and if the cause of death was unknown the government mandated an autopsy. Davies conducted a survey of eleven of the nation's most highly trained pathologists, and they all said the same thing: sudden unexplained infant deaths were exceedingly rare. In fact, Davies learned that of the fifteen SIDS babies from 1980 to 1984, only twelve were Chinese.

Davies's curiosity was piqued. Chinese parents had virtually no experience with SIDS. And this was despite the fact that a number of conditions—such as very crowded housing, extremely low breastfeeding rates, and "abound[ing]" rates of respiratory illness—would have predicted high SIDS incidence according to western research. Admitting that his speculations were entirely observational, Davies posited that cultural factors were at work. "I wonder," he ruminated, "whether the possible influences of life-style and caretaking practices on [SIDS] are being underestimated in preference for more exotic and esoteric explanations." Sleeping position stood out to Davies—most Chinese parents put their infants to sleep on their backs. Davies thought babies laying on their stomachs might reasonably "be expected to obstruct their airways more easily" than babies laying on their backs, either because their nostrils were squished or because if they spit up, their breathing passages might become blocked by vomit.[56]

Over time, Davies became more convinced of his supposition. He spearheaded a prospective study of SIDS in China and reported his team's preliminary findings in 1988. In the project's first full year, twenty-one SIDS episodes occurred (an incidence rate of 0.29 per thousand live births). Davies and his colleagues compared the cases against controls and examined a number of potential factors; "the one," they said, "that showed a significant difference was the usual posture in which the baby was placed to sleep."[57] This looked compelling.

A host of investigators in other countries retreated to epidemiological surveys to see if Davies' idea carried any weight. In the summer of 1988, *The Lancet* released two more reports. Researchers in the U.K. studied 265 SIDS babies and found that 42 percent slept prone; in the control group of comparable size, only 25 percent of babies slept prone.[58] Physician Susan Beal reviewed nine separate studies from around the globe—all of them revealed a preponderance of SIDS cases among babies who slept on their stomachs. In South Australia and in France, in the Netherlands, the U.K., Hong Kong, and Ireland, more SIDS babies had slept prone.[59]

The Netherlands offered a particularly influential quasi-natural experiment. Prior to the 1970s, the nation boasted one of the lowest SIDS rates in the western world. At the time, only about 1 percent of babies generally slept on their stomachs. Then, in 1971, at the International Pediatric Congress held in Vienna, two researchers suggested that prone sleeping had physiological advantages. Among some of the presumed benefits of stomach sleeping, they intimated that it might prevent gastroesophageal reflux, reduce babies' energy expenditure, confer orthopedic advantages (such as precluding infantile scoliosis or misshapen skulls), and reduce colic. In response, the Dutch medical field and media began promoting stomach sleeping for babies. The reversal resulted in a deathly turnaround: when the nation adjusted its sleep positioning practices, SIDS rates more than doubled (from less than 0.5 per thousand live births to 1.31 per thousand). The marked increase, scientists determined, "cannot be explained by certification errors alone."[60] In 1987, after the international medical community started to grow concerned about prone sleeping, the national Dutch medical organization reversed its advice and recommended non-prone sleeping postures for babies. The next year, SIDS mortality dropped by nearly 40 percent.[61]

Initially, not everyone was convinced. To be sure, the data from different countries was consistent. In a 1991 review study of nineteen case-controlled research projects exploring the relationship between prone sleeping and SIDS (none of which were conducted in the U.S.), authors Susan Beal and C. F. Finch reported that "every study . . . found a higher percentage of SIDS infants sleeping prone."[62] No researchers argued that prone sleeping caused SIDS on its own—they pointed to prone sleeping as a possible, and preventable, trigger in the SIDS complex.[63]

But more than a few researchers were concerned about jumping to conclusions. They worried about the reliability of data obtained retrospectively from distressed parents.[64] And they were uncertain about confounding factors, including low birth weight and maternal education.[65] Plus, no projects had measured the correlation in the United States; "cultural differences in infant-care practices," explained Dr. Susan Orenstein, "make it hazardous to transfer conclusions from other populations to an unexamined population, even if the studies upon which the conclusions are based were impeccable."[66] Others feared back sleeping might be subtly detrimental to babies' development in unknown ways, and they wanted a full explanation before recommending changes. Researchers speculated that prone sleeping factored into SIDS by blocking airways, predisposing babies to rebreathing excess exhaled air, or becoming overheated, but no one knew for sure. If prone sleeping mattered, doctors wanted to know why.

Intriguingly, the positioning intervention sparked a professional divide that echoed similar elements as the debate regarding the apnea monitoring intervention. In one camp were doctors who thought the associative evidence between stomach sleeping and SIDS was substantive enough to warrant public health interventions promoting supine sleeping. These physicians thought withholding information that might help prevent SIDS would be highly unethical. On the opposite side of the fence were practitioners who thought it was too soon to act based on available evidence. Doubters expressed concerns about the effects of publicizing the message that prone sleeping was implicated in SIDS (and that supine sleeping was protective against it). First, they thought it might have unanticipated physical consequences. Second, they thought it could unnecessarily instigate feelings of guilt in SIDS parents or in parents who struggled to implement or maintain supine sleeping for any reason. "Are we justified," asked Carl Hunt and Daniel Shannon, "in creating a new responsibility for parents to supervise maintenance of the 'right' sleeping position, especially when the potential hazards of prone sleeping are as yet undefined in the US?"[67] Hunt and Shannon advocated delay before recommending changes to the public at large.

They wanted more research, and just as Abraham Bergman had done in critiquing apnea monitors, they expressed that "medical history is unfortunately replete with examples of precipitous action based on preliminary data and resulting in harm."[68]

Most of the skeptics soon became converts. Studies showing a correlation between SIDS and prone sleeping were one thing, but studies indicating that SIDS declined as prone sleeping declined tipped the scale. Around 1990, several nations started to advise parents against prone sleeping, and the effects were startling. By 1991, four nations had watched their SIDS rates drop notably after medical professionals advised against prone sleeping. In Avon County, England, for example, prone sleeping rates decreased from 56 to 28 percent, and SIDS incidence promptly fell from 3.7 to 2 per thousand live births. This kind of evidence, suggestive of causality, eventually convinced even the most dubious critics.[69] Campaigns promoting supine sleeping in New Zealand, Norway, Britain, and Denmark all precipitated marked declines in SIDS.[70] In addition, the first prospective study (which surveyed parents about how their babies slept before SIDS, rather than after) corroborated the results of retrospective analyses. Researchers in Tasmania interviewed the parents of more than three thousand perceived high-risk babies about a multitude of factors, including those most suspected of confounding the prone sleeping correlation: infant birth weight, maternal age, and maternal smoking habits. After adjusting to control for all such variables, the prone sleeping association still stood firm.[71] Plus, no evidence that supine sleeping was hazardous ever came to light.

In the middle of 1992, American medical periodicals jumped on the bandwagon. In May, *JAMA* featured a review article on prone sleeping and SIDS. Its two authors, one of whom (Warren Guntheroth) had initially "discounted" the suggestion that prone sleeping might have something to do with SIDS, announced that "without exception, all studies demonstrated an increased risk for SIDS associated with the prone sleeping position." Furthermore, they explained, "publicity against the use of the prone position has been associated with reduction of SIDS by 20% to 67%, paralleling the reduction in the use of the prone position, with no increase in deaths from aspiration or in other diagnostic categories."[72] The single most influential factor known to reduce SIDS had been lying in front of families and physicians all along.

CRIB SAFETY

When investigators started to key into the association with prone sleeping, some clinical journals began reporting on the potentially fatal dangers of unsafe infant sleep environments. Pediatric literature had advised mothers how to arrange their babies' cribs, bassinettes, or cradles since the turn of the century. Initially, as long as a baby slept in a well-ventilated room with clean bedding, pediatricians voiced few preferences. Over time, they started to favor cribs over cradles or bassinettes because they were rooted in place, which ideally would help parents enact separate sleeping.[73] Professionals' directions for crib preparations also started to look increasingly spartan as decades passed. In the early 1900s pillows had been acceptable, if occasionally discouraged. By the mid-1900s, pillows were no longer advisable—"no pillow of any kind should be put under the baby's head"—and could no longer be employed as infants' mattresses because they were too soft. Blankets should not impede a baby's neck or head in any way.[74]

In the 1970s, crib considerations met an American public alert to consumer rights and consumer protection. In the late 1960s President Lyndon Johnson had appointed seven members to a National Commission on Product Safety charged with assessing the nation's consumer safety legislation. The Commission's conclusions were disappointing; one of its findings was that more than two hundred crib strangulations were reported nationwide each year. No legislation regulated the design of cribs or other "infant furniture."[75] Media pieces began taking note of reported crib accidents; in 1972, the Consumer Product Safety Commission was created, and shortly thereafter it issued regulations for standard crib measurements.[76] These themes did not escape pediatricians' notice.

One of the first medical accounts that specifically addressed crib safety, relatively isolated at the time, was published in 1977; its authors estimated that more than six hundred American babies died every year as a direct result of unsafe sleep conditions. The researchers extrapolated this estimate from their count of sixteen such deaths in Wayne County, Michigan, and described the mortalities as "accidental asphyxial deaths." This echoed Harold Abramson's portrayal of accidental mechanical suffocation in the 1940s. They explained that most cases were associated with "loose, pliable, plastic coverings of bed articles," and that they were entirely preventable. The best advice they could offer parents was to use a firm mattress that fit snuggly into their baby's crib, ensure the crib had no gaps or corners in which the baby could get stuck, and make sure the crib was completely empty of and distanced from any kind of rope-like materials. Importantly, since the subjects had died from an identifiable, presumably preventable cause, the authors specified that the deaths were "exclusive of" SIDS. They further asserted that mislabeling similar cases as SIDS would result in the diagnosis "losing its significance for all parties concerned."[77] In differentiating SIDS from suffocation and accident cases, the article broached a philosophical issue surrounding the SIDS diagnosis—when a possible cause of death is located, the case is no longer considered SIDS.

Almost a decade later, coinciding with the spike in international surveillance of sleep positioning, interest in these kinds of details deepened. Authors started to draw attention to characteristic unsafe conditions for babies: water beds, cushy pillows, polystyrene pillows, and too many blankets.[78] A number of studies found that prone sleeping combined with certain environmental factors, such as overheating (from excessive blankets or bundling), was particularly dangerous.[79] These evaluations, both indirectly and directly, called the SIDS diagnosis into question. If sudden infant mortality was composed of cases of "suffocation" or "rebreathing" caused by babies' bedding, what did that mean about SIDS?[80] A physician at the University of California even suggested "that SIDS is a death from suffocation," caused mostly by breathing blockages in stomach-sleeping babies. He granted that SIDS was a "very convenient" label that helped comfort grieving families but proposed that the term "positional suffocation" might be more useful in describing the sudden deaths of babies discovered facedown.[81]

Research into safe sleep branched out to explore the nature of infants' sleeping surfaces—including the presence of any bedfellows—more broadly. In 1978 one investigator in Washington, DC, reviewed 92 SIDS deaths from earlier in the decade. He found that 44 of the cases were "instances of bed-sharing," and also remarked that "a disproportionate percentage of bed-sharing cases occurred on weekends."[82] In the 1980s, more reports wondered why SIDS was more likely to occur on weekends than weekdays, just as many had with regards to overlaying one hundred years earlier. One, in Auckland, New Zealand, submitted that higher weekend rates might "represent deficiencies in maternal access or utilisation of primary care," or might "be related to lower standards of maternal care and supervision at the weekend than during the week."[83] Like so many other pieces of information, the significance of a possible weekend correlation escaped medicine. As was the case with research into infant sleep positioning, international perspective refined the scholarship on customary sleeping arrangements. But whereas looking at studies on infant body position from multiple nations and cultures ultimately produced a stable, evidence-based recommendation for how parents should lay babies to sleep, the outcomes related to bed-sharing and co-sleeping were far more controversial.

SHARED SLEEP

The international data collected from sleep positioning studies looked confusing in regards to co-sleeping. In the United States and most western cultures, the separation mandate (that children sleep alone on separate sleeping surfaces in separate rooms from their parents) was so culturally engrained in the twentieth century as to be almost taken for granted. Around 1900, advice literature had started to caution parents against sleeping with their children. But in the same way that medicine never critically examined the health advantages or disadvantages of side, back, or stomach sleeping, for most of the twentieth century it conducted virtually no formal research on shared sleeping. In the late 1980s, though, professionals began to key into the topic after social scientists started trumpeting the virtues of "co-sleeping" and more Americans seemed to be partaking. Medicine then became invested in silencing the "alternative" medical advice that shared sleeping had health benefits. But the data dividing organized medicine's solitary sleeping advice from social scientists' submission that shared sleeping be taken seriously was, in reality, cloudy.

In 1976, anthropology student Tine Thevenin published the first edition of *The Family Bed*, a book intent to break the "taboo" on co-family sleeping. Thevenin appeared on *Oprah* as well as the *Phil Donahue Show* three times, always paired against opposing physicians. By the time of her death in 2010, Thevenin's book had gone through a second printing and sold some 150,000 copies.[84] Thevenin, a mother herself, was frustrated about societal pressure to practice solitary sleeping (she described meeting parents who "confessed" to letting their children sleep in bed with them). Thevenin pointed to family sleeping as a welcome alternative to the detached modern custom of separate sleeping. She described family sleeping as making a "comeback," and compared it to breastfeeding and natural childbirth, two practices that also witnessed renewed interest and numbers around the same time.[85] In 1984, one of the first studies on co-sleeping habits in the U.S. indicated that the practice might be more common among Americans than was generally acknowledged, just as Thevenin suggested. In a sample of 150 families in the Cleveland area, 35 percent of white families and 70 percent of black families reported that co-sleeping was a "routine and recent practice" in their homes.[86]

Thevenin shared the testimony of families committed to shared sleeping. Her approach was not limited to infancy but rather fit into a more general child-centric parenting strategy rooted in family togetherness. Thevenin decried separate sleep as an artificial by-product of modernity; "the breakdown in family sleeping parallels the alienation, depersonalization and dehumanization that have followed the development of industrialization," she said. Co-family sleeping was a more natural behavior that provided children and parents with physical and emotional closeness. In almost all nonwestern, traditional cultures, she described, babies customarily slept with their mothers until their first birthday, and many slept between both parents. Thevenin described that such arrangements had many varied benefits, ranging from improved and prolonged breastfeeding to better sleep and enhanced psychological development and security. Thevenin acknowledged the reputed connections between SIDS and co-sleeping, but she was critical. She suggested that simply placing a baby's cradle next to the parental bed until the child was a little older would grant families concerned about "overlaying" similar benefits of co-sleeping without the risks.[87]

Other scholars studied sleeping patterns from the vantage of evolutionary medicine, a field that uses the theory of evolution to understand and interpret health and disease in humans.[88] Proponents, many of whom are anthropologists, point to infant development, and in particular to infant sleep behaviors and SIDS, as one of their field's "striking success stor[ies]."[89] Evolutionary medical anthropologists argued that in the past, human infants slept with their parents and did not practice the kind of consolidated, nighttime sleep common in most American homes. They held that shared sleeping arrangements offered evolutionary advantages modern science may have overlooked, and that most babies in the past did not sleep by themselves or for extended, regularized periods of time. As they explained, human babies are programmed to provoke and maximize maternal responsiveness. The complex, often unconscious ways in which mothers and infants who sleep together interact—including frequently arousing one another—may have been beneficial in terms of natural selection.[90] The evolutionary approach to pediatric sleep understood solitary sleeping as a modern, western practice actuated by changes such as single-family homes with multiple bedrooms, bottle-feeding, and middle-class consumerism.[91] Separate sleeping, evolutionary scientists argued, prioritized western cultural values of independence over the "fundamentally normal and evolutionarily adaptive behaviors" of the past. "To tell non-western mothers that infants should be placed alone, in an enclosed pen, in a darkened room, and allowed to cry themselves to sleep would not only be met with astonishment," they noted, "but would be characterized as child abuse in much of the world."[92] When this outlook on infant sleeping collided with the international work on SIDS and infant sleep positioning, the topic of co-sleeping exploded in medical and lay publications.

The cross-cultural data on co-sleeping and sudden infant death is aggravatingly complicated. A few cultures that practiced co-sleeping, such as the Maori in southern New Zealand, had astronomically high SIDS rates. But many cultures (most notably in Asia) in which co-sleeping was normative experienced lower rates. In three cities in Japan, for example, SIDS rates measured only 0.15 per thousand births (Tokyo), 0.053 per thousand births (Fukuoka), and 0.22 per thousand births (Saga).[93] Often, however, co-sleeping-normative societies had no modern mechanisms in place for diagnosing SIDS and measuring rates. Most cultures that practiced co-sleeping also had very different sleep settings compared to those in traditional western societies, including the United States. For example, many families slept on flat, hard surfaces rather than cushy mattresses, slept without pillows or blankets, or were more inclined to favor supine sleeping. Even leading researchers in favor of co-sleeping permitted that low SIDS rates in shared-sleeping societies were not necessarily indicative of anything and were extremely difficult to maneuver.

These discrepancies illustrate that although evolutionary medicine acknowledges the profound influence of culture, the exact role of culture in evolutionary health is not entirely clear.[94] Furthermore, historical practices are neither intrinsically "natural" nor superior; as Roger Byard quipped in 1994, "it could be argued that sleeping several feet above a floor on a soft mattress covered by layers of synthetic material does not necessarily replicate traditional tribal or animal behaviour."[95] Evolutionary medicine is much more sophisticated than academic nostalgia for times past, but it is not implicitly accurate; the approach has its foibles. Marlene Zuk, a professor who studies behavioral ecology and evolutionary biology at the University of Minnesota, writes compellingly about evolutionary medicine's strengths and weaknesses. She highlights that understanding human health and behavior from an evolutionary outlook demands examining the environment and context in which evolution occurred.[96]

As Zuk explains, the field of evolutionary pediatrics contends that modern infants suffer from a mismatch between their evolutionarily determined biological needs and modern society.[97] Anthropologist James McKenna's research is emblematic of this concept. In the 1980s, McKenna researched infant sleep from an evolutionary standpoint with gusto. His work reached an audience beyond academia, and his committed stance on the benefits of co-sleeping has made him a controversial and fascinating figure in the history of SIDS. McKenna was highly critical of SIDS research, deriding the field as western-centric, biased, and single-minded. SIDS researchers, McKenna contended, made faulty assumptions about infant development that constricted their research and clouded their findings. He was particularly emphatic that infants' bodies and development be studied in coordination with, rather than isolated from, their social and physical surroundings. Discounting infants' tandem physiological and societal evolutions, McKenna urged, was shortsighted; babies' physical and social worlds were "inseparable."[98]

McKenna was bothered by formal medicine's overall approach to SIDS. He found it problematic that scientists conducting SIDS research relied on solitary sleeping arrangements as their baseline control. "The clinical picture of the normative development of infant sleep behavior," said McKenna, "is derived from studies of infants sleeping alone in sleep laboratories. These data," he explained, "in addition to the experiences of middle-class American parents who do not sleep with their infants, have given rise to a conceptualization of infant sleep that may be at odds with what infants have actually experienced throughout prehistoric and most of historic time."[99] Research on SIDS was biased, he said, towards solitary, nocturnal, consolidated sleep, and it negated the much more highly varied evolutionary patterns of sleeping. For McKenna, these blinders resulted in major distortions and a "serious gap in existing knowledge."[100]

McKenna did not see himself as offering a new hypothesis for SIDS—he said he was synthesizing interdisciplinary work and "rethinking . . . the SIDS puzzle"—but as an enthusiastic proponent of co-sleeping, his work carried a divergent message.[101] McKenna proposed that human babies' uniquely slow postnatal development made them vulnerable to SIDS. He proposed that parent-infant co-sleeping might have positive—rather than negative—outcomes in both the short and long term. Animal studies on parent-infant separation already suggested as much. Results showed that separating nonhuman infant primates from their parents, even for brief periods of time, elicited immediate physiological effects; physical contact helped the infants regulate body temperature and heart rate, while the absence of contact correlated with increased heart rates, apneas, and decreased smiling.[102]

McKenna's own research in humans seriously questioned contemporary pediatric sleep conventions. Evolution, McKenna asserted, suggested that "nocturnal physical contact with a parent [would] provide some physiological benefits."[103] As he described, parents' breathing and proximity helped babies develop effective respiratory patterns.[104] The physical closeness afforded by co-sleeping was crucial, McKenna said, in helping babies establish successful breathing. "There may be no more fundamental form of parent-infant interactional synchrony than the response of parents and infants to each other's breathing cues which, while cosleeping, may move toward a form of complementary breathing," McKenna stated.[105] Babies responded to and learned from their parents' rhythmic breathing patterns; a range of "sensory exchanges," including touching, smelling, and breathing, potentially diminished a baby's chances of experiencing a "respiratory crisis."[106] The exchange of carbon dioxide gases, for example, might aid babies struggling to breathe—some research suggested that infants were able to smell CO_2 and that CO_2-heavy air stimulated "reflexive breathing."[107] By extension, infants sleeping with their mothers tended to arouse more frequently, which could be advantageous.[108]

Furthermore, solitary sleeping environments might "deprive infants of sensory cues" of variable (and unpredictable) significance to each individual infant's healthy growth.[109] In some studies, infants who were more isolated from their mothers had lower I.Q. scores than those who experienced "extensive contact" with their mothers right after birth. Mothers who were constantly close with their infants, McKenna observed, seemed to have higher levels of "affection" for their children and improved caretaking experiences.[110]

It did not take long for McKenna to bridge his own work with the contemporary SIDS research investigating apnea and infant sleep. McKenna did not recommend that all American infants sleep in their parents' beds, he did not argue that separate sleeping caused SIDS, and he did not claim that co-sleeping would eliminate SIDS.[111] Nor was he fundamentally anti-technology, even expressing excitement when one study indicated that placing mechanically breathing teddy bears in cribs could elicit the same stabilizing effects on a baby's breathing as its parents.[112] McKenna acknowledged that overlaying was a possibility when considering co-sleeping. But so too, he pointed out, were deadly accidents in cribs—both catastrophes were equally improbable risks.[113] Still, the message that co-sleeping could be protective for human babies was confrontational to formal medicine, and responses to McKenna's work generally fell into two categories—ignorance or opposition.

Over time, McKenna further refined his argument to account for the fact that infants sleep in a wide variety of environments. He distinguished between two kinds of co-sleeping: bed-sharing, in which parents and babies sleep in the same bed, and room-sharing, in which parents and babies sleep in the same room. (McKenna thus articulated that bed-sharing was only one type of co-sleeping.) Although he did not recommend bed-sharing across the board, McKenna was clearly discouraged with the "universal recommendations" against it and the ways in which it was demonized. "Mothers' bodies," he bemoaned, "whether offering breast milk or not and independent of sobriety, continue to be regarded as potentially lethal weapons—wooden rolling pins, if you will, over which neither mothers nor their infants have control during sleep."[114] In fact, room-sharing did gain currency as a decidedly advantageous bedtime arrangement. In the early twenty-first century, McKenna argued vehemently in favor of room-sharing, explaining that multiple studies documented a 50 percent reduction in the chances of SIDS when a "committed caregiver, usually the mother, sleeps in the same room but not in the same bed with their infant."[115]

Spanning the sciences, the evidence on bed-sharing was mixed: some suggested it was beneficial, while some indicated it may be a risk factor for infant mortality.[116] "To share one's bed with an infant is to invite tragedy," one Johns Hopkins physician opined in the *New England Journal of Medicine*.[117] Many studies considered bed-sharing in relation to overlaying directly. In 2001, a piece in a major academic journal for forensic pathologists set out to study a case series of infant deaths with unclear causes. One of its chief concerns was sorting out "overlaying." Kim Collins, the pathologist who ran the study, defined overlaying as a type of mechanical asphyxia that occurs when an adult or older child smothers an infant in bed and suffocates it. Her analysis indicated that overlaying and SIDS were difficult to distinguish pathologically, and she concluded that "overlaying is a true entity" that could be prevented by constructing safe sleeping environments.[118] When they reviewed data on overlaying from the late 1800s, one group of scientists reiterated the dangers of bed-sharing but still concluded that given the difficulty of differentiating between SIDS and overlaying, the safety of bed-sharing was "unlikely" to ever be "unequivocally settled."[119] Perhaps they were right. Juxtaposed against literature from the 1800s, this more recent conversation about overlaying suggests that even though a great deal changed in the intervening century, overlaying and SIDS remained intimately connected denominations. Ultimately, in the late 1980s and 1990s, the safe-sleep-environment approach to SIDS reconsidered the nineteenth-century premise of overlaying.

BACK TO SLEEP

In 1992, the AAP formally recommended that healthy babies be placed to sleep on their sides or backs. The Academy acknowledged striations in sleeping customs but asserted that the international evidence was "convincing."[120] The questions of why and how were still unanswered, but supine sleeping reduced the risk of SIDS. A representative speculation about prone sleeping's relation to SIDS explained that it could make babies more susceptible to other variables, such as soft mattresses, mild infections, or overheating: prone sleeping "allow[ed] other risk factors . . . to become active."[121] At a press conference in June 1994, a group of national and private organizations formally announced the launch of a U.S. public health intervention to implement the AAP's 1992 sleeping recommendations. The Back to Sleep campaign relied on the same research that had compelled the Academy to revise its policy two years prior: continued studies conducted in the United States, Australia, Britain, New Zealand, the Netherlands, Norway, and Sweden between 1980 and 1992 all indicated that declines in prone infant sleeping correlated with notable reductions in SIDS rates. NICHD director Duane Alexander explained that Back to Sleep was devised to "reverse" the practice of most American parents to position babies on their stomachs, with the goal of reducing the percentage of prone-sleeping babies from an estimated 75 percent to just 10 percent. The campaign was aimed at both the public and physicians, and planners used radio, television, and print media.[122] The results were startling. From 1992 to 2005, prone sleeping rates in the U.S. declined from 70 percent to 13 percent; the SIDS rate during those years was cut more than in half (from 1.2 deaths per thousand live births to 0.54).[123]

In a curious twist, evolutionary scientists and medical scientists both claimed the advantages of supine sleeping as evidence testifying to the supremacy of their approach. The AAP couched its sleeping recommendations as irreconcilable with any approach dissenting from solitary sleeping. But anthropologists who favor shared sleeping claim that supine sleeping makes perfect sense—"breastfeeding mothers do not need slogans to tell them how to place their babies in bed."[124] This claim may contain truth in a cultural vacuum, but it certainly was not the case in the modern western world; in America, breastfeeding mothers *did* need slogans to advise them how to lay their babies to sleep. Medical anthropologists argued that the pediatricians who for decades advised parents to place infants to sleep on their stomachs were dangerously oblivious to evolutionary wisdom. "The supine sleep position evolved in tandem with both breast feeding and mother-infant co-sleeping," McKenna asserted. "It was only after breast feeding was replaced with bottle-feeding and solitary infant sleep environments replaced maternal-infant social sleep that recommendations to place infants prone for sleep made sense, or was even possible. But it was a tragic mistake that led to the deaths of thousands of Western babies from SIDS."[125] Yet sudden infant deaths were not unknown before the rise of bottle-feeding and solitary sleeping around 1900. The historical record of overlaying cases that stretches back hundreds of years at the very least complicates the evolutionary argument.

Plus, recent investigations reiterate that these issues cannot be considered independent of social circumstances. In 2013, SIDS rates in the U.S. were 83 percent higher among black families and 95 percent higher among American Indian or Alaskan native families.[126] The circumstantial risk factors for SIDS that science identified in the 1980s and beyond—supine sleeping, safe sleep environments, and even breastfeeding in the first decade of the 2000s—were never isolated decisions.[127] Each one circumscribed a behavioral component that reflected families' complex social circumstances. Most often, strategies for minimizing risk were more customary among middle- and upper-class families and less likely to be adopted by lower-class families. Lower-class families may not have realistically been able to "opt" to breastfeed or to afford an infant crib, for example. In 2015, younger, minority, and poor families had higher rates of prone sleeping and bed-sharing, were more likely to use unsafe bedding materials, and had lower rates of breastfeeding.[128] These functional risk factors have never been equally calibrated across class.

The broader evolutionary framework should not be taken for granted. Evolutionary medicine is vulnerable to an abstraction Marlene Zuk describes as a "paleofantasy"—it risks assuming that humans "were at some point perfectly adapted." When? This notion, of course, is not true. Evolution is always underway, and pointing to any given time or practice in the past as ideal would be highly problematic for many reasons.[129] Advocating for behaviors such as co-sleeping merely on the grounds that they are "more natural" would be dangerous. McKenna's studies illustrate a more nuanced approach because he takes cultural forces into account (indeed, part of what distinguishes McKenna's work is that he has contextualized his claims to apply to the modern world), but the extensive variability among human environments and behaviors make widespread evolutionarily based childcare directives "risky."[130] Perhaps these issues have contributed to the inaccurate representation of the co-sleeping divide as antithetical.

But to believe that medical anthropologists like James McKenna and pediatricians who support the AAP's infant sleep policies are fundamentally at odds misses an important opportunity. Evolutionary science and organized medicine might have more in common than they do in conflict. McKenna's underlying premise—that certain manageable environmental factors are relevant in pre-cluding SIDS—was the same underlying premise for the AAP's supposedly oppositional safe sleeping guidelines. The AAP always stood firmly against bed-sharing, but in 2005 it began recommending that babies sleep "separate but proximate" to their parents—in cribs in parents' rooms.[131] That suggestion was a marked change even from the late 1980s, when formal literature advised that babies sleep in a separate room from their parents. The fresh advice fit with McKenna's perspective—both saw room-sharing as the most widely applicable way to advise parents and babies to sleep. Formal pediatric and evolutionary medicine differed in terms of which circumstances they chose to emphasize, and would challenge one another on the permissibility and risks of bed-sharing, but the lines of reasoning buttressing their frameworks are actually remarkably similar. The distorted portrayal of the co-sleeping debate in the lay sphere and in organized medicine as a polarized dichotomy has been a gross oversimplification of the available evidence.

More research suggested that differentiating between room-sharing and bed-sharing was indeed a critical measure. Room-sharing poses no special risk for SIDS. Bed-sharing can pose an increased risk of SIDS—but not in and of itself. Rather, bed-sharing in combination with other risk factors poses an increased risk of SIDS. It is particularly dangerous for mothers who smoke, for example, or for parents under the influence of alcohol. SIDS also occurs disproportionately when bed-sharing takes place on couches or takes place non-routinely (when parents who do not habitually practice bed-sharing sleep with their baby). Evidence suggests that "the associations between bedsharing and SIDS risk vary greatly depending on the circumstances under which bedsharing occurs." As Peter Fleming, a professor of infant health and developmental physiology in the U.K., conveys, "for mothers who wish to breastfeed, do not smoke, do not take recreational drugs or drink alcohol, and are aware of the importance of maintaining a safe sleep environment around their baby at night, there is no good evidence that choosing to share their bed with their baby puts the baby at increased risk of unexpected death."[132]

The public health message in the United States, meanwhile, has maintained that bed-sharing is always dangerous. (Unlike social scientists, for whom "the question of where and with whom babies sleep does not have a right or wrong answer," public health professionals were invested in classifying "appropriate" and "inappropriate" kinds of infant sleep.[133]) One suggestion for reconciling some of the discrepancies about the relationship between SIDS and bed-sharing came from Roger Byard, a forensic pathologist in Australia who has published extensively on SIDS. Byard submitted that SIDS babies who die alone in beds are different, and need to be recorded differently, from babies who die in beds with adults. "Shared sleeping deaths are different [than] SIDS deaths in solitary sleepers . . . [and] are undoubtedly a separate group," he says. "Lumping them all together under the rubric of SIDS does nothing to help us develop an understanding of the different lethal mechanisms that may be involved."[134] Byard's proposal might hold promise—just as developing a more nuanced understanding of different types of co-sleeping did—but it also poses serious threats for parents. A separate category of SIDS reserved for cases of shared sleeping would almost implicitly condemn parents. In many ways, this tease—a partial resolution sullied by undesired effects—is emblematic of SIDS history.

CONCLUSION

The historical record of SIDS research strongly supports the recommendation for supine sleeping. Studies dating back even into the first half of the twentieth century did log an association between stomach sleeping and sudden infant death. Indeed, many projects found that SIDS victims were frequently discovered in a facedown position, but as Richard Naeye reflected, that "never seemed a likely explanation for very many SIDS deaths."[135]

Even though epidemiological investigations observed associations between prone sleeping and sudden infant death in the 1960s, the very notion of sleep positioning as a cause of death seemed aberrant. In the first place, the fact that most American babies slept on their stomachs obfuscated the issue. Additionally, prone sleeping as a potential cause for SIDS did not square with contemporary convictions about sudden infant mortality. Prone sleeping implied suffocation, and researchers starting in the late 1940s were intent on refuting the idea of suffocation as a cause for sudden infant death. They pointed to a published anecdotal report (authored by Paul Woolley in the 1940s) as sure-fire proof that babies were capable of adjusting their faces to the side if need be in order to breathe. As journalist Jane Brody wrote in the *New York Times* in 1978, "Careful research has shown that it is just about impossible for a healthy infant to suffocate in his bedclothes."[136] Initial researchers were also wedded to the notion that babies who died suddenly were normal. Since prone sleeping clearly did not cause infant deaths uniformly, the theory insinuated abnormality. Even after investigators became more accepting of abnormalities as factors in SIDS in the 1970s, they still were dismissive of sleep positioning as a relevant factor because it was so simple. As one group of medical scientists summarized, the proposition that sleep positioning was a relevant factor in sudden infant death was "not just inconsistent with the biological evidence. It was actually counterintuitive . . . [and] hard to accept." The same authors also pointed out that the contemporary focus on apnea monitoring, near-miss SIDS, and high-risk babies distracted researchers' attention from weighing the effects of less complicated interventions, such as sleeping posture, that applied to *all* infants.[137] Although the evidence regarding co-sleeping lends to less prominent conclusions, it underscores the same themes as the evidence regarding supine sleeping.

American parents, doctors, and researchers were able to implement the first demonstrated measure to reduce the risk of SIDS in the 1990s as a direct result of international medical research and interdisciplinary perspectives on disease etiology. The enumeration and enactment of safe sleep protocols for babies succeeded in precipitously reducing SIDS rates in America as well as other nations. In so doing, however, they also taught American parents that even the most seemingly simple decisions—laying a baby on its stomach or its back—could be critical factors, matters of life and death. And Americans, especially those impacted by SIDS, must have wondered how something so vital went unnoticed for so long. Medical counsel about providing babies with safe sleep yielded drops in infant mortality, but it still did not make bedtime rituals any less stressful for parents. With the understanding that every detail surrounding how and where a baby sleeps might matter, many parents still do not rest easy.

CONCLUSION:
"THE DISEASE OF THEORIES"[1]
Discovering SIDS

It would be entirely possible to tell the story of SIDS as one of advancement and improvement. The risk-reduction campaigns instituted in the U.S. and other countries starting around 1990—which centered primarily on prone sleeping but also addressed other factors such as maternal smoking and breastfeeding—occasioned real, measurable reductions in SIDS rates. After the American Academy of Pediatrics endorsed non-prone sleeping in 1992, tens of thousands of American parents stopped laying their babies to sleep on their stomachs. Infant prone sleeping rates fell from 70 percent in 1992, to around 25 percent in 1996, to about 15 percent in 1999.[2] SIDS rates fell by half, from 1.2 deaths per thousand live births to 0.53 per thousand by the end of the 1990s.[3] Elsewhere around the globe, similar public health campaigns resulted in similar outcomes; in most nations, SIDS rates dropped by more than 50 percent.[4] The marked global decline in SIDS incidence in the 1990s was undoubtedly a major achievement, and parents could take solace in the fact that SIDS was rarer than ever before.

Yet even accounting for this triumph, the history of SIDS can be characterized neither by progression nor declension. As tends to be the case with SIDS, close scrutiny reveals complexity. SIDS reductions were not evenly distributed. In 2005, SIDS incidence worldwide ranged from between 0.1 and 0.8 deaths per thousand live births—a wide discrepancy. Countries employed varying SIDS definitions that stipulated different age brackets and death-scene investigation protocols, making it difficult to ascertain uniform statistics.[5] Even after the long downtrend in SIDS triggered by supine sleeping, the U.S. still had one of the highest SIDS rates on the planet.[6] In 2014 the Centers for Disease Control assessed that the U.S. ranked twenty-seventh among wealthy nations for infant mortality, with rates nearing six deaths per thousand live births; SIDS remained the fourth leading cause of infant death. The Back to Sleep campaign did not reach Americans uniformly. Many minority caretakers either did not receive or were resistant to its message because supine sleeping conflicted with cultural parenting traditions. SIDS continued to affect Native American, Alaskan Native, and African American families more than white families.[7] In 2003, blacks and American Indians experienced SIDS rates of 1.08 and 1.24 per thousand live births, respectively, compared to a rate of 0.51 per thousand live births for white babies. One decade later, the statistics were still dismal: SIDS rates were 83 percent higher among blacks and 95 percent higher among American Indians or Alaskan Natives. The disparity was so great that a standard encyclopedic entry on SIDS reviewed in 2014 chose to list "black race" as a risk factor for the syndrome.[8] Identification as African American, Alaskan Native, or Native American was similarly deemed a separate risk factor for SIDS in an extensive initiative designed to distribute cribs and provide information about safe sleep to high-risk families.[9]

Furthermore, some physicians called the legitimacy of SIDS declines in the U.S. after 1999 into question. They contended, quite compellingly, that "diagnostic shift," rather than true case reductions, accounted for the diminishing SIDS incidence from 1999 onward. From that year until 2001, SIDS dropped by 17.4 percent while post-neonatal mortality at large held steady. Even though there were fewer cases of SIDS, in other words, the same numbers of babies were dying. Reviewers suggested that medical examiners and coroners simply used the SIDS label less frequently and instead ascribed more infant deaths to suffocation, strangulation in bed, or cause unknown/unspecified. When they combined deaths classified as suffocation, unknown, or unspecified with deaths classified as SIDS for the period from 1999 to 2001, researchers compiled a data report that indicated a "nonsignificant decline in SIDS."[10]

In one of the studies that most forcefully asserted this conclusion, authors reviewed relevant data between 1989 and 2001. They determined that the decline in SIDS in the 1990s was "genuine" and directly resulted from the proliferation of the supine sleeping intervention. But between 1999 and 2001, reductions in SIDS were a fabrication spun by data. The investigators located a concurrent increase in infant deaths reported as unknown/unspecified and a near doubling of infant deaths attributed to accidental suffocation and strangulation in bed; in these categories, furthermore, they found that epidemiological profiles mirrored SIDS associations. An additional piece of evidence supporting these researchers' claim was that since 1999, prone sleeping rates in the U.S. had barely changed. Most of the decrease in SIDS rates since 1999, the authors reported, was "not true decline."[11] All of this thorny data helps demonstrate how the story of SIDS is more circuitous than sequential, that the diagnosis's legacy is as pendulous as its historical evolution. SIDS is a mixed bag.

In the twenty-first century, the origins of the SIDS diagnosis in the nineteenth-century conception of overlaying are plainly clear. Doctors perceived the problem of overlaying as simple suffocation caused by mothers who lacked maternal aptitude. They saw overlaying as a preventable loss that occurred as a direct result of inferior environmental circumstances, namely overtired, inebriate, or reckless caregivers. Around the turn of the twentieth century, medicine examined alternative explanations for overlaying, entertaining the enlarged thymus theory and AMS before working to establish the SIDS diagnosis. Each represented a new way of interpreting sudden infant death, but they sustained suspicions about parents' possible roles in their babies' deaths. SIDS, more than anything else, marked an attempt to extinguish lingering concerns about parents' part in sudden infant mortality—its construction was motivated by medicine's desires to remedy a problem and to relieve its survivors.

The SIDS construction stemmed from earlier attempts to explain what was happening to babies who died suddenly or unexpectedly, but SIDS still clearly represented an effort to deal with a condition whose "first and only symptom is death" in a new way. In other words, although SIDS was one of Americans' many reinterpretations of the overarching problem of sudden infant death, it still differed notably from the frameworks that preceded it. SIDS was the first explanation for sudden unexpected infant death to offer a targeted, formalized medical diagnosis unique to sudden infant mortality; to define the problem of sudden infant mortality by its inexplicability; and to be plainly steered by parents' feelings. The SIDS label completely redefined Americans' conceptions of sudden infant death; it transformed sudden, unexpected infant mortality from a topic of scattered medical inquiry into a more coherent and "worthy" medical dilemma.

And yet SIDS did not solve the manifold problems of sudden infant mortality, and it was not a clean slate. Although the diagnosis was conceived in large part to erase earlier notions of understanding, it was unable to do so effectively and thoroughly. In particular, SIDS did not eradicate the unwanted allusions to parental culpability that were tied especially to overlaying and to accidental mechanical suffocation—it simply reintroduced them in fresh ways. SIDS reapportioned some of the blame parents felt, scattering fault among mothers, medicine, monitors, and society. The SIDS label thus did not fully achieve one of its creators' predominant goals—exonerating parents.

However, by offering new language and by bringing sudden infant mortality into the light, it did bring distraught parents together. The SIDS category enabled affected parents to find one another and unify; their fellowship, manifest through networks like the National SIDS Foundation, appreciably relieved their hardships. The SIDS label facilitated channels for peer support and activism, which served as outlets for parents and contributed to their making SIDS a more "mainstream" diagnosis in American society. SIDS equipped parents working to revise their neighbors' and family members' perceptions of sudden infant mortality with language they desperately needed to do so. It helped parents advance broader social and medical awareness and acceptance of unexpected infant loss as an inexplicable fate that could happen to anyone—even the most upstanding, responsible, and loving parents. That in the twenty-first century most readers likely approached this history with a preexisting understanding of SIDS as a devastating tragedy, and did not need to be convinced of it as a tormenting experience, testifies to parents' success in this regard. By bringing affected Americans together, SIDS did alleviate some of the personal and social stigma and pain attached to sudden infant death. The SIDS diagnosis was arguably most influential for the collaborations it actuated.

But SIDS is a heartrending example of the limitations of modern medicine. Once it was named, American medicine tried to pinpoint what caused SIDS with almost no success. The American medical establishment was unable to either clearly discern the causes of SIDS or definitively disprove disagreeable explanations such as overlaying or homicide. These defeats contributed to the perpetuation of long-standing misgivings about sudden infant mortality. American medicine never realized its intention of burying the entangled notions of suffocation, infanticide, and overlaying; medicine never entirely laid to rest the issue of parental culpability. Although the SIDS definition officially discounted the notion of suffocation, it continued to be read between the lines in medical and popular literature.

The prospect of suffocation—whether accidental or purposeful—remained embedded in SIDS scholarship and public health initiatives. At the end of the twentieth century, some of the enduring questions about overlaying, infanticide, and accidental suffocation reappeared as experts debated the possible connections between safe sleeping and SIDS. In a sort of diagnostic renaissance, many professionals directly revived use of terms such as "suffocation in bed" or "overlaying." In fact, between 1984 and 2004, infant death rates attributed to "accidental suffocation or strangulation bed" more than quadrupled, from 0.028 deaths per thousand live births to 0.125.[12] The new umbrella category of sudden unexpected infant death (SUID), devised in the early 2000s, accounts not only for SIDS but also for all ill-defined and unspecified causes of infant mortality, including strangulation and accidental suffocation in bed. In 2013, there were more than 3,400 documented SUIDs in the U.S.[13] Meanwhile, safe sleep advice to parents also deepened the historical ties between SIDS and suffocation. In 2010, a highly contested public health campaign in Milwaukee denounced bed-sharing by depicting adult bed headboards as babies' tombstones and displaying images of babies laying in plush bedding on their stomachs adjacent to butcher knives. The message clearly conveyed to parents—that bed-sharing was profoundly dangerous and irresponsible—implied that parents' poor decision-making caused SIDS.

The correlate to the fact that qualms about suffocation persistently beset the SIDS diagnosis was that they continued to harass SIDS families. Because the SIDS construction failed to invalidate the broad premise of suffocation, Americans were never wholly persuaded that SIDS was always entirely inexplicable and unpreventable. The mere possibility that parents might be able to engage in risk minimization strategies, whether they be high-tech monitoring or crafting a safe sleep environment, continued to sow doubts about parents' roles in SIDS.

Beyond these considerations, the particular delineations of SIDS in the second half of the 1900s may have been, medically speaking, restraining. The profile of SIDS, and the purposes that motivated its creation, likely clouded researchers' vision. Physicians understood SIDS as a complex medical phenomenon definitively unrelated to suffocation. Most SIDS researchers were so intent to controvert suffocation that they were loath to consider causes or strategies they perceived as connected to suffocation. Because they were operating within a particular framework of understanding for sudden infant mortality, in other words, scientists working to solve SIDS were less likely to notice certain details and to interpret them as significant, and may have been unwittingly dismissive of relevant evidence.

Furthermore, when doctors started to become more comfortable with the idea that SIDS might result from various different causes, many of which were also probably multifactorial, SIDS began to appear even more problematic as a concept. If SIDS was a stand-in for multiple separate types of death, what good was it to researchers? Encapsulating this notion, one group of pathologists wrote in 1988 that "the unitary concept of SIDS has been unproductive. Advances in understanding the causes and in the prevention of these deaths will come from breaking the deaths down into groups that can be specifically investigated."[14] Another physician explained in 1995 that SIDS was, to a certain extent, "more of a 'diagnostic dustbin' into which are placed a variety of unrelated entities . . . It is also likely that the aetiology of SIDS is heterogeneous and that the term SIDS is not so much a diagnosis but a term covering a variety of mechanisms which result in a common lethal outcome."[15] Medicine's strategy of approaching all unexpected, sudden infant mortality via the SIDS category may have hamstrung scientists by constraining them to its elements instead of freeing them to explore multiple variable avenues of possible causation.

Finally, these manifold limitations—of both medical science and of the SIDS diagnosis itself—offer insight into the concepts of diagnosis and medicalization. Firstly, SIDS speaks to the power of diagnosis in American society in the twentieth century to imbue meaning. It illustrates how medical classifications serve dually as scientific tools and social scripts. The SIDS label shaped a unique American medical venture and fashioned a new schema for how individuals, medical professionals, families, and society should respond to sudden infant death. It is further noteworthy that the SIDS label, which is fundamentally based on the premise of inexplicability, derived from similarly presenting incidents that doctors explained with ease. The origins and history of the diagnosis suggest that Americans, starting in the middle of the twentieth century, became deeply uncomfortable conversing about the potential role of parenting decisions in sudden infant mortality. The question of whether or not parents, and medicine, could have done (or refrained from doing) anything to prevent sudden unexpected infant fatalities is at the core of SIDS, but it is an intensely prickly and sensitive quandary. Medical professionals engaged in that debate quite willingly early in the twentieth century, but they hastily retreated from it in the family-centeredness of the postwar era. The SIDS diagnosis was a way for medicine and society to try to address the problem of sudden infant mortality while also invalidating the conversation about whether parenting activities might be involved in it. Towards the end of the 1900s, doctors and laypeople began to reopen that discussion, and their renewed willingness to debate parental culpability indicates that SIDS was partially de-medicalized at the dawn of the twenty-first century.

SIDS underscores that medicalization does not implicitly demonize or pathologize; the process is not intrinsically objectionable. In 2006 Charles Rosenberg suggested that "what some sociologists and social critics have for decades called 'medicalization' is in practice the use of time- and place-specific vocabularies of disease entities as a tool for at once conceptualizing and managing behavior and feelings."[16] Americans aimed to medicalize sudden infant mortality via SIDS in large part as a strategy for vindicating parents—SIDS located a problem, conceptualized it as the worst kind of tragedy that was *devoid* of pathology, and patterned fresh strategies for responding to families with empathy. When Americans began to invoke "new" language for SIDS (a vocabulary preoccupied with suffocation) around 2000, the diagnosis began to lose some of its footing in the medical realm, and this resulted in once again shifting the functionality and connotations of the diagnosis.

CONCLUSION

Each time Americans reinvented sudden infant death and reconceived of its causes, they tried to stamp out old ideas. SIDS was the mid-late twentieth-century generation's way of explaining sudden infant death—it was not the first explanation and it was not the last. In the 1980s, some researchers sardonically dubbed SIDS the "disease of theories," because professionals had so many different ideas about the syndrome, and the history of SIDS really bears this categorization out.[17] SIDS was a disease of theories, but the theme underlying that designation runs even deeper—sudden infant mortality was itself a problem, a phenomenon of theories, and SIDS was just one of those. The SIDS construction was not entirely novel, since it reflected ideas from the past, but it was unique in that it offered a categorical diagnosis, defined the problem as unexplainable, and took parents' feelings into account. Transition to the "SIDS version" of sudden infant mortality also elicited important shifts. It gave unexpected infant mortality a name, and most Americans became familiar with it. SIDS medicalized sudden infant death and retooled it as an exceptionally distressing and confusing loss of life—again, that twenty-first century readers already know this and believe it illustrates how SIDS achieved this goal of social recognition. But the conception failed to yield comprehensive answers or solutions to the problem it represented.

In reference to rubella, in her book *Dangerous Pregnancies*, historian Leslie Reagan intimated that the "discovery of disease was not a moment but a process."[18] SIDS is a powerful illustration of this truism. Americans spent the entire twentieth century "discovering" SIDS; America's fraught historical relationship with SIDS has been a delicate balancing act, a story of foundering. Sudden infant death syndrome did not emerge as much as it unfolded in American society and medicine, and its story is still very much ongoing. Americans are still discovering SIDS, and will continue doing so in the future.

ACKNOWLEDGMENTS

I am indebted to the History Department at the University of Cincinnati in more ways than one. The department's funding supported my education and research, and enabled me to travel to numerous academic conferences and research libraries. The Taft Center at UC helped me to take advantage of multiple professional opportunities, including numerous archival visits. I also received support from the Graduate Student Governance Association, the University Research Council, and the Roger Daniels Fellowship, all at UC. Support from the UCLA Library and the Huntington Library helped me to travel and work in their archives.

Multiple individuals at UC helped bring this project to fruition. Thanks to Maura O'Connor and Chris Phillips, who saw the beginnings of this project in research seminars; both encouraged me to pursue the topic and pushed me to "think bigger" even when I didn't want to. Hope Earls was the ultimate advocate for graduate students, and I am glad to have gotten the chance to work with her and get to know her. Thanks to Alyssa McClanahan and to Nicole Lyon Roccas for their editing, comradery, and friendship.

I owe others a special debt of gratitude. Besides being a terrific and honest teacher, Isaac Campos has a knack for editing; his suggestions occasioned drastic improvements in my writing, and his support gave me conviction even when I had doubts. Wendy Kline introduced me to the history of medicine and helped me feel at home in the field. She has continued to be a fountain of encouragement, advice, and mentorship. David Stradling's insights significantly improved this project. He is, quite simply, a model advisor. Lastly, I was honored that Janet Golden's eyes met my work, and it benefitted greatly from her having read it.

When I wrote to Carolyn Szybist Sodini, I hoped I had written to the right person—as it turned out, nothing could be closer to the truth. In Carolyn I found a literal and metaphorical archive, and I am so grateful to her for sharing her story, and her life, with me.

Peter Mickulas has been a fantastic editor—his patience, feedback, and guidance were a welcome introduction to the world of publication, and he made the process plainly enjoyable. My two readers offered invaluable insights which challenged me to rework several areas that needed clarification and expansion—many thanks for their suggestions and reflections.

I could not have finished this book without my family. I am fortunate to call my siblings my best friends. Andrew: we've seen each other through college, grad school, and residency; I hope I've reciprocated even a small fraction of the support and loyalty you show me and my family every day. Cullen: you have been an unpredicted source of confidence and a (predicted) well of humor. Thank you for all of your pilgrimages north, and for helping me successfully escape from my work during numerous weekend frivolities. Mary: What can I say? You've walked with me more miles than I can count, and helped me navigate more decisions than I can remember. You are the best. And, though not in name, Sarah Bell and Tina Hubbard are sisters to me, and I am beyond grateful to have them in my life.

My parents' generosity is overwhelming. Dan: despite an overwhelmingly challenging and hectic schedule, you somehow manage to make peace of mind look easy. You exemplify dedication, and not a day has passed that I haven't benefitted from your hard work, love, support, and happiness. Patty: you are an anchor. It is impossible to tally all of the ways in which you contributed to this book, much less my everyday life and well-being. You unfailingly put everyone before yourself; this book is dedicated to you.

Joshua: you show me every day what it means to work well (and play well). Without your support and love, your proclivity for intellectual exploration and outdoor recreation, and your literally (yes, literally) unswerving faith in me, this project would still be long in the making (and it definitely would have been less fun). Thank you for knowing I could do this; thank you for everything.

And lastly, thank you to James, for breathing life into this project.

NOTES

INTRODUCTION

1. National Center for Chronic Disease Prevention and Health Promotion Division of Reproductive Health, Centers for Disease Control, "Achievements in Public Health, 1900–1999: Healthier Mothers and Babies," *CDC Morbidity and Mortality Weekly Report* 48, no. 38 (October 1999): 849–58.

2. Rima D. Apple, *Perfect Motherhood: Science and Childrearing in America* (New Brunswick, NJ: Rutgers University Press, 2006), 94; Peter N. Stearns, *Anxious Parents: A History of Modern Childrearing in America* (New York: New York University Press, 2003); Cecelia M. Dobrish, "The Double Miracle That's Saving High Risk Newborns," *Parent's Magazine and Better Homemaking,* June 1977; Eileen Stukane, "Medical Miracles Save Newborns in Trouble," *Parent's Magazine and Better Family Living,* November 1972; Harry Schwartz, "What Health Crisis?" *New York Times,* October 18, 1971.

3. "Baby Crib Deaths Up, Philadelphia Reports," *New York Times,* July 7, 1963; Harold Schmeck, "10,000 Babies Die of Unknown Causes, Yearly Report Says," *New York Times,* October 29, 1964.

4. This was a common phrase; John F. Kennedy's assistant secretary of Health, Education, and Welfare, for example, used it in the early 1960s to describe U.S. medical prowess. Elena Conis, *Vaccine Nation: America's Changing Relationship with Immunization* (Chicago: University of Chicago Press, 2015), 35.

5. Gopal K. Singh and Stella M. Yu, "Infant Mortality in the United States: Trends, Differentials, and Projections, 1950 through 2010," *American Journal of Public Health* 85, no. 7 (July 1995): 957, 958.

6. David Rutstein, "Why Do We Let These Babies Die?" *Reader's Digest,* August 1964, 2, box 126, folder 8, Maternity Center Association Records, Archives and Special Collections, Columbia University Health Sciences Library (hereafter, MCA Records); Singh and Yu, "Infant Mortality in the United States," 960, 961.

7. Quoted in Conis, *Vaccine Nation,* 53.

8. Richard Firstman and Jamie Talan, *The Death of Innocents: A True Story of Murder, Medicine, and High-Stakes Science* (New York: Bantam Books, 1997), 205–6.

9. "'Crib' Death: The Mysterious Killer," Proceedings and Debates of the 91st Congress, Second Session, Congressional Record (Washington, DC: U.S. Senate, January 19, 1970), box 7, folder 6, Lester Adelson Papers, Dittrick Medical History Center Archives, Case Western Reserve University, Cleveland, Ohio (hereafter, Adelson Papers).

10. Abraham Bergman, J. Bruce Beckwith, and C. George Ray, eds., *Sudden Infant Death Syndrome: Proceedings of the Second International Conference on Causes of Sudden Death in Infants* (Children's Orthopedic Hospital and Medical Center and University of Washington School of Medicine, Seattle: University of Washington Press, 1969), 18.

11. "'Crib' Death: The Mysterious Killer."

12. D. L. Russell-Jones, "Sudden Infant Death in History and Literature," *Archives of Disease in Childhood* 60 (1985): 280; Todd L. Savitt, "Sudden Infant Death Syndrome," *The Cambridge Historical Dictionary of Disease* (Cambridge: Cambridge University Press, 2003); Abraham

Bergman, *The "Discovery" of Sudden Infant Death Syndrome: Lessons in the Practice of Political Medicine* (New York: Praeger, 1986), v, xi; "Vital and Health Statistics: Trends in Infant Mortality by Cause of Death and Other Characteristics, 1960–88," Data from the National Vital Statistics System, 20 (Hyattsville, MD: U.S. Department of Health and Human Services, Public Health Service, January 1993), 1, 9.

13. Quoted in Marion Steinman, "Crib Death: Too Many Clues?" *New York Times*, May 16, 1976.

14. Charles E. Rosenberg, *Explaining Epidemics and Other Studies in the History of Medicine* (New York: Cambridge University Press, 1992), 305, 310.

15. This approach mirrors and attests to other scholarship on disease in society. In her analysis of anxiety in twentieth-century America, for example, historian Andrea Tone expressly treats anxiety as "something at once real and historically rooted; an actual experience inseparable from the constellation of ideas, individuals, and events that gave it meaning." Sociologist Peter Conrad, in his series of case studies on medicalization, similarly emphasizes the value of working to unpack "the viability of medical designation" rather than the "validity of diagnosis." Andrea Tone, *The Age of Anxiety: A History of America's Turbulent Affair with Tranquilizers* (New York: Basic Books, 2009), xii; Peter Conrad, *The Medicalization of Society: On the Transformation of Human Conditions into Treatable Disorders*, Baltimore: Johns Hopkins University Press, 2007, 4.

16. Sheila Rothman, *Living in the Shadow of Death: Tuberculosis and the Social Experience of Illness in American History* (Baltimore: Johns Hopkins University Press, 1994); Charles Rosenberg, *The Cholera Years: The United States in 1832, 1849, 1866* (Chicago: University of Chicago Press, 1962); David Oshinsky, *Polio: An American Story* (Oxford: Oxford University Press, 2005); Janet Golden, *Message in a Bottle: The Making of Fetal Alcohol Syndrome* (Cambridge: Harvard University Press, 2005); Siddhartha Mukherjee, *The Emperor of All Maladies: A Biography of Cancer* (New York: Scribner Books, 2010); Leila Rupp, *A Desired Past: A Short History of Same-Sex Love in America* (Chicago: University of Chicago Press, 1999); Judith Houck, *Hot and Bothered: Women, Medicine, and Menopause in Modern America* (Cambridge: Harvard University Press, 2006); Judith Leavitt, *Brought to Bed: Childbearing in America, 1750–1950* (New York: Oxford University Press, 1986); Christian Warren, *Brush with Death: A Social History of Lead Poisoning* (Baltimore: Johns Hopkins University Press, 2000).

17. D. A. Smith, "Sudden Infant Death Syndrome—A Valid Diagnosis?" *Medical Hypotheses* 36 (1991): 183.

18. Elaine Tyler May, *Barren in the Promised Land: Childless Americans and the Pursuit of Happiness* (Boston: Harvard University Press, 1995), 138; Elaine Tyler May, *Homeward Bound: American Families in the Cold War Era*, 3rd ed. (New York: Basic Books, 2008), 3.

19. Barron H. Lerner, *The Breast Cancer Wars: Hope, Fear, and the Pursuit of a Cure in Twentieth-Century America* (Oxford: Oxford University Press, 2001); Allan Brandt, *The Cigarette Century: The Rise, Fall, and Deadly Persistence of the Product That Defined America* (New York: Basic Books, 2007); Elizabeth Siegel Watkins, *On the Pill: A Social History of Oral Contraceptives, 1950–1970* (Baltimore: Johns Hopkins University Press, 1998); Elizabeth Siegel Watkins, *The Estrogen Elixir: A History of Hormone Replacement Therapy in America* (Baltimore: Johns Hopkins University Press, 2007); Phil Brown, *No Safe Place: Toxic Waste, Leukemia, and Community Action* (Berkeley: University of California Press, 1990); Warren, *Brush with Death*; Paul Starr, *The Social Transformation of American Medicine: The Rise of a Sovereign Profession and the Making of a Vast Industry* (New York: Basic Books, 1982), 379, 408.

20. "Sudden Infant Death Syndrome: Joint Hearing Before Certain Subcommittees of the Committee on Post Office and Civil Service and the Committee on Energy and Commerce

and the Select Committee on Children, Youth, and Families," § House of Representatives, Congress (1985), 15.

21. This is in reference to Fred Dore, Judy Choate, and Robert Redford.

22. Sherwin B. Nuland, *How We Die: Reflections on Life's Final Chapter* (New York: Alfred A. Knopf, 1994), 106.

23. Quoted in Judy Klemesrud, "A Tragedy with an Aftermath of Guilt," *New York Times*, June 19, 1972.

CHAPTER 1 "DEATHS OF INFANTS IN BED": THE HISTORICAL ORIGINS OF SIDS

1. William Wynn Westcott, "Inebriety in Women and the Overlaying of Infants," *British Journal of Inebriety* 1, no. 2 (October 1903): 1209.

2. "The Prevention of Overlaying," *The Lancet* 145, no. 3729 (April 1895): 1073.

3. Charles Templeman, "Two Hundred and Fifty-Eight Cases of Suffocation of Infants," *Edinburgh Medical Journal* 38 (December 1892): 322–39.

4. William L. Langer, "Infanticide: A Historical Survey," *History of Childhood Quarterly* 1, no. 3 (1974): 360, 361.

5. Daniel Rodgers, *Atlantic Crossings: Social Politics in a Progressive Age* (Boston: Harvard University Press, 1998); Richard Meckel, *Save the Babies: American Public Health Reform and the Prevention of Infant Mortality* (Baltimore: Johns Hopkins University Press, 1990).

6. Kings 3:16–27, *King James Bible*.

7. Catherine Damme, "Infanticide: The Worth of an Infant Under Law," *Medical History* 22, no. 1 (January 1978): 3–4; Langer, "Infanticide: A Historical Survey," 356.

8. Langer, "Infanticide: A Historical Survey," 356–57; Damme, "Infanticide: The Worth," 3–4; Kathryn L. Moseley, "The History of Infanticide in Western Society," *Issues in Law and Medicine* 1, no. 5 (1986): 356.

9. Todd Savitt, "The Social and Medical History of Crib Death," *Journal of the Florida Medical Association* 66, no. 8 (August 1979): 856.

10. For some examples across genres, see Margaret Barnard, "Sudden Infant Death Syndrome," *Medico-Legal Bulletin*, bulletin no. 224, 20, no. 12 (December 1971): 1; J. Bruce Beckwith, "The Sudden Infant Death Syndrome," *Current Problems in Pediatrics* 3, no. 8 (June 1973): 7; Eileen Hasselmeyer and Jehu Hunter, "The Sudden Infant Death Syndrome," *Obstetrics and Gynecology Annual* 4 (1975): 214; Gail Grenier Sweet, "Sudden Infant Death Syndrome: A Personal View," *Mothering*, Summer 1981, 105, box 3, folder 14, Wisconsin Bureau of Community Health and Prevention: Sudden Infant Death Syndrome Project Records, Wisconsin State Historical Society Archives (hereafter, WSIDSP Records); D. L. Russell-Jones, "Sudden Infant Death in History and Literature," *Archives of Disease in Childhood* 60 (1985): 278; Giulia Ottaviani, *Crib Death: Sudden Unexplained Death of Infants—The Pathologist's Viewpoint* (Milan, Italy: Springer, 2007), 2; "Facts About Sudden Infant Death Syndrome" (U.S. Department of Health, Education, and Welfare, Public Health Service, National Institutes of Health, n.d.), box 12, file #1, John Milton Adams Papers (Collection 1293), Department of Special Collections, Charles E. Young Research Library, University of California, Los Angeles (hereafter, Adams Papers).

11. Golden further explains that "what was seen in the past was not FAS. The clinical features of [alcohol-related birth defects] noted by eighteenth-, nineteenth-, and early twentieth-century observers unquestionably resemble those offered by late twentieth-century physicians because they were looking at the same physiological phenomenon. However, the meaning of those features was different because of the vantage point—historical, medical, and cultural—of those who described the particular infants and their parents." Janet Golden, *Message in a Bottle: The Making of Fetal Alcohol Syndrome* (Cambridge: Harvard University Press, 2005), 34, 16, 13.

12. Robert William Fogel and Stanley L. Engerman, *Time on the Cross: The Economics of American Negro Slavery*, 1989th ed. (New York: W. W. Norton, 1974), 124, quote from 125.

13. Savitt reasserted his argument four years later in a piece specifically addressing the history of sudden infant death syndrome. Todd Savitt, "Smothering and Overlaying of Virginia Slave Children: A Suggested Explanation," *Bulletin of the History of Medicine* 49, no. 3 (Fall 1975): 400, 401; Savitt, "The Social and Medical History of Crib Death," 856.

14. Michael P. Johnson, "Smothered Slave Infants: Were Slave Mothers at Fault?" *Journal of Southern History* 47, no. 4 (November 1981): 495–96, 499, 501.

15. Ibid., 494, 514–15, 518–19, 510.

16. Deborah Gray White, *Ar'n't I a Woman?: Female Slaves in the Plantation South* (New York: W. W. Norton, 1985), 88–89.

17. Ariane Kemkes, "'Smothered' Infants: Neglect, Infanticide or SIDS?: A Fresh Look at the Nineteenth-Century Mortality Schedules," *Human Ecology* 37 (2009): 394, 400.

18. Previously, vital statistics were the purview of religious bodies, recorded through the sacraments (christenings, marriages, burials). George C. Alter and Ann G. Carmichael, "Classifying the Dead: Toward a History of the Registration of Causes of Death," *Journal of the History of Medicine* 54 (April 1999): 115–17; Halbert L. Dunn and National Office of Vital Statistics, eds., "Chapter 1: History and Organization of the Vital Statistics Program," in *Vital Statistics of the United States, 1950*, vol. 1 (Washington, DC: United States Government Printing Office, 1954), 2, 5, http://www.cdc.gov/nchs/data/vsus/vsus_1950_1.pdf. For an in-depth analysis of the piecemeal reports on mortality figures before 1900, see Samuel H. Preston and Michael R. Haines, eds., *Fatal Years: Child Mortality in Late Nineteenth-Century America* (Princeton, NJ: Princeton University Press, 1991).

19. *Ninth Census*, vol. 2, "The Vital Statistics of the United States" (Washington, DC: Government Printing Office, 1872), 18–21.

20. Suffocation rates—ranging from 2.5 to 4 per thousand—mirrored later SIDS rates. John S. Billings, "Report on the Mortality and Vital Statistics of the United States as Returned at the Tenth Census (June 1, 1880)," Census (Washington, DC: Department of the Interior, 1886), 372, 354; John S. Billings, "Report on the Mortality and Vital Statistics of the United States as Returned at the Tenth Census (June 1, 1880)," Census (Washington, DC: Department of the Interior, 1885), 22; John S. Billings, "Report on Vital and Social Statistics in the United States at the Eleventh Census: 1890," Census (Washington, DC: Department of the Interior, 1894), 22; *Vital Statistics: A Memorial Volume of Selections from the Reports and Writings of William Farr* (London: Offices of the Sanitary Institute, 1885), 203.

21. Myron E. Wegman, "Infant Mortality in the Twentieth Century, Dramatic but Uneven Progress," *Journal of Nutrition* 131, no. 2 (February 1, 2001): 401S; Gregory Davis, "Mind Your Manners: Part I: History of Certification and Manner of Death Classification," *American Journal of Forensic Medicine and Pathology* 18, no. 3 (September 1997): 219–23.

22. Preston and Haines, *Fatal Years*, 50; Milton Kotelchuck, "Safe Mothers, Healthy Babies: Reproductive Health in the Twentieth Century," in *Silent Victories: The History and Practice of Public Health in Twentieth-Century America*, ed. John W. Ward and Christian Warren (Oxford: Oxford University Press, 2007), 106; Davis, "Mind Your Manners"; quote from William G. Rothstein, *Public Health and the Risk Factor: A History of an Uneven Medical Revolution* (Rochester, NY: University of Rochester Press, 2003), 32.

23. "Country Comparison: Infant Mortality Rate," in *The World Factbook* 2013–14 (Washington, DC: Central Intelligence Agency, 2013), https://www.cia.gov/library/publications/the-world-factbook/rankorder/2091rank.html.

24. Elizabeth A. Reedy, *American Babies: Their Life and Times in the Twentieth Century* (Westport, CT: Praeger Publishers, 2007), 4.

25. Preston and Haines, *Fatal Years*, 52.

26. Rosie Findlay, "More Deadly Than the Male . . . ? Mothers and Infanticide in Nineteenth-Century Britain," *Cycnos* 23, no. 2 (n.d.): 2, http://revel.unice.fr/cycnos/document.html?id=763.

27. Nancy Schrom Dye and Daniel Blake Smith, "Mother Love and Infant Death, 1750–1920," *Journal of American History* 73, no. 2 (September 1, 1986): 344.

28. Sylvia D. Hoffert, "'A Very Peculiar Sorrow': Attitudes Toward Infant Death in the Urban Northeast, 1800–1860," *American Quarterly* 39, no. 4 (Winter 1987): 601, 602, 603, 606.

29. Peter N. Stearns, *Anxious Parents: A History of Modern Childrearing in America* (New York: New York University Press, 2003), 38.

30. Thomas Cone, *History of American Pediatrics* (Boston: Little, Brown, 1979), 70; Reedy, *American Babies*, 39; Preston and Haines, *Fatal Years*, 13; Alexandra Minna Stern and Howard Markel, eds., *Formative Years: Children's Health in the United States, 1880–2000* (Ann Arbor: University of Michigan Press, 2002), 7.

31. Dye and Smith, "Mother Love and Infant Death," 343.

32. Jan Lewis, "Mother's Love: The Construction of an Emotion in Nineteenth-Century America," in *Mothers and Motherhood: Readings in American History*, ed. Rima Apple and Janet Golden (Columbus: Ohio State University Press, 1997), 56; Margaret Marsh, "Motherhood Denied: Women and Infertility in Historical Perspective," in *Mothers and Motherhood: Readings in American History*, ed. Apple and Golden, 222, quote from 221.

33. Rima Apple, "Constructing Mothers: Scientific Motherhood in the Nineteenth and Twentieth Centuries," in *Mothers and Motherhood: Readings in American History*, ed. Apple and Golden, 93.

34. William Chafe, *The Paradox of Change: American Women in the Twentieth Century* (Oxford: Oxford University Press, 1991), 5, 16.

35. John Burnham, "Why Did the Infants and Toddlers Die?: Shifts in Americans' Ideas of Responsibility for Accidents—From Blaming Mom to Engineering," *Journal of Social History* 29, no. 4 (Summer 1996): 819; Marsh, "Motherhood Denied," 222.

36. Viviana Zelizer, *Pricing the Priceless Child: The Changing Social Value of Children* (New York: Basic Books, 1985), 25, 32, 23.

37. Dye and Smith, "Mother Love and Infant Death," 347.

38. Meckel, *Save the Babies*, 154.

39. Dye and Smith, "Mother Love and Infant Death," 349, 330–31, 352; Zelizer, *Pricing the Priceless Child*, 23, 28.

40. Jacqueline Wolf, *Don't Kill Your Baby: Public Health and the Decline of Breastfeeding in the Nineteenth and Twentieth Centuries* (Columbus: Ohio State University Press, 2001), 45.

41. "American Association for the Study and Prevention of Infant Mortality: First Annual Meeting, Held at Baltimore, Nov. 9–11, 1910," *JAMA* 55, no. 26 (December 1910): 2260.

42. Meckel, *Save the Babies*, 112.

43. Ibid., 5–6.

44. George Newman, *Infant Mortality: A Social Problem* (London: Methuen, 1906); Jacqueline Wolf, *Deliver Me from Pain: Anesthesia and Birth in America* (Baltimore: Johns Hopkins University Press, 2009), 225–26; Kotelchuck, "Safe Mothers, Healthy Babies," 107.

45. Meckel, *Save the Babies*, 5–6.

46. Ibid., 100, 220, 152.

47. Dye and Smith, "Mother Love and Infant Death," 343.

48. Kotelchuck, "Safe Mothers, Healthy Babies," 109.

49. Dye and Smith, "Mother Love and Infant Death," 352.

50. Apple, "Constructing Mothers"; quote from Rima D. Apple, *Perfect Motherhood: Science and Childrearing in America* (New Brunswick, NJ: Rutgers University Press, 2006), 94.

51. This newfound attention was partly the result of eugenic concerns about national degeneration, partly the result of a "tremendous outpouring of public and official concern with child welfare," and also partly stemmed from greater familiarity with infant mortality rates. Meckel, *Save the Babies*, 101, 102–3.

52. National Center for Chronic Disease Prevention and Health Promotion Division of Reproductive Health, Centers for Disease Control, "Achievements in Public Health, 1900–1999: Healthier Mothers and Babies," *CDC Morbidity and Mortality Weekly Report* 48, no. 38 (October 1999): 849–58.

53. Kwang-Sun Lee, "Infant Mortality Decline in the Late 19th and Early 20th Centuries: The Role of Market Milk," *Perspectives in Biology and Medicine* 50, no. 4 (Autumn 2007): 586; Kotelchuck, "Safe Mothers, Healthy Babies," 113.

54. Christian Warren, *Brush with Death: A Social History of Lead Poisoning* (Baltimore: Johns Hopkins University Press, 2000), 41.

55. Savitt, "The Social and Medical History of Crib Death," 855.

56. Rodgers, *Atlantic Crossings*.

57. William Wynn Westcott, "The Overlaying of Infants," *British Medical Journal* 2, no. 2236 (November 1903): 1208.

58. Westcott, "Inebriety in Women and the Overlaying of Infants," 68; "Medical Progress: The Overlaying of Infants," *Medical News* 83, no. 25 (December 19, 1903): printed in the New York Times.

59. Arthur Newsholme, *The Elements of Vital Statistics* (London: Swan Sonnenschein, 1889), 107–8; Arthur P. Luff, *Text-Book of Forensic Medicine and Toxicology*, vol. 2 (London: Longmans, Greene, 1895), 146; T. N. Kelynack, ed., *The Drink Problem: In Its Medico-Sociolegal Aspects* (London: Methuen, 1907), 135, 168.

60. Newman, *Infant Mortality*, 42, 211.

61. James M. Adams, "Case of Asphyxia in an Infant, From Being Overlain in Bed," *The Lancet* 40, no. 1033 (1843): 401, 402.

62. "Suffocation of Infants," *The Lancet* 131, no. 3373 (April 1888): 788.

63. "Infancy: Food and Sleep," in *Cassell's Book of the Household: A Work of Reference on Domestic Economy*, vol. 3 (London: Cassell, 1890), 132.

64. W. H. Willcox, "Infantile Mortality from 'Overlaying,'" *British Medical Journal* 2, no. 2282 (September 1904): 754.

65. Quote from "Drink in England," *New York Times*, April 8, 1888.

66. For examples, see Warren G. Guntheroth, *Crib Death: The Sudden Infant Death Syndrome* (Mount Kisco, NY: Futura Publishing, 1989), 6; Jean Golding, Sylvia Limerick, and Aidan Macfarlane, *Sudden Infant Death: Patterns, Puzzles, and Problems* (Seattle: University of Washington Press, 1985), 7; "Sudden Death in Infancy," *The Lancet* 259, no. 6722 (June 1952): 1291; J. Bruce Beckwith, "The Sudden Infant Death Syndrome," 9; Hasselmeyer and Hunter, "The Sudden Infant Death Syndrome," 215; S. R. Kendeel and J. A. Ferris, "Sudden Infant Death Syndrome: A Review of the Literature," *Journal of Forensic Science Society* 17, no. 4 (October 1977): 223; Russell-Jones, "Sudden Infant Death in History and Literature," 279.

67. For unclear reasons, Templeman only observed a portion of the total 399 reported cases. The questions of insurance and illegitimacy were often referenced but infrequently alleged directly as causative in overlaying. As Charles Paget explained in a presentation at the International Congress of Hygiene and Demography in 1891, the connection between overlaying and infant insurance was uncertain; overlaying's "true cause," he reflected, "may be simply recklessness or ignorance." Templeman, "Two Hundred and Fifty-Eight Cases," 323, 325; C. E. Shelly, ed., *Transactions of the Seventh International Congress of Hygiene and Demography, London, August 10th-17th, 1891*, vol. 4 (London: Eyre and Spottiswoode, 1892), 68.

68. D. L. Thomas, "On Infantile Mortality," *Public Health* 11 (1898): 812.

69. Quoted in "The Overlying of Children," *The Lancet* 165, no. 4254 (March 1905): 660.

70. Mrs. M. A. Baines, "The Rearing of Our Children: A Series of Valuable Papers by Distinguished American Women: On the Prevention of Excessive Infant Mortality," *Herald of Health and Journal of Physical Culture* 14, no. 1 (July 1869): 6.

71. Arthur Leared, "Infant Mortality and Its Causes," *Reprinted from the "English Woman's Journal,"* 1862, 7.

72. Willcox, "Infantile Mortality from 'Overlaying'" (1904), 754–55.

73. "The Overlying of Children," *The Lancet* 165, no. 4254 (March 1905): 660.

74. Westcott, "Inebriety in Women and the Overlaying of Infants," 68.

75. "Drink in England," *New York Times*, April 8, 1888.

76. Henry Enos Tuley, "The Newborn," *Archives of Pediatrics* 26 (1909): 582.

77. "The Prevention of Overlaying."

78. "The Overlying of Children," *The Lancet* 165, no. 4254 (March 1905): 660.

79. Westcott, "Inebriety in Women and the Overlaying of Infants," 67.

80. "A Penalty for Overlaying," *The Lancet* 135, no. 3472 (March 1890): 613; "The Mortality of Children from Overlying or Accidental Burning," *The Lancet* 168, no. 4333 (September 1906): 749.

81. "The Overlaying of Infants," *British Medical Journal* 2, no. 2236 (November 1903): 1231; Westcott, "The Overlaying of Infants."

82. Thomas, "On Infantile Mortality," 813.

83. Westcott also credited Germany and France with low overlaying rates and thought that the main reason was that "the thin red and white wines of France and the light beers of Germany do not make women drunkards." (He neglected to account for the how the "deadly intoxicant" of absinthe in Paris might influence overlaying in that country.) Willcox, "Infantile Mortality from 'Overlaying'" (1904), 755; "The Mortality of Children from Overlying or Accidental Burning," 750; Westcott, "Inebriety in Women and the Overlaying of Infants," 68.

84. W. H. Willcox, "Infantile Mortality from Overlaying," *St. Mary's Hospital Gazette*, February 1905, 16.

85. Willcox, "Infantile Mortality from 'Overlaying'" (1904), 755.

86. Westcott, "Inebriety in Women and the Overlaying of Infants," 68.

87. G. Ernest Herman, *First Lines in Midwifery: A Guide to Attendance on Natural Labour for Medical Students and Midwives*, Manuals for Students of Medicine (London: Cassell, 1895), 181; Marian Humfrey, *A Manual of Obstetric Nursing*, vol. 2 (London: Sampson Low, Marston and Company, 1895), 161.

88. Honnor Morten, *The Midwives' Pocket Book and Guide to the London Obstetrical Society's Examination* (London: Scientific Press, 1897), 85.

89. Henry Arthur Allbutt, *Every Mother's Handbook: A Guide to the Management of Her Children* (London: Simpkin, Marshall, Hamilton, Kent and Co., 1897), 47.

90. Andrew Wilson, ed., *The Modern Physician: Being a Complete Guide to the Attainment and Preservation of Health*, vol. 5 (London: Caxton Publishing, 1904), 97, 175.

91. Willcox, "Infantile Mortality from 'Overlaying'" (1904), 755; "The Etiology of Overlaying," *The Lancet* 192, no. 4970 (November 1918): 755.

92. C. O. Hawthorne, *Forensic Medicine and Toxicology: A Manual for Students*, 2nd ed. (Glasgow: A. Stenhouse, College, Gate, and Hillhead, 1897), 46.

93. "Abstracts," *Pediatrics* 16 (1904): 254.

94. "Correspondence: London Letter," *American Practitioner and News* 8, no. 2 (July 1889): 51; "Notes and Queries," *American Practitioner and News* 9, no. 1 (January 1890): 28–32; quote from "Current Literature: Hygiene and Therapeutics," *Archives of Pediatrics* 22, no. 9 (1905): 640; "Infantile Mortality from 'Overlaying,'" *The Critique* 13, no. 9 (September 1906): 343.

95. George T. Elliot Jr., "The Hygiene of Infancy," *Chicago Medical Examiner* 10 (January 1869): 28.

96. James Moores Ball, ed., *Tri-State Medical Journal*, vol. 3 (St. Louis: James Moores Ball, 1896), 211.

97. Massachusetts Medico-Legal Society, "Transactions of the Massachusetts Medico-Legal Society" 3, no. 1 (1899): 10–11.

98. "Medical Progress: Medicine," *Medical News* 83, no. 25 (December 19, 1903): 1172; Louis Starr and Thompson S. Westcott, "Pediatrics," *American Journal of the Medical Sciences* 127, no. 2 (February 1904): 359; "Abstracts," *Pediatrics* 16 (1904): 254.

99. Edwin Graham, "Infant Mortality," *JAMA* 51, no. 13 (1908): 1048.

100. Edmund Cautley, *The Diseases of Infants and Children* (New York: Paul B. Hoeber, 1912), 102.

101. "The Anti-Alcohol Exhibit at the International Congress on Hygiene," *Scientific Temperance Journal* 22, no. 2 (October 1912): 18.

102. For the year 1897, the report notes that four of the seven infant suffocation cases occurred on Saturday or holiday nights. Rhode Island State Board of Health, "Report of the State Board of Health of the State of Rhode Island, for the Year Ending December 31, 1894" (Providence, RI, 1896), 17, 176; Rhode Island State Board of Health, "Report of the State Board of Health of the State of Rhode Island, for the Year Ending December 31, 1895" (Providence, RI, 1897), 176; Rhode Island State Board of Health, "Annual Report of the State Board of Health of the State of Rhode Island for the Year Ending December 31, 1897" (Providence, RI, 1899), 180, 261; Rhode Island State Board of Health, "Report of the State Board of Health of the State of Rhode Island, for the Year Ending December 31, 1899" (Providence, RI, 1903), 192; Rhode Island State Board of Health, "Report of the State Board of Health of the State of Rhode Island, for the Year Ending December 31, 1902" (Providence, RI, 1910), 188; Rhode Island State Board of Health, "Report of the State Board of Health of the State of Rhode Island, for the Year Ending December 31, 1903" (Providence, RI, 1911), 188; Rhode Island State Board of Health, "Report of the State Board of Health of the State of Rhode Island for the Year Ending December 31, 1904" (Providence, RI, 1911), 190.

103. Massachusetts Medico-Legal Society, "Transactions of the Massachusetts Medico-Legal Society" 2 (1898): 8.

104. "Accidental Suffocation and Sudden Death," *Medical and Surgical Reporter* 63, no. 6 (August 9, 1890): 176.

105. Graham, "Infant Mortality," 1048; Hermann M. Briggs and William T. Jenkins, "Accidental Suffocation and Sudden Death," *Medical and Surgical Reporter* 63, no. 6 (August 9, 1890): printed in the *New York Times*.

106. Briggs and Jenkins, "Accidental Suffocation and Sudden Death."

107. This was suggested, for example, in one Philadelphia study that recorded 210 of 864 children's deaths as due to "unknown causes." Graham, "Infant Mortality," 1048.

108. "Miscellany: Overlying of Infants," *New York Medical Journal and Philadelphia Medical Journal* 80, no. 21 (November 1904): 1007.

109. "Foreign Miscellany," *Christian Advocate and Journal* 37, no. 23 (June 5, 1862): 183; "Child Murder," *The Spectator* 38 (August 5, 1865): 859; "Crime in England: Statistics of the Past Year," *New York Observer and Chronicle*, August 31, 1865, 277.

110. For representative examples, see "Two Cases of Suffocation," *New York Times*, June 5, 1882; "Smothered to Death in Bed," *New York Times*, January 21, 1896.

111. M.D.C., "Correspondence: London," *The Round Table: A Saturday Review of Politics, Finance, Literature, Society, and Art* 2 (September 16, 1865): 26.

112. Westcott, "The Overlaying of Infants," 1209.

CHAPTER 2   CAUSE OF DEATH: SIDS

1. "Proceedings: Conference on Sudden Death in Infancy" (Public Health Service, November 30, 1949), 2, box 12, file # 1, Adams Papers.

2. Edwin Graham, "Infant Mortality," *JAMA* 51, no. 13 (1908): 1048.

3. "Proceedings: Conference on Sudden Death in Infancy," 1949, 26.

4. Abraham Bergman, J. Bruce Beckwith, and C. George Ray, eds., "Sudden Infant Death Syndrome: Proceedings of the Second International Conference on Causes of Sudden Death in Infants" (Children's Orthopedic Hospital and Medical Center and University of Washington School of Medicine, Seattle: University of Washington Press, 1969), 18.

5. Sherwin B. Nuland, *How We Die: Reflections on Life's Final Chapter* (New York: Alfred A. Knopf, 1994), 105.

6. Suzanne Harris, "To Keep Infants Alive: The Struggle to Solve the Mystery of Crib Death," *Washington Post*, November 29, 1970, box 132, folder 6, MCA Records.

7. Ann Dally, "Status Lymphaticus: Sudden Death in Children from 'Visitation of God' to Cot Death," *Medical History* 41 (1997): 74.

8. Mizuki Nishino et al., "The Thymus: A Comprehensive Review," *RadioGraphics* 26, no. 2 (2006): 335–36, 337.

9. Abraham Bergman, *The "Discovery" of Sudden Infant Death Syndrome: Lessons in the Practice of Political Medicine* (New York: Praeger, 1986), 4; Todd Savitt, "The Social and Medical History of Crib Death," *Journal of the Florida Medical Association* 66, no. 8 (August 1979): 856, 857; Warren G. Guntheroth, "The Thymus, Suffocation, and Sudden Infant Death Syndrome: Social Agenda or Hubris?" *Perspectives in Biology and Medicine* 37, no. 1 (1993): 3.

10. Edith Boyd, "The Weight of the Thymus Gland in Health and in Disease," *American Journal of Diseases of Children* 43, no. 5, part 1 (May 1932): 1163; Dally, "Status Lymphaticus," 76; Guntheroth, "The Thymus, Suffocation, and Sudden Infant Death Syndrome," 4, 6–7; Alton Goldbloom and F. W. Wiglesworth, "Sudden Death in Infancy," *Canadian Medical Association Journal* 38, no. 2 (February 1938): 119; Thomas Cone, *History of American Pediatrics* (Boston: Little, Brown, 1979), 193.

11. Quoted in Guntheroth, "The Thymus, Suffocation, and Sudden Infant Death Syndrome," 9.

12. The same motive was also true of SIDS.

Dally, "Status Lymphaticus," 70–71, 72; Guntheroth, "The Thymus, Suffocation, and Sudden Infant Death Syndrome," 6, 7; W. J. McCardie, "Status Lymphaticus in Relation to General Anaesthesia," *British Medical Journal* (January 1908): 196.

13. Guntheroth, "The Thymus, Suffocation, and Sudden Infant Death Syndrome," 7.

14. Charles A. Parker, "Surgery of the Thymus Gland. Thymectomy. Report of Fifty Operated Cases," *American Journal of Diseases of Children* 5, no. 2 (February 1913): 110, 121.

15. Dally, "Status Lymphaticus," 74, 77.

16. Boyd, "The Weight of the Thymus Gland," 1163; M. Todd Jacobs, Donald P. Frush, and Lane F. Donnelly, "The Right Place at the Wrong Time: Historical Perspective of the Relation of the Thymus Gland and Pediatric Radiology," *Radiology* 210, no. 1 (January 1999): 14.

17. Dally, "Status Lymphaticus," 78.

18. Reuben Peterson and Norman F. Miller, "Thymus of New-Born and Its Significance to the Obstetrician," *JAMA* 83, no. 4 (July 1924): 237, 238.

19. Enlarged thymuses were initially diagnosed through symptomology and percussion but then increasingly by X-ray.

Sidney Farber, "Fulminating Streptococcus Infections in Infancy as a Cause of Sudden Death," *New England Journal of Medicine* 211, no. 4 (July 1934): 158; Dally, "Status Lymphaticus," 79.

20. As two researchers stated, "What we have been regarding as a pathological entity under the name of status thymicolymphaticus is only an expression of the normal state of the lymphatic system in the well nourished actively growing child . . . in spite of repeated affirmation no proof has ever been brought forward that it is the cause of sudden death in infants."

Bergman, *The "Discovery" of Sudden Infant Death Syndrome*, 4; Boyd, "The Weight of the Thymus Gland," 1171; Goldbloom and Wiglesworth, "Sudden Death in Infancy," 120, footnote quote on 122; Dally, "Status Lymphaticus," 74.

21. Cone, *History of American Pediatrics*, 193.

22. Dally, "Status Lymphaticus," 80, 81; Herbert C. Archibald, "Sudden Unexplained Death in Childhood—Can It Be Prevented?" *Archives of Pediatrics* 59 (January 1942): 59.

23. Boyd, "The Weight of the Thymus Gland," 1207.

24. Edward H. Campbell, "Causes of Death in Status Lymphaticus," *American Journal of Diseases of Children* 44, no. 6 (December 1932): 1297.

25. Jesse L. Carr, "Status Thymico-Lymphaticus: Part I: Historical Background and Consideration of Normal Thymic Weight," *Journal of Pediatrics* 27, no. 1 (July 1945): 1; Archibald, "Sudden Unexplained Death in Childhood," 59.

26. Goldbloom and Wiglesworth, "Sudden Death in Infancy," 120, 122.

27. Dally, "Status Lymphaticus," 84, 83, 71.

28. J. Bruce Beckwith, "The Sudden Infant Death Syndrome," *Current Problems in Pediatrics* 3, no. 8 (June 1973): 9.

29. Siddhartha Mukherjee, *The Emperor of All Maladies: A Biography of Cancer* (New York: Scribner Books, 2010), 18, 19; John Craig, "Profiles in Pediatrics: Sidney Farber," *Journal of Pediatrics* 128, no. 1 (January 1996): 160.

30. Farber, "Fulminating Streptococcus Infections," 154, 156, 157.

31. Richard Smith, a physician in Boston, also called thymic death "an easy escape for us [pathologists] when a sudden death occurs which we cannot adequately explain." He challenged physicians to "stand up in our boots" and reject it.

Ibid., 156, 157, 158.

32. Ibid., 157, 158.

33. Gafafer lamented that "the references in the medical literature to this cause of death [AMS] are not as voluminous as might be thought. This is especially true," he noted, "with respect to articles with adequate statistical support." William M. Gafafer, "Time Changes in the Mortality from Accidental Mechanical Suffocation among Infants under 1 Year Old

in Different Geographic Regions of the United States, 1925–32: Studies on the Fatal Accidents of Childhood No. 4," *Public Health Reports (1896–1970)* 51, no. 48 (November 1936): 1641.

34. Ibid., 1644, 1646.

35. Harold Abramson, "Accidental Mechanical Suffocation in Infants," *Journal of Pediatrics* 25 (1944): 404, 405, 411.

36. The remaining 15 percent of cases were not associated with either supine or prone sleeping; the babies were found in an adult's bed and determined to have been "overlaid." Ibid., 410, quote from 404.

37. Ibid., 410–11.

38. Archibald, "Sudden Unexplained Death in Childhood," 57.

39. Paul V. Woolley, "Mechanical Suffocation During Infancy: A Comment on Its Relation to the Total Problem of Sudden Death," *Journal of Pediatrics* 26, no. 6 (June 1945): 572.

40. Ibid., 573.

41. Woolley identified this responsibility as "a duty secondary in importance only to saving the patient." Ibid., 572, 573.

42. Ibid., 573.

43. Bradley T. Thach, "Sudden Infant Death Syndrome: Old Causes Rediscovered?" *New England Journal of Medicine* 315, no. 2 (1986): 127; James S. Kemp and Bradley T. Thach, "Sudden Death in Infants Sleeping on Polystyrene-Filled Cushions," *New England Journal of Medicine* 324, no. 26 (June 1991): 1862.

44. Woolley, "Mechanical Suffocation During Infancy," 573, 575.

45. Valdes-Dapena, Marie, "Sudden and Unexpected Death in Infancy: A Review of the World Literature, 1954–1966," *Pediatrics* 39, no. 1 (January 1967): 129.

46. Susan Swoiskin, "Sudden Infant Death: Nursing Care for the Survivors," *Journal of Pediatric Nursing* 1, no. 1 (February 1986): 34.

47. Thach, "Sudden Infant Death Syndrome: Old Causes Rediscovered?" 127; Roger Byard and Henry Krous, eds., *Sudden Infant Death Syndrome: Problems, Progress and Possibilities* (New York: Oxford University Press, 2001), 142.

48. W. H. Davison, "Accidental Infant Suffocation," *British Medical Journal* 2, no. 4416 (August 1945): 251, 252.

49. Ibid., 251.

50. Ibid., 252.

51. David J. Rothman, *Strangers at the Bedside: A History of How Law and Bioethics Transformed Medical Decision Making* (New York: Basic Books, 1991), 122–23.

52. Allan Brandt and Martha Gardner, "The Golden Age of Medicine?" in *Companion to Medicine in the Twentieth Century*, ed. Roger Cooter and John Pickstone (London: Harwood Academic Publishers, 2000), 23–24, 28, 29.

53. Michael P. Johnson and Karl Hufbauer, "Sudden Infant Death Syndrome as a Medical Research Problem since 1945," *Social Problems* 30, no. 1 (October 1, 1982): 66.

54. Jacob Werne and Irene Garrow, "Sudden Deaths of Infants Allegedly Due to Mechanical Suffocation," *American Journal of Public Health* 37, no. 6 (June 1947): 675.

55. Ibid., 676, 677.

56. Ibid., 677, 683.

57. Ibid., 684, 675, 686.

58. "Sudden Death in Infancy," *The Lancet* 240, no. 6214 (October 1942): 403.

59. Letitia Fairfield, "Accidental Death from Suffocation in Infants," *Medico-Legal Journal* 16, no. 4 (1948): 146.

60. Savitt, "The Social and Medical History of Crib Death," 858.

61. "Proceedings: Conference on Sudden Death in Infancy," 1949, Adams Papers.
62. Ibid., 4, 14.
63. Ibid., 2, 3, 19, 18, 26.
64. Ibid., 20.
65. Ibid., 32.
66. Edith Stern, "Babies Don't Smother," *McCalls*, 1952, 44, 118, box 7, folder 14, Adelson Papers; Johnson and Hufbauer, "Sudden Infant Death Syndrome as a Medical Research Problem," 68.
67. Louise Bruner, "Babies Rarely Smother," *Today's Health*, July 1952, 72, box 7, folder 14, Adelson Papers.
68. "Infant Deaths from Suffocation," *JAMA* 142, no. 6 (April 1950): 1296–97.
69. Karl Hufbauer, "Federal Funding and Sudden Infant Death Research," *Social Studies of Science* 16, no. 1 (February 1986): 70–71.
70. Werne had signed off on a number of autopsies that had in fact been performed by others in his department. In the midst of his demise, Werne continued to propound that AMS was unjustified. Two years after his dismissal, Werne hanged himself on his bedroom door. Almost twenty years later, in 1978, a colleague remarked that Werne's suicide was rumored to have been "because nobody wanted to believe" his sudden infant death research. Jacob Werne and Irene Garrow, "Sudden Apparently Unexplained Death During Infancy: I. Pathologic Findings in Infants Found Dead," *American Journal of Pathology* 29, no. 4 (August 1953): 633; Jacob Werne and Irene Garrow, "Sudden Apparently Unexplained Death During Infancy: II. Pathologic Findings in Infants Observed to Die Suddenly," *American Journal of Pathology* 29, no. 5 (1953): 817; "City Is Investigating Autopsies in Queens," *New York Times*, October 27, 1953; "Autopsies Inquiry Is Made City-Wide," *New York Times*, November 3, 1953; "Jury Urges Shift in Autopsy Policy," *New York Times*, March 19, 1954; "Infant Deaths Analyzed: Medical Examiner Casts Doubt on Suffocation as Cause," *New York Times*, February 28, 1953; Colin Evans, *Blood on the Table: The Greatest Cases of New York City's Office of the Chief Medical Examiner* (New York: Berkeley, 2008), 101–2; John M. Adams, letter to the editor, November 21, 1978, 1, box 13, SIDS/Crib Death folder, Adams Papers.
71. David Dolinak and Elizabeth K. Balraj, "In Memoriam: Lester Adelson, MD (1914–2006)," *American Journal of Forensic Medicine and Pathology* 27, no. 3 (September 2006): 283.
72. James Weston, "Abstract: The Effects of SIDS Information and Counseling Projects on Medicolegal Death Investigative Studies" (Fourth National SIDS Conference: The Medico-Legal Aspects of SIDS—Approaches to a Death Investigation System via a SIDS Model, Minneapolis, 1980), 4, box 3, folder 4, WSIDSP Records.
73. Pathologists, especially in large metropolitan centers, dominated the first generation of sudden infant death experts—they were the physicians actually confronting cases. Alternative groups of doctors who might be interested, such as pediatricians or emergency room physicians, had less experience since most cases to which they would respond were already "over." Pathologists in smaller cities were also unlikely to encounter enough cases to either spark much interest or conduct research. Lester Adelson, "A Forensic Pathologist Looks at Sudden and Unexpected Death in Infancy and Childhood . . . A Personal Statement" (Research Conference on SIDS, Children's Hospital, Columbus, Ohio, September 1976), 2, 14, box 7, folder 1, Adelson Papers.
74. Lester Adelson, letter to Page Hudson, September 20, 1969, box 7, folder 5, Adelson Papers.
75. Lester Adelson and Eleanor Roberts Kinney, "Sudden and Unexpected Death in Infancy and Childhood," *Pediatrics* 17, no. 5 (1956): 663–64, 665.

76. Ibid., 694, 677.

77. Ibid., 694.

78. "'Suffocation' in Infancy," *The Lancet* 255, no. 6600 (February 1950): 357.

79. George J. Carroll, "Sudden Death in Infants," *Current Medical Digest*, January 1955, quote from 51; Keith Bowden, "Sudden Death or Alleged Accidental Suffocation in Babies," *Medical Journal of Australia* 1, no. 3 (January 1950): 71, 72.

80. "'Suffocation' in Infancy," *The Lancet* 255, no. 6600 (February 1950): 357.

81. Carroll, "Sudden Death in Infants," 409.

82. George J. Carroll, "Sudden Death in Infants," *The Journal of Pediatrics* 45, no. 4 (October 1954): 411.

83. Carroll, "Sudden Death in Infants," 51, 52.

84. C. P. Handforth, "Sudden Unexpected Death in Infants," *Canadian Medical Association Journal* 80 (June 1959): 872.

85. Ralph J. Wedgwood and Earl P. Benditt, eds., "Sudden Death in Infants: Proceedings of the Conference on Causes of Sudden Death in Infants," Public Health Service Publication No. 1412 (Conference on Causes of Sudden Death in Infants, Seattle, Washington: National Institute of Child Health and Human Development, 1963), 132.

86. Ibid., 86, 81.

87. Ibid., 70, 71.

88. Ibid., 127, 34.

89. Ibid., 11.

90. Ibid., 32.

91. Ibid., 37, 14–15.

92. Ibid., 14, 27.

93. Only 33 of 99 polled coroners' officers in London felt there was "any risk at all" that these children suffocated. Ibid., 140, 143.

94. Ibid., 11.

95. Bergman, Beckwith, and Ray, "Proceedings of the Second International Conference on Causes of Sudden Death in Infants," 47.

96. Analysis also indicated that a number of factors had no apparent association with SIDS, including parental age, sleep position, milk consumption, birth order, family illness, and familial medical history. Robert Strimer, Lester Adelson, and Robert Oseasohn, "Epidemiological Features of 1,134 Sudden, Unexpected Infant Deaths: A Study in the Greater Cleveland Area from 1956–1965," *JAMA* 209 (September 1969): 1497; Bergman, Beckwith, and Ray, "Proceedings of the Second International Conference on Causes of Sudden Death in Infants," 48–52, quote on 49.

97. Bergman, Beckwith, and Ray, "Proceedings of the Second International Conference on Causes of Sudden Death in Infants," 49; Strimer, Adelson, and Oseasohn, 1496, 1494; "Crib Death," *Medical World News*, October 7, 1966, 155, box 7, folder 7, Adelson Papers.

98. Strimer, Adelson, and Oseasohn, 1496.

99. National Foundation for Sudden Infant Death, "NFSID News Letter IV," Summer 1969, 1, box 12, file #1, Adams Papers.

100. Bergman, Beckwith, and Ray, "Proceedings of the Second International Conference," 3, ix.

101. Beckwith was referring to Students for a Democratic Society.

102. The absence of the term "unexplained" from the SIDS label did not sidestep this problem, since the notion that death must be unexplained was still embedded in the definition. Bergman, Beckwith, and Ray, "Proceedings of the Second International Conference," 14–16.

103. Ibid., 18.

104. Ibid., 40–41, 55, 64–66.

105. Valdes-Dapena, Marie et al., "Sudden Unexpected Death in Infancy: A Statistical Analysis of Certain Socioeconomic Factors," *Journal of Pediatrics* 73, no. 3 (1968): 388, 390.

106. National Foundation for Sudden Infant Death, "NFSID News Letter IV," Summer 1969, 3, box 12, file #1, Adams Papers.

107. Bergman, Beckwith, and Ray, "Proceedings of the Second International Conference," 216.

108. Bergman, Beckwith, and Ray, "Proceedings of the Second International Conference," 25–31, 73.

109. Ibid., 74–75.

110. Ibid., 83, 87, 120–21.

111. Ibid., 154, 157, 175.

112. Ibid., 210, 223.

113. Similar questions were apparently met with disdain in 1963. Warren Guntheroth commended his colleagues at the 1969 conference for cultivating a "much more congenial atmosphere than we had in 1963, when one of Dr. Wedgwood's compatriots got almost violent about the thought that this syndrome might be reversible." (Unfortunately, the 1963 proceedings give no hint as to this exchange.) Ibid., 199.

114. Ibid., 71, 210, 202–3.

115. Ibid., 210.

116. Adelson, "A Forensic Pathologist Looks at Sudden and Unexpected Death in Infancy and Childhood," 1.

CHAPTER 3   THE THEORY OF THE MONTH CLUB: CONDUCTING RESEARCH ON SIDS

1. "Sudden Death in Infancy," *Lancet* 2, no. 7681 (1970): 1021, 1022.

2. Subcommittee on Health and Subcommittee on Child and Youth, "Sudden Infant Death Syndrome," § Committee on Labor and Public Welfare (1973), 93rd Congress, First Session, 21.

3. Anne L. Wright, "Models of Mystery: Physician and Patient Perceptions of Sudden Infant Death Syndrome," *Social Science and Medicine* 26, no. 6 (1988): 589; for example, Clyde Chamberlain, "Sample Letter from Dane County Coroner," n.d., box 3, folder 2, WSIDSP Records; J. L. Emery, "Is Sudden Infant Death Syndrome a Diagnosis? Or Is It Just a Diagnostic Dustbin?" *British Medical Journal* 299 (1989): 1240.

4. U.S. Public Health Services, "Sudden Infant Death Syndrome," *Nosology Guidelines: Supplement to the Cause of Death Coding Manual*, April 1975, 2–4; "Nosology Guidelines: Supplement to the Cause-of-Death Coding Manual," Sudden Infant Death Syndrome (Rockville, MD: U.S. Department of Health, Education, and Welfare, April 1975), box 7, folder 14, Adelson Papers; Centers for Disease Control, "Perspectives in Disease Prevention and Health Promotion: Premature Mortality Due to Sudden Infant Death Syndrome," *CDC Morbidity and Mortality Weekly Report* 35, no. 11 (1986): 170; Centers for Disease Control, "Sudden Infant Death Syndrome: U.S., 1980–1988," *CDC Morbidity and Mortality Weekly Report* 41, no. 28 (July 1992): 515–17.

5. Nicholas Wade, "Crib Death: Foremost Baby Killer Long Ignored by Medical Research," *Science* 184, no. 4135 (April 1974): 447.

6. "1972: More Infants Lived, and Could Expect to Live Longer," *JAMA* 225, no. 6 (August 6, 1973): 568.

7. National Center for Chronic Disease Prevention and Health Promotion Division of Reproductive Health, Centers for Disease Control, "Achievements in Public Health, 1900–1999: Healthier Mothers and Babies," *CDC Morbidity and Mortality Weekly Report* 48, no. 38 (October 1999): 849–58.

8. Paul Starr, *The Social Transformation of American Medicine: The Rise of a Sovereign Profession and the Making of a Vast Industry* (New York: Basic Books, 1982), 335.

9. Wade, "Crib Death," 448; Michael P. Johnson and Karl Hufbauer, "Sudden Infant Death Syndrome as a Medical Research Problem since 1945," *Social Problems* 30, no. 1 (October 1, 1982): 75; J. Geoff Gregory, "Citation Study of a Scientific Revolution: Sudden Infant Death Syndrome," *Scientometrics*, 2, 3, 5 (1983): 323.

10. "Sleep Studies and Sudden Infant Death: Apnea Discoveries Stir Optimism in the Etiologic Quest," *Medical World News*, October 5, 1973, box 7, folder 7, Adelson Papers; Lester Adelson, "A Forensic Pathologist Looks at Sudden and Unexpected Death in Infancy and Childhood . . . A Personal Statement" (presented at the Research Conference on S.I.D.S., Children's Hospital, Columbus, Ohio, 1976), 9, box 7, folder 1, Adelson Papers.

11. Marie Valdes-Dapena, "Sudden and Unexpected Death in Infants: The Scope of Our Ignorance," *Pediatric Clinics of North America*, August 1963, 693.

12. The association between SIDS and feeding resurfaced decades later; in the twenty-first century, breastfeeding is an accepted strategy for reducing SIDS risk. See, for example, W. G. Guntheroth, "The Significance of Pulmonary Petechiae in Crib Death," *Pediatrics* 52, no. 4 (1973): 601; C. George Ray et al., "Studies of the Sudden Infant Death Syndrome in King County, Washington 1. The Role of Viruses," *JAMA* 211, no. 4 (January 1970): 619–23.

13. Clara Raven, "Sudden Infant Death Syndrome: An Epidemiologic Study," *Journal of the American Medical Women's Association* 29, no. 3 (March 1974): 131; John M. Adams, letter to the editor, November 21, 1978, box 13, SIDS/Crib Death folder, Adams Papers; John M. Adams, "Sudden Unexpected Death in Infants," n.d., 5–6, box 12, file #1, Adams Papers.

14. Raven, "Sudden Infant Death Syndrome," 131.

15. Joan L. Caddell et al., "The Magnesium Load Test: III. Correlation of Clinical and Laboratory Data in Infants from One to Six Months of Age," *Clinical Pediatrics* 14, no. 5 (May 1975): 478–84; D.F.L. Money, "Vitamin E and Selenium Deficiencies and Their Possible Etiological Role in the Sudden Death in Infants Syndrome," *Journal of Pediatrics* 77, no. 1 (1970): 165–66; "Doc Claims Vitamin C Can Eliminate Crib Deaths," *Midnight*, n.d., box 7, folder 7, Adelson Papers; "A Biochemist Links Crib Death to Low Level of Sugar in Blood," *New York Times*, July 5, 1975; Harold Schmeck, "Botulism Poisonings Are Linked to Several Cases of 'Crib Death,'" *New York Times*, June 20, 1977; Victor Cohn, "Risk of Botulism in Feeding Honey to Infants Under 1 Year," *Washington Post*, July 6, 1978; A.M.W. Porter, "Sudden and Unexpected Death in Infancy," *The Lancet* 296, no. 7687 (1970): 1358; Richard Naeye et al., "Selected Hormone Levels in Victims of the Sudden Infant Death Syndrome," *Pediatrics* 65, no. 6 (June 1980): 1134–36; "Crib Deaths Linked to Hormone Levels in Autopsy Study," *New York Times*, November 6, 1981; "Crib Death: A Piece of New Evidence," *Newsweek*, November 16, 1981; Cristine Russell, "Maryland Researchers Link Thyroid Hormone to 'Crib Death,'" *Washington Post*, November 7, 1981; Howard L. Golub and Michael Corwin, "Infant Cry: A Clue to Diagnosis," *Pediatrics* 69, no. 2 (February 1982): 197–201; Virginia Adams, "Babies' Cries Viewed as Clues to Diseases," *New York Times*, June 13, 1979.

16. Donald R. Peterson, "Sudden Unexpected Deaths in Infants: Incidence in Two Climatically Dissimilar Metropolitan Communities," *American Journal of Epidemiology* 95, no. 2 (February 1972): 98; Mark A. Greenberg, Kenrad E. Nelson, and Bertram W. Carnow, "A Study

of the Relationship Between Sudden Infant Death Syndrome and Environmental Factors," *American Journal of Epidemiology* 98, no. 6 (1973): 412–22.

17. Wyeth recalled the rest of vaccination lot 64201 in response to an FDA request. As David Geier and Mark Geier describe, drug companies learned from the situation and "took measures of their own to ensure against future recalls. After the Tennessee incident, pertussis manufacturers arranged that entire lots would never again be sent to single areas of the country . . . The small lot plan meant that no one region of the country would have enough adverse reactions to a single lot of whole-cell pertussis vaccine to alert the clinicians in that region to the fact that they were using a highly reactogenic lot." Geraldine Norris, "Memorandum to SIDS Information and Counseling Projects on SIDS Episodes and DPT Immunization," April 20, 1979, box 1, folder 13, WSIDSP Records; "Vaccine for Infant Recalled After Deaths of 4 Babies," *New York Times*, March 22, 1979; "Four Infants' Deaths Probed," *Washington Post*, April 27, 1979; Richard Naeye, "Sudden Infant Death Syndrome, Is the Confusion Ending?" *Modern Pathology* 1, no. 3 (1988): 172; David Geier and Mark Geier, "A True Story of Pertussis Vaccination: A Sordid Legacy?" *Journal of the History of Medicine* 57 (July 2002): 271.

18. Roger H. Bernier et al., "Diphteria-Tetanus Toxoids-Pertussis Vaccination and Sudden Infant Deaths in Tennessee," *Journal of Pediatrics* 101, no. 3 (September 1982): 420–21.

19. James D. Cherry, "Historical Review of Pertussis and the Classical Vaccine," *Journal of Infectious Diseases* 174, supplement 3 (1996): S260–61.

20. Geier and Geier, "A True Story of Pertussis Vaccination," 258, 259, 260.

21. Arthur Allen, *Vaccine: The Controversial Story of Medicine's Greatest Lifesaver* (New York: W. W. Norton, 2007), 258–61; Elena Conis, *Vaccine Nation: America's Changing Relationship with Immunization* (Chicago: University of Chicago Press, 2015), 94–95.

22. Geier and Geier, "A True Story of Pertussis Vaccination," 258, 259, 260.

23. Ibid., 260.

24. T. Allen Merritt and Marie Valdes-Dapena, "SIDS Research Update," *Pediatric Annals* 13, no. 3 (March 1984): 194–95; Centers for Disease Control, "DTP Vaccination and Sudden Infant Deaths—Tennessee," *Morbidity and Mortality Weekly Report* 28, no. 11 (March 23, 1979): 131; "North Eastern Ohio Chapter of the National Sudden Infant Death Syndrome Foundation, Statement of Medical Research Board of the NSIDSF," n.d., Adelson Papers, box 7, folder 6, Dittrick Archives; Cristine Russell, "Doctors Challenge Evidence Connecting Crib Death, Shots," *Washington Post*, May 1, 1982.

25. Geier and Geier, "A True Story of Pertussis Vaccination," 272; Allen, *Vaccine*, 251, 255.

26. Cherry, "Historical Review," S261.

27. Paul S. Pierson, Patricia Howard, and Herbert Kleber, "Sudden Deaths in Infants Born to Methadone-Maintained Addicts," *JAMA* 220, no. 13 (June 1972): 1733–34; Abraham Bergman and Lisa A. Wiesner, "Relationship of Passive Cigarette-Smoking to Sudden Infant Death Syndrome," *Pediatrics* 58, no. 5 (November 1976): 665, 667; Marie Valdes-Dapena, "The Pathologist and the Sudden Infant Death Syndrome," *American Journal of Pathology* 106, no. 1 (January 1982): 127.

28. Gary A. Giovino, "Epidemiology of Tobacco Use in the United States," *Oncogene* 21, no. 48 (2002): 7330, 7333; David E. Nelson et al., "Cigarette Smoking Prevalence by Occupation in the United States: A Comparison Between 1978 to 1980 and 1987 to 1990," *Journal of Occupational Medicine* 36, no. 5 (1994): 518.

29. Valdes-Dapena, "The Pathologist and the Sudden Infant Death Syndrome," 127; Bengt Haglung and Sven Cnattingius, "Cigarette Smoking as a Risk Factor for Sudden Infant Death Syndrome: A Population-Based Study," *American Journal of Public Health* 80, no. 1 (January 1990): 29–31; Michael H. Malloy, Howard J. Hoffman, and Donald R. Peterson, "Sudden

Infant Death Syndrome and Maternal Smoking," *American Journal of Public Health* 82, no. 10 (October 1992): 1380–82; Kenneth C. Schoendorf and John L. Kiely, "Relationship of Sudden Infant Death Syndrome to Maternal Smoking During and After Pregnancy," *Pediatrics* 90, no. 6 (December 1992): 905.

30. Leslie Reagan, *Dangerous Pregnancies: Mothers, Disabilities, and Abortion in Modern America* (Berkeley: University of California Press, 2010); Janet Golden, *Message in a Bottle: The Making of Fetal Alcohol Syndrome* (Cambridge: Harvard University Press, 2005); Jane Brody, "Personal Health," *New York Times*, January 6, 1982.

31. U.S. Department of Health and Human Services, "The Health Consequences of Smoking—50 Years of Progress: A Report of the Surgeon General" (Atlanta: U.S. Department of Health and Human Services, Centers for Disease Control and Prevention, National Center for Chronic Disease Prevention and Health Promotion, Office on Smoking and Health, 2014), 84, 86; Joel Greenberg, "U.S. Advises Total Abstinence From Drinking for Pregnant Women," *New York Times*, July 18, 1981; "Study Says Smoking Perils Baby Even if Halted before Pregnancy," *New York Times*, January 17, 1979; "Bad News for Women Smokers," *Newsweek*, January 28, 1980; "Prenatal Factors in Crib Death," *New York Times*, June 29, 1982.

32. Peter Lyons and Barbara Rittner, "The Construction of the Crack Babies Phenomenon as a Social Problem," *American Journal of Orthopsychiatry* 68, no. 2 (April 1998): 313–20.

33. Todd Rosen and Helen L. Johnson, "Drug-Addicted Mothers, Their Infants, and SIDS," *Annals of the New York Academy of Sciences* 533 (August 1988): 89, 93.

34. Sally L. Davison Ward et al., "Sudden Infant Death Syndrome in Infants of Substance-Abusing Mothers," *Journal of Pediatrics* 117, no. 6 (December 1990): 878–79.

35. In the 1950s, Pickwickian syndrome was largely treated as a symptom of obesity. Robert W. Clark and Helmut S. Schmidt, "Sleep Apnea: Neurological and Neuro Endocrinological Aspects of SIDS" (Research Conference on SIDS, Children's Hospital, Columbus, Ohio, 1976), 37, box 7, folder 1, Adelson Papers.

36. Amy Olson and Clifford Zwillich, "The Obesity Hypoventilation Syndrome," *American Journal of Medicine* 118 (2005): 948–49; Matthew J. Wolf-Meyer, *The Slumbering Masses: Sleep, Medicine, and Modern American Life* (Minneapolis: University of Minnesota Press, 2012), 28, 40.

37. John W. Shepard et al., "History of the Development of Sleep Medicine in the United States," *Journal of Clinical Sleep Medicine* 1, no. 1 (January 2005): 6, 11, 37.

38. Abraham Bergman, J. Bruce Beckwith, and C. George Ray, eds., *Sudden Infant Death Syndrome: Proceedings of the Second International Conference on Causes of Sudden Death in Infants* (Children's Orthopedic Hospital and Medical Center and University of Washington School of Medicine, Seattle: University of Washington Press, 1969), 182–83, 193.

39. Three babies were referred for apnea and two siblings were then incorporated into the group.

40. Alfred Steinschneider, "Prolonged Apnea and the Sudden Infant Death Syndrome: Clinical and Laboratory Observations," *Pediatrics* 50, no. 4 (October 1972): 651–52, 647.

41. Ibid., 652, 646; J. Bruce Beckwith, "The Sudden Infant Death Syndrome" (Rockville, MD: U.S. Department of Health, Education, and Welfare, 1976), 26, box 7, folder 4, Adelson Papers; Alfred Steinschneider, "Nasopharyngitis and Prolonged Sleep Apnea," *Pediatrics* 56, no. 6 (December 1975): 967–71.

42. Journalists Richard Firstman and Jamie Talan document this fascinating episode in detail (though, regrettably, without detailed citations). Richard Firstman and Jamie Talan, *The Death of Innocents: A True Story of Murder, Medicine, and High-Stakes Science* (New York: Bantam Books, 1997); William J. R. Daily, Marshall Klaus, and H. Belton P. Meyer, "Apnea

in Premature Infants: Monitoring, Incidence, Heart Rate Changes, and an Effect of Environmental Temperature," *Pediatrics* 43, no. 4 (April 1969): 516; Ruthmary Deuel, "Polygraphic Monitoring of Apneic Spells," *Archives of Neurology* 28, no. 2 (February 1973): 74.

43. In his analysis in 1983, Geoff Gregory observed that this "level of citations was many times what would be expected" for *Pediatrics*. Gregory, "Citation Study of a Scientific Revolution." Abraham Bergman, "Wrong Turns in Sudden Infant Death Syndrome Research," *Pediatrics* 99, no. 1 (January 1997): 119; Gregory, "Citation Study of a Scientific Revolution," 319.

44. Deuel, "Polygraphic Monitoring of Apneic Spells," 76, 74.

45. According to one article, a normal three-month-old baby would experience some eighty breathing pauses during every one hundred minutes, most of which lasted less than ten seconds. Toke Hoppenbrouwers et al., "Polygraphic Studies of Normal Infants During the First Six Months of Life: III. Incidence of Apnea and Periodic Breathing," *Pediatrics* 60, no. 4 (October 1977): 418, 425; "Sleep Apnoea in Children," *British Medical Journal* 1, no. 6126 (June 1978): 1506.

46. J. L. Unger, "Sudden Death Syndrome: Recurrent Apnea," *Journal of the Kansas Medical Society* 75, no. 4 (1974): 122.

47. Matt Clark, "Clues to Crib Death," *Newsweek*, January 5, 1976, 53.

48. "Abstract of Presentation to Council of Chapter Presidents NFSID," March 18, 1976, 1, box 1, folder 19, WSIDSP Records.

49. Contemporary experts recognized and highlighted this reappraisal. In 1983, J. G. Gregory completed a fascinating citation review study of SIDS. He contextualized this major shift in SIDS research as an example of a Kuhnian scientific revolution, because the prevailing paradigm of normality was upset and replaced. (Gregory described the replacement paradigm as the "respiratory abnormality paradigm.") He argued that the transition occurred "through the sleep apnea hypothesis." Marie Valdes-Dapena, "Sudden Unexplained Infant Death, 1970 Through 1975: An Evolution in Understanding," *Pathology Annual* 12, no. 1 (1977): 117; Richard Naeye, "The Sudden Infant Death Syndrome: A Review of Recent Advances," *Archives of Pathology and Laboratory Medicine* 101, no. 4 (April 1977): 165; Gregory, "Citation Study of a Scientific Revolution," 314, 325.

50. "Final Report of a Study: 'The Management of Sudden Infant Death Syndrome (SIDS) in the United States,'" in "Sudden Infant Death Syndrome," pub. L, no. 93–56, § Subcommittee on Public Health and Environment of the Committee on Interstate and Foreign Commerce (1973), 61.

51. Eileen Hasselmeyer and Jehu Hunter, "The Sudden Infant Death Syndrome," *Obstetrics and Gynecology Annual* 4 (1975): 229.

52. "Final Report of a Study," in "Sudden Infant Death Syndrome," 71–72.

53. "Rights of Children, Part 1: Examination of the Sudden Infant Death Syndrome," § Subcommittee on Children and Youth of the Committee on Labor and Public Welfare (1972), 17.

54. Council on Scientific Affairs, "Autopsy: A Comprehensive Review of Current Issues," *JAMA* 258, no. 3 (July 1987): 364, 366; Edwin Diamond, "Are We Ready to Leave Our Bodies to the Next Generation?" *New York Times*, April 21, 1968.

55. Illinois Sudden Infant Death Syndrome Commission, "Infant Survival: 'New Hope for the Family . . . ,'" Report and Recommendation of the Sudden Infant Death Syndrome (SIDS) Study Commission of the State of Illinois to the Members of the 78th General Assembly (Illinois, 1974), Appendix II, Figure 6a, Loose Materials, Sudden Infant Death Syndrome Study Commission, "Administrative Files," Record Series 572.001, Illinois State Archives (hereafter, Illinois SIDS Commission Records); "Final Report of a Study," in "Sudden Infant Death Syndrome," 62.

56. "Final Report of a Study," in "Sudden Infant Death Syndrome," 75; "Until Crib Death Problem Is Solved, Victims' Parents Need More Help," *JAMA* 226, no. 11 (December 10, 1973): 1299.

57. "Rights of Children, Part 1," 72.

58. Noel S. Weiss, Delray Green, and Dean E. Krueger, "Problems in the Use of Death Certificates to Identify Sudden Unexpected Infant Deaths," *Health Services Reports* 88, no. 6 (July 1973): 555–58.

59. "Sudden Infant Death Syndrome," pub. L, no. 93–56, § Subcommittee on Public Health and Environment of the Committee on Interstate and Foreign Commerce (1973), 55.

60. Burt A. Folkart and Robert W. Welkos, "Dr. Theodore Curphey Dies; 1st County Doctor-Coroner," *Los Angeles Times*, December 3, 1986.

61. "Grand Jury Will Investigate Coroner's Office Next Week: Decision Welcomed by Curphey," *Los Angeles Times*, November 20, 1958.

62. Theodore J. Curphey, "Curriculum Vitae," n.d., 3–4, box 17, folder 7, Theodore J. Curphey Papers, Huntington Library, San Marino, California (hereafter, Curphey Papers).

63. Although it was not accepted for publication, Curphey's study suggested that deaths were the result of interrelated breakdowns in the respiratory and cardiac systems. Theodore J. Curphey, "Cardiac Fuchsinophilia in Sudden Deaths in Children," 1964, 12, box 17, folder 2, Curphey Papers.

64. Paul F. Wehrle, "Joint Public Health Committee American Academy of Pediatrics Southern California Chapter and Los Angeles Pediatric Society, Minutes," July 22, 1964, box 17, folder 7, Curphey Papers; "Minutes of Meeting of Planning Group for Studies of Sudden Deaths in Infants and Children," June 21, 1964, 2–3, box 17, folder 7, Curphey Papers; Gerald Lieberman et al., "Abstract Reproduction: An Epidemiologic Study of Sudden Death in Infancy," 1965, box 17, folder 7, Curphey Papers.

65. Beryl S. Graham, letter to Theodore Curphey, June 28, 1962, box 16, folder 3, Curphey Papers.

66. National Foundation for Sudden Infant Death, "National Foundation for Sudden Infant Death (SID) Epidemiological Investigation," March 1967, box 17, folder 3, Curphey Papers.

67. Margaret R. Pomeroy, "Sudden Death Syndrome," *American Journal of Nursing* 69, no. 9 (September 1969): 1866.

68. Only two families declined home visits. Ibid., 1888.

69. Beyond the presumption of smothering or suffocation, other typical misconceptions included that the child had choked on its own aspirated vomit and that the child was ill and could have been saved if he had visited a doctor. Alternatively, if the child had seen a doctor, some parents were concerned the physician had "missed something." Ibid., 1887–88.

70. J. Bruce Beckwith, *The Sudden Infant Death Syndrome* (Rockville, MD: U.S. Department of Health, Education, and Welfare, 1976), 29, box 7, folder 4, Adelson Papers.

71. Marie Valdes-Dapena, "Sudden, Unexpected and Unexplained Death in Infancy—A Status Report, 1973," *New England Journal of Medicine* 289, no. 22 (November 1973): 1196.

72. J. Bruce Beckwith, "The Sudden Infant Death Syndrome," *Current Problems in Pediatrics* 3, no. 8 (June 1973): 31.

73. Jane Brody, "Personal Health," *New York Times*, March 29, 1978.

74. "Notes, Milwaukee County PH Nursing Seminar," September 4, 1980, box 2, folder 19, WSIDSP Records.

75. Sandy Rovner, "SIDS: Overcoming the Sense of Blame," *Washington Post*, November 20, 1985.

76. Morris Green, "Psychological Aspects of Sudden Unexpected Death in Infants and Children: Review and Commentary," *Pediatric Clinics of North America* 21, no. 1 (1974): 114.

77. Abraham Bergman, "Sudden Infant Death Syndrome," *Postgraduate Medicine* 51, no. 7 (June 1972): 156.
78. Committee on Infant and Preschool Child, "The Sudden Infant Death Syndrome," *Pediatrics* 50, no. 6 (December 1972): 964.
79. Robert A. Hoekelman, "A New Perspective on Sudden Infant Death Syndrome," *American Journal of Diseases of Children* 130, no. 11 (November 1976): 1191–92.
80. Abraham Bergman, "Psychological Aspects of Sudden Unexpected Death in Infants and Children: Review and Commentary," *Pediatric Clinics of North America* 21, no. 1 (February 1974): 118–19.
81. Colin Parkes Murray, "Grief: Lessons from the Past, Visions for the Future," *Psychologica Belgica* 50, no. 1 and 2 (2010): 9–10; Elizabeth A. Doughty and Wendy J. Hoskins, "Death Education: An Internationally Relevant Approach to Grief Counseling," *Journal for International Counselor Education* 3 (2011): 26–27; Berthold P. R. Gersons and Ingrid V. E. Carlier, "Post-Traumatic Stress Disorder: The History of a Recent Concept," *British Journal of Psychiatry* 161 (1992): 745–46; Elisabeth Kübler-Ross, *On Death and Dying: What the Dying Have to Teach Doctors, Nurses, Clergy, and Their Own Families* (New York: Scribner, 1969).
82. Zoe Smialek, "Observations on Immediate Reactions of Families to Sudden Infant Death," *Pediatrics* 62, no. 2 (August 1978): 161; Harold J. May and Frederick J. Breme, "SIDS Family Adjustment Scale: A Method of Assessing Family Adjustment to Sudden Infant Death Syndrome," *Omega: Journal of Death and Dying* 13, no. 1 (1982): 61–62.
83. Abraham Bergman, "Sudden Infant Death Syndrome," *American Family Physician* 8, no. 1 (July 1973): 100.
84. Ruth Maxwell, Lewis H. Roht, and Paul Callen, "Incidence of Sudden Infant Death Syndrome in Texas, 1969–1972; Estimation by the Surrogate Method," *Texas Medicine* 72 (October 1976): 58.
85. Stanford Friedman, "Psychological Aspects of Sudden Unexpected Death in Infants and Children," *Pediatric Clinics of North America* 21, no. 1 (February 1974): 105.
86. David A. Baptiste, "Time-Elapsed Marital and Family Therapy with Sudden Infant Death Syndrome Families," *Family Systems Medicine* 1, no. 3 (1983): 47; Bradley H. Zebal and Susan F. Woolsey, "SIDS and the Family: The Pediatrician's Role," *Pediatric Annals* 13, no. 3 (March 1984): 238.
87. Lee Salk, "Sudden Infant Death: Impact on Family and Physician," *Clinical Pediatrics* 10, no. 5 (1971): 248.
88. Lester Adelson quoted in Inette Miller Conte, "Doctors Probe Babies' Crib Deaths," *Cleveland Press*, n.d., box 7, folder 6, Adelson Papers.
89. Ralph Franciosi, "Sudden Infant Death Syndrome," *Minnesota Medicine* 58, no. 9 (September 1975): 683.
90. Dorte M. Christiansen, Ask Elklit, and Miranda Olff, "Parents Bereaved by Infant Death: PTSD Symptoms up to 18 Years after the Loss," *General Hospital Psychiatry* 35 (2013): 606, 608–9.
91. Pomeroy, "Sudden Death Syndrome," 1889.
92. Abraham Bergman, "Sudden Infant Death Syndrome: An Approach to Management," *Primary Care* 3, no. 1 (March 1976): 5.
93. These effects could extend beyond the immediate family, to babysitters and physicians. Sharon Aadalen, "Coping with Sudden Infant Death Syndrome: Intervention Strategies and a Case Study," *Family Relations* 29, no. 4 (October 1980): 587; Baptiste, "Time-Elapsed Marital and Family Therapy," 56; Pomeroy, "Sudden Death Syndrome," 1888; quote from "North Eastern Ohio Chapter of the National Sudden Infant Death Syndrome Foundation Newsletter,"

Spring 1986, box 7, folder 12, Adelson Papers; Salk, "Sudden Infant Death," 249; Frederick Mandell, Mary McClain, and Robert Reece, "Sudden and Unexpected Death: The Pediatrician's Response," *Archives of Pediatric and Adolescent Medicine* 141, no. 7 (1987): 748–50; Gertrude R. Friedman, Ralph Franciosi, and Robert M. Drake, "The Effects of Observed Sudden Infant Death Syndrome (SIDS) on Hospital Staff," *Pediatrics* 64, no. 4 (October 1979): 538, 540.

94. For example, see "Seminar on SIDS" (Rockville, MD: U.S. Department of Health, Education, and Welfare, Public Health Service, Maternal and Child Health Service, March 1973), 3, box 7, folder 6, Adelson Papers; Bergman, "Sudden Infant Death Syndrome: An Approach to Management," 6; May and Breme, "SIDS Family Adjustment Scale," 64; Baptiste, "Time-Elapsed Marital and Family Therapy," 56; Linda A. Chernus, "Marital Treatment Following Early Infant Death," *Clinical Social Work Journal* 10, no. 1 (1982): 28–38; Victoria Lee Judson, "The Effects of Sudden Infant Death Syndrome" (University of Texas at Arlington, School of Social Work, Thesis, 1987); Carolyn Szybist, "Autobiography" (college course paper requirement, National Louis University, Evanston, Illinois, Fall 1979), 11–12; Coleman McCarthy, "Neither Predictable Nor Preventable: The Sudden Infant Death Mystery," *Washington Post*, December 31, 1971; Janet Michel Nakushian, "Restoring Parents' Equilibrium after Sudden Infant Death," *American Journal of Nursing* 76, no. 10 (October 1976): 1604.

95. "Presentation for Wisconsin SIDS Program," October 1979, 3, box 1, folder 9, WSIDSP Records.

96. "Sudden Infant Death Syndrome: Joint Hearing before Certain Subcommittees of the Committee on Post Office and Civil Service and the Committee on Energy and Commerce and the Select Committee on Children, Youth, and Families," § House of Representatives, Congress (1985), 97, 100.

97. One dissenting paper reported that based on a survey of seventy-five SIDS mothers in Oklahoma, more than half described "increased marital closeness during the period after the death of their child." Max Price et al., "Maternal Perceptions of Sudden Infant Death Syndrome," *Children's Health Care* 14, no. 1 (1985): 26; Marion Steinman, "Crib Death: Too Many Clues?" *New York Times*, May 16, 1976; Pat Hensel, "Infant Death: A Mystery," *Milwaukee Journal*, October 14, 1979, box 1, folder 1, WSIDSP Records; Judy Klemesrud, "A Tragedy with an Aftermath of Guilt," *New York Times*, June 19, 1972; "Sudden Infant Death Syndrome," pub. L, 10; Pat Valenta, "Letter of Support, Wisconsin SIDS Project Progress Report," January 1981, box 1, folder 1, WSIDSP Records; Marilyn Kirk, "National Sudden Infant Death Syndrome Minnesota Chapter," n.d., 1, box 1, folder 19, WSIDSP Records; National Sudden Infant Death Syndrome Foundation, Minnesota Chapter, "Minnesota S.I.D.S. Newsletter," vol. 1, no. 2 (May 1981), 1, box 2, folder 26, WSIDSP Records; National Sudden Infant Death Syndrome Foundation, Southeastern Wisconsin Chapter, "National Sudden Infant Death Syndrome Foundation, Southeastern Wisconsin Chapter: Newsletter," Summer 1982, 3, box 1, folder 6, WSIDSP Records; Janice Mendoza, letter to Beryl Graham, August 17, 1962, box 16, folder 3, Curphey Papers; Szybist, "Autobiography."

98. For example, see Pomeroy, "Sudden Death Syndrome," 1888; Janice Greene, "Killer Disease: Sudden Infant Death Syndrome," *Nursing Care* 8, no. 4 (April 1975): 20; Jehu Hunter, "Fact Sheet: What Is SIDS?" (National Institute of Child Health and Development & SIDS Clearinghouse, n.d.), box 1, folder 6, WSIDSP Records; "Facts about Sudden Infant Death Syndrome" (U.S. Department of Health, Education, and Welfare, Public Health Service, National Institutes of Health, n.d.), 7–8, box 12, file #1, Adams Papers.

99. Pomeroy, "Sudden Death Syndrome," 1889.

100. Bergman, "Sudden Infant Death Syndrome: An Approach to Management," 6; Margaret Pomeroy, "The Nurse's Visit to SIDS Families," ed. J. Bruce Beckwith (National

Foundation for Sudden Infant Death Syndrome, n.d.), 1, box 2, folder 18, WSIDSP Records; Sally M. Nikolaisen and Reg Arthur Williams, "Parent's View of Support Following the Loss of Their Infant to Sudden Infant Death Syndrome," *Western Journal of Nursing Research* 2, no. 3 (1980): 594.

101. Frederick Mandell, Elizabeth McAnulty, and Robert M. Reece, "Observations of Paternal Response to Sudden Unanticipated Infant Death," *Pediatrics* 65, no. 2 (February 1980): 222, 224.

102. Baptiste, "Time-Elapsed Marital and Family Therapy," 53–54.

103. Nakushian, "Restoring Parents' Equilibrium," 1604.

104. "Evaluation of SIDS Workshop," October 3, 1979, box 1, folder 9, WSIDSP Records.

105. Ibid.

106. M.J.J. O'Reilly and M. K. While, "Clinical Insights in Pediatrics: Sudden Death Syndrome," July 13, 1968, box 12, file #1, Adams Papers.

107. Robert R. Robinson, ed., *SIDS 1974: Proceedings of the Francis E. Camps International Symposium on Sudden and Unexpected Deaths in Infancy* (Toronto: Canadian Foundation for the Study of Infant Deaths, 1974), xix.

108. "Ohio Chapter: National Sudden Infant Death Syndrome Foundation Newsletter," Spring 1980, 1, box 7, folder 2, Adelson Papers.

109. Quoted in D. L. Russell-Jones, "Sudden Infant Death in History and Literature," *Archives of Disease in Childhood* 60 (1985): 280.

110. Lester Adelson, "A Forensic Pathologist Looks at Sudden and Unexpected Death in Infancy and Childhood . . . A Personal Statement" (Research Conference on SIDS, Children's Hospital, Columbus, Ohio, 1976), 15.

111. Robinson, *SIDS 1974*, 341.

112. Ibid., 65, 66.

CHAPTER 4   RISKY BABIES

1. "Sudden Infant Death Syndrome: Joint Hearing Before Certain Subcommittees of the Committee on Post Office and Civil Service and the Committee on Energy and Commerce and the Select Committee on Children, Youth, and Families," § House of Representatives, Congress (1985), (hereafter, SIDS Joint Hearing 1985) 14.

2. Marie Valdes-Dapena, "Can Crib Death Be Prevented?" *Journal of Forensic Sciences* 24, no. 3 (July 1979): 539; Marie Valdes-Dapena, "Abstract: Up-Date SIDS Research" (presented at the Fourth National SIDS Conference: The Medico-Legal Aspects of SIDS—Approaches to a Death Investigation System via a SIDS Model, Minneapolis, 1980), 1, box 2, folder 4, WSIDSP Records.

3. D. A. Smith, "Sudden Infant Death Syndrome—A Valid Diagnosis?" *Medical Hypotheses* 36 (1991): 183.

4. Naeye's control group consisted of seventy-five infants accidentally killed. He found that "the pulmonary arteries of SIDS babies were thicker; the periadrenal tissue of SIDS babies showed more brown fat; the liver of SIDS babies contained more red blood cells; and the muscle of the right ventricle was thicker in SIDS victims." Additionally, Naeye found that "infants who became SIDS victims had lower Apgar scores, more neurologic and feeding difficulty and more respiratory distress during the neonatal period than infants dying from other causes." Richard Naeye, "Pulmonary Arterial Abnormalities in the Sudden-Infant-Death Syndrome," *New England Journal of Medicine* 289, no. 22 (November 1973): 1167; "Abstract of Presentation to Council of Chapter Presidents NFSID," March 18, 1976, 1, box 1, folder 19,

WSIDSP Records, box 1, folder 19; "Differences Seen in Infant Victims: Studies Link Sudden Deaths in Heart, Blood Cell Production," *New York Times*, March 20, 1976; "Research Planning Workshops on the Sudden Infant Death Syndrome: 12. Metabolic Factors" (Bethesda, MD: National Institute of Child Health and Human Development, Perinatal Biology and Infant Mortality Branch, U.S. Department of Health, Education, and Welfare, March 1976), 4, 6; Ruth Maxwell, Lewis H. Roht, and Paul Callen, "Incidence of Sudden Infant Death Syndrome in Texas, 1969–1972; Estimation by the Surrogate Method," *Texas Medicine* 72 (October 1976): 61.

5. Robert A. Hoekelman, "A New Perspective on Sudden Infant Death Syndrome," *American Journal of Diseases of Children* 130, no. 11 (November 1976): 1191; J. Geoff Gregory, "Citation Study of a Scientific Revolution: Sudden Infant Death Syndrome," *Scientometrics* 5 (1983): 314.

6. Marie Valdes-Dapena, "Sudden Unexplained Infant Death, 1970 Through 1975: An Evolution in Understanding," *Pathology Annual* 12, no. 1 (1977): 120.

7. Quoted in "Differences Seen in Infant Victims: Studies Link Sudden Deaths in Heart, Blood Cell Production," *New York Times*, March 20, 1976.

8. Richard Naeye, "The Sudden Infant Death Syndrome: A Review of Recent Advances," *Archives of Pathology and Laboratory Medicine* 101, no. 4 (April 1977): 165.

9. This was not new in the 1970s—it simply gained a more general following. In 1956, Lester Adelson had suggested that "hunting for one abnormality" was a gross "oversimplification." Multifactorial causation was also a leading topic of discussion at the 1969 conference in Seattle. Saul and Sylvia Goldberg, parent-founders of the Guild for Infant Survival, even explained after the meeting that "no single factor seems to be the answer for sudden infant death. Most of those present agree that a combination of several factors acting under a certain set of circumstances could result in sudden infant death." Lester Adelson and Eleanor Roberts Kinney, "Sudden and Unexpected Death in Infancy and Childhood," *Pediatrics* 17, no. 5 (1956): 685; Guild for Infant Survival, "Report on Second International Conference on Sudden Death Syndrome of Infancy" (Baltimore, MD, 1969), box 7, folder 6, Adelson Papers.

10. J. Bruce Beckwith, "The Sudden Infant Death Syndrome," *Current Problems in Pediatrics* 3, no. 8 (June 1973): 30.

11. Toke Hoppenbrouwers et al., "Sudden Infant Death Syndrome: Sleep Apnea and Respiration in Subsequent Siblings," *Pediatrics* 66, no. 2 (August 1980): 213.

12. Marie Valdes-Dapena, "Sudden Infant Death Syndrome: Morphology Update for Forensic Pathologists—1985," *Forensic Science International* 30 (1986): 184.

13. Carl E. Hunt and Robert T. Brouillette, "Sudden Infant Death Syndrome: 1987 Perspective," *Journal of Pediatrics* 110, no. 5 (May 1987): 670; quote from "Science Watch: Sudden Infant Death," *New York Times*, April 3, 1979.

14. Naeye, "The Sudden Infant Death Syndrome: A Review of Recent Advances," 165; Gregory, "Citation Study of a Scientific Revolution," 324.

15. "Younger" mothers indicated women who birthed their first child before turning twenty. Ruth E. Little and Donald R. Peterson, "Sudden Infant Death Syndrome Epidemiology: A Review and Update," *Epidemiologic Reviews* 12 (1990): 243, 244; The Centers for Disease Control, "Sudden Infant Death Syndrome: United States, 1983–1994," *Morbidity and Mortality Weekly Report* 45, no. 40 (October 11, 1996): 859–63; Dorothy Kelly and Daniel C. Shannon, "Sudden Infant Death Syndrome and Near Sudden Infant Death Syndrome: A Review of the Literature, 1964 to 1982," *Pediatric Clinics of North America* 29, no. 5 (October 1982): 1241, 1243, 1245; Roger Byard and Henry Krous, "Sudden Infant Death Syndrome: Overview and Update," *Pediatric and Developmental Pathology* 6 (2003): 113–14.

16. The scale individually weighted and combined scores from eight factors: (1) mother's age, (2) mother's number of previous pregnancies, (3) duration of the mother's second-stage labor, (4) mother's blood group, (5) baby's weight, (6) whether the baby was a twin, (7) whether the baby was bottle- or breastfed, and (8) whether the mother ever experienced a urinary tract infection during her pregnancy. R. G. Carpenter et al., "Prevention of Unexpected Infant Death: Evaluation of the First Seven Years of the Sheffield Intervention Programme," *The Lancet* 321, no. 8327 (April 1983): 723–24; Robert R. Robinson, ed., *SIDS 1974: Proceedings of the Francis E. Camps International Symposium on Sudden and Unexpected Deaths in Infancy* (Toronto: Canadian Foundation for the Study of Infant Deaths, 1974), 98–99, 100, 105.

17. Carpenter et al., "Prevention of Unexpected Infant Death: Evaluation of the First Seven Years of the Sheffield Intervention Programme," 724, 727, 726.

18. R. G. Carpenter et al., "Prevention of Unexpected Infant Death: A Review of Risk-Related Intervention in Six Centers," *Annals of the New York Academy of Sciences* 533 (February 1988): 102.

19. Marie Valdes-Dapena, "Sudden Infant Death Syndrome: A Review of the Medical Literature 1974–1979," *Pediatrics* 66, no. 4 (October 1980): 602–3; Robinson, *SIDS 1974*, 186–87.

20. SIDS Joint Hearing 1985, 19, 20, 21; Valdes-Dapena, "Sudden Infant Death Syndrome: Morphology Update for Forensic Pathologists—1985," 178–79.

21. SIDS Joint Hearing 1985, 15, 41, 49.

22. Little and Peterson, "Sudden Infant Death Syndrome Epidemiology," 243.

23. Sandy Rovner, "SIDS: Debating the Value of Home Monitors," *Washington Post*, October 7, 1986.

24. Risk factor methodologies became customary around 1960. Quote from "Risk Factors: A Misleading Concept," *Public Health* 97, no. 5 (1983): 245; William G. Rothstein, *Public Health and the Risk Factor: A History of an Uneven Medical Revolution* (Rochester, NY: University of Rochester Press, 2003), 2.

25. Valdes-Dapena, "Sudden Unexplained Infant Death, 1970 Through 1975," 124–25.

26. Marc Bulterys, "High Incidence of Sudden Infant Death Syndrome Among Northern Indians and Alaska Natives Compared with Southwestern Indians: Possible Role of Smoking," *Journal of Community Health* 15, no. 3 (June 1990): 185–87; "Sudden Infant Death Syndrome—United States, 1980–1988," *JAMA* 268, no. 7 (August 1992): 856; Roger Byard, "Sudden Infant Death Syndrome: A 'Diagnosis' in Search of a Disease," *Journal of Clinical Forensic Medicine* 2 (1995): 122; Eileen Hasselmeyer and Jehu Hunter, "The Sudden Infant Death Syndrome," *Obstetrics and Gynecology Annual* 4 (1975): 216; Hiroshi Shiono et al., "Sudden Infant Death Syndrome in Japan," *American Journal of Forensic Medicine and Pathology* 9, no. 1 (1988): 7.

27. Lehman Black et al., "Effects of Birth Weight and Ethnicity on Incidence of Sudden Infant Death Syndrome," *Journal of Pediatrics* 108, no. 2 (February 1986): 212, 213; Marie Valdes-Dapena, "Sudden Infant Death Syndrome: Overview of Recent Research Developments from a Pediatric Pathologist's Perspective," *Pediatrician* 15, no. 4 (1988): 224; Hasselmeyer and Hunter, "The Sudden Infant Death Syndrome," 217–18.

28. Valdes-Dapena, Marie et al., "Sudden Unexpected Death in Infancy: A Statistical Analysis of Certain Socioeconomic Factors," *Journal of Pediatrics* 73, no. 3 (1968): 392.

29. John Wanzenried, "'What to Say' and 'What Not to Say' to the Sudden Infant Death Syndrome Parent," n.d., 2–3, box 2, folder 26, WSIDSP Records.

30. Attachment D, "SIDS Regional Center, Loyola University of Chicago Stritch School of Medicine, Renewal Application," 1977, Illinois SIDS Commission Records; Connie Guist, "Letter and Data Sheet Sent to Public Health Nurse Following a Telephoned SIDS Referral,"

November 1980, box 1, folder 1, WSIDSP Records; "Wisconsin Sudden Infant Death Syndrome Project: Home Visit Questionnaire," n.d., box 1, folder 1, WSIDSP Records.

31. Case report, February 9, 1960, "Lettergram to Theodore Curphey," box 16, folder 1, Curphey Papers; case report, January 15, 1962, "Lettergram to Theodore Curphey," box 16, folder 1, Curphey Papers; M. Renate Dische, "The Enigma of Sudden Infant Death," *Ladies' Home Journal*, March 1965, Curphey Papers, box 17, folder 3, Huntington Library.

32. Case report, January 29, 1959, "Lettergram to Theodore Curphey," box 16, folder 1, Curphey Papers; Neiswander, letter to Beryl Graham, October 11, 1962, box 16, folder 3, Curphey Papers.

33. L. M. Schulman, letter to Beryl Graham, April 15, 1963, box 16, folder 3, Curphey Papers.

34. Dische, "The Enigma of Sudden Infant Death."

35. Beryl S. Graham, "Lettergram to Theodore J. Curphey," October 1, 1958, box 16, folder 1, Curphey Papers.

36. For example, Beryl S. Graham, "Lettergram to Theodore J. Curphey," October 25, 1960, box 16, folder 2, Curphey Papers; quote from Beryl S. Graham, letter to Theodore Curphey, April 18, 1962, box 16, folder 3, Curphey Papers.

37. Margaret R. Pomeroy, "Sudden Death Syndrome," *American Journal of Nursing* 69, no. 9 (September 1969): 1890.

38. In the SIDS group, 54 percent of mothers apparently had "below average" intelligence, compared with only 39 percent in a separate group. I.D. Richards and H. T. McIntosh, "Confidential Inquiry into 226 Consecutive Infant Deaths," *Archives of Diseases in Childhood* 47, no. 255 (1972): 705.

39. Robinson, *SIDS 1974*, 135, 145, 350.

40. David Ralph, "Sudden Infant Death: Causes Remain Unknown," *Monroe Evening Times*, April 14, 1981, box 1, folder 6, WSIDSP Records.

41. The piece generated lively correspondence, with some writers challenging the validity of its conclusions (saying that "inappropriate diagnosis of these deaths as accidental or homicidal is detrimental to the emotional well-being of the parents of children who die of SIDS and also hampers research in the field"), and others praising the work as a momentous body of findings. Millard Bass, Richard E. Kravath, and Leonard Glass, "Death-Scene Investigation in Sudden Infant Death," *New England Journal of Medicine* 315, no. 2 (July 10, 1986): 102; "Crib Deaths Often Due to Accidents," *Plain Dealer*, July 10, 1986, box 7, folder 2, Adelson Papers; "Investigation of SIDS," *New England Journal of Medicine* 315, no. 26 (December 1986): 1676–77.

42. For example, Bruce Beckwith stated at the same meeting, "smart people, extremely competent and well trained and experienced mothers lose their babies the same way." Robinson, *SIDS 1974*, 341.

43. Autopsy costs varied substantially depending on facilities and location. For example, in 1977, costs in Wisconsin were estimated between $230 and $250 per infant, but could be as low as $125 in metropolitan areas like Dane County and as high as $400 in outlying areas of Milwaukee County. "Sudden Infant Death Syndrome," Pub. L. No. 93–56, § Subcommittee on Public Health and Environment of the Committee on Interstate and Foreign Commerce (1973), 81–83; "Until Crib Death Problem Is Solved, Victims' Parents Need More Help," *JAMA* 226, no. 11 (December 10, 1973): 1299; "Management of Sudden Death in Infants Is Termed 'Disgrace,'" *Hospital Tribune*, June 25, 1973, box 7, folder 7, Adelson Papers; "Bill Analysis," February 23, 1977, box 2, folder 29, WSIDSP Records.

44. Illinois Sudden Infant Death Syndrome Commission, "Infant Survival: 'New Hope for the Family...,'" Report and Recommendation of the Sudden Infant Death Syndrome (SIDS)

Study Commission of the State of Illinois to the Members of the 78th General Assembly (Illinois, 1974), appendix II, figure 10, Illinois SIDS Commission Records.

45. Abraham Bergman and J. Bruce Beckwith, "Sudden Death Syndrome of Infancy," in *Ambulatory Pediatrics*, ed. Morris Green and Robert Haggerty (Philadelphia: W. B. Saunders, 1968), 142; "SIDS Regional Center, Loyola University of Chicago Stritch School of Medicine, Renewal Application," 1977, 18; Wayne Welch, "Crib Death Tragedy: How Parents Adjust to Baby's Mysterious Disease," *San Francisco Chronicle*, October 5, 1971, box 12, File #1, Adams Papers; John Niemitz, letter to Joseph Corbine, April 3, 1980, box 3, folder 5, WSIDSP Records; "SIDS Progress Report," n.d., Exhibit XXVII, 2, C, Renewal Application for Ill. Dept. of Public Health Sudden Infant Death Syndrome Information and Counseling Center, Illinois SIDS Commission Records.

46. "Sleep Studies and Sudden Infant Death: Apnea Discoveries Stir Optimism in the Etiologic Quest," *Medical World News*, October 5, 1973, 60, box 7, folder 7, Adelson Papers.

47. "Until Crib Death Problem Is Solved, Victims' Parents Need More Help," 1299.

48. Lower-class and minority families were both grossly underrepresented in the study population. (Seventy-nine percent of the families were white.) Illinois Sudden Infant Death Syndrome Commission, "Infant Survival: 'New Hope for the Family . . . ,'" appendix II, figure 11; Subcommittee on Health and Subcommittee on Child and Youth, "Sudden Infant Death Syndrome," § Committee on Labor and Public Welfare (1973) (hereafter, SIDS Hearings, 1973), 50, 77.

49. SIDS Hearings, 1973, 50.

50. Beckwith, "The Sudden Infant Death Syndrome," 29.

51. SIDS Hearings, 1973, 48.

52. Ibid., 47, 54–62.

53. SIDS Hearings, 1973, 47; Abraham Bergman, "Unexplained Sudden Infant Death," *New England Journal of Medicine* 287, no. 5 (August 1972): 254–55.

54. Milton Helpern, "Medical Examiners and Infant Deaths," *New England Journal of Medicine* 287, no. 20 (November 1972): 1050–51.

55. Milton Helpern, letter to Minnesota senator Walter F. Mondale, August 15, 1972, 1–3, box 17, folder 5, Curphey Papers.

56. SIDS Hearings, 1973, 47; Richard Maschal, "Dad Was Held in Jail as Baby Son Was Buried," *Charlotte Observer*, August 10, 1972, 53.

57. For example: "Crib Deaths Linked to Normal Causes, Not Parental Neglect," *New York Times*, October 27, 1968.

58. Sandra Grant, "'Crib Deaths' Answer Seen Imminent," *Evening Sun*, April 27, 1970; Suzanne Harris, "Sudden Infant Death Causes Uncovered," *Plain Dealer*, December 20, 1970; "A Biochemist Links Crib Death to Low Level of Sugar in Blood," *New York Times*, July 5, 1975; "Antibodies Found in Lungs of SIDS Victims," *Medical Center News*, March 8, 1978, box 13, SIDS/Crib Death folder, Adams Papers; Jane Brody, "California Researchers Report They Have Identified a Bacterium Linked to Crib Deaths," *New York Times*, June 25, 1978.

59. For example, Benjamin Weiser, "Arlington Woman Is Charged With 1971 Slaying of Infant," *Washington Post*, August 17, 1979; "Father Charged in Death of Baby," *Washington Post*, May 29, 1980; "Baby Sitter Arrest Came After 5 Deaths in 2 Years," *New York Times*, July 26, 1982; "Crib Death Study Says Don't Bundle," *Plain Dealer*, November 27, 1984, box 7, folder 11, Adelson Papers; "Crib Deaths Often Due to Accidents," *Plain Dealer*, July 10, 1986, box 7, folder 2, Adelson Papers.

60. For examples, see SIDS Joint Hearing 1985, 11; Judy Klemesrud, "A Tragedy with an Aftermath of Guilt," *New York Times*, June 19, 1972.

61. Carla Cantor, "SIDS: 'We Don't Know Why Your Baby Died,'" *New York Times*, March 13, 1988.

62. Abraham Bergman, "Sudden Infant Death Syndrome: An Approach to Management," *Primary Care* 3, no. 1 (March 1976): 3.

63. Lester Adelson, "A Forensic Pathologist Looks at Sudden and Unexpected Death in Infancy and Childhood . . . A Personal Statement," (Research Conference on SIDS, Children's Hospital, Columbus, Ohio, 1976), 9, box 7, folder 1, Adelson Papers.

64. Richard Naeye, "Preventing the Sudden Infant Death Syndrome," *Paediatric and Perinatal Epidemiology* 4, no. 1 (1990): 17.

65. Warren G. Guntheroth, "Sudden Infant Death Syndrome (Crib Death)," *American Heart Journal* 93, no. 6 (June 1977): 785.

66. Marie Valdes-Dapena, "The Pathologist and the Sudden Infant Death Syndrome," *American Journal of Pathology* 106, no. 1 (January 1982): 121.

67. Stewart Asch, "Crib Deaths: Their Possible Relationship to Post Partum Depression and Infanticide," *Journal of Mt. Sinai Hospital* 35, no. 3 (1968): 214, 216–17, 218, 219.

68. Walter Kukull and Donald R. Peterson, "Sudden Infant Death and Infanticide," *American Journal of Epidemiology* 106, no. 6 (1977): 485, 486.

69. Abraham Bergman, letter to all chapters of the NSIDSF, September 28, 1977, box 7, folder 14, Adelson Papers.

70. Alan W. Cashell, "Homicide as a Cause of the Sudden Infant Death Syndrome," *American Journal of Forensic Medicine and Pathology* 8, no. 3 (1987): 256, 258.

71. A subdural hematoma is a pooling of blood just outside the brain. It usually results from a traumatic head injury and is dangerous because as blood collects on the brain's surface, blocked against the skull, it puts undue pressure on the brain, which in turn can lead to severe problems and even death. John Caffey, "Multiple Fractures in the Long Bones of Infants Suffering from Chronic Subdural Hematoma," *Clinical Orthopaedics and Related Research*, reprint (originally published in the *American Journal of Roentgenology*, 1946), 469 (2011): 755; John E. B. Myers, "A Short History of Child Protection in America," *Family Law Quarterly* 42, no. 3 (Fall 2008): 454–55.

72. Caffey further noted that in one case, "the infant was clearly unwanted by both parents and this raised the question of intentional ill-treatment of the infant," although he said evidence was "inadequate to prove or disprove this point." Caffey, "Multiple Fractures," 756, quote on 757.

73. Myers, "A Short History of Child Protection in America," 455.

74. Ibid.

75. C. Henry Kempe et al., "The Battered-Child Syndrome," *Child Abuse and Neglect*, reprint (originally published in the *Journal of the American Medical Association*, 1962), 9 (1985): 145–46.

76. Etienne G. Krug et al., eds., "Child Abuse and Neglect by Parents and Other Caregivers," in *World Report on Violence and Health* (Geneva: World Health Organization, 2002), 67, 68.

77. Myers, "A Short History of Child Protection in America," 456–57; Theodore J. Curphey et al., "The Battered Child Syndrome: Responsibilities of the Pathologist," *California Medicine* 102, no. 2 (February 1965): 102.

78. "Final Report of a Study: 'The Management of Sudden Infant Death Syndrome (SIDS) In the United States,' (1972)," SIDS Hearings, 1973, 88. This same notion was conveyed in Katherine K. Christoffel, Edward J. Zieserl, and Janet Chiaramonte, "Should Child Abuse and Neglect Be Considered When a Child Dies Unexpectedly?" *American Journal of Diseases of*

Children 139 (September 1985): 876–80; Bob Greene, "A Healthy Baby Is Found Dead," n.d., box 2, folder 23/24, WSIDSP Records.

79. A.M.B. Minford, "Child Abuse Presenting as Apparent 'Near-Miss' Sudden Infant Death Syndrome," *British Medical Journal* 282 (February 1981): 521.

80. "How to Distinguish Between SIDS and Child Abuse and Neglect," n.d., box 1, folder 6, WSIDSP Records.

81. Theodore J. Curphey, letter to David Chadwick, January 26, 1966, box 17, folder 10, Curphey Papers.

82. Marian Eskin, *Child Abuse and Neglect: A Literature Review and Selected Bibliography*, ed. Marjorie Kravitz (Washington, DC: U.S. Department of Justice, 1980), 5, 15.

83. Andrea J. Sedlak and Diane D. Broadhurst, *Executive Summary of the Third National Incidence Study of Child Abuse and Neglect* (Washington, DC: U.S. Department of Health and Human Services, 1996), accessed at https://www.childwelfare.gov/pubs/statsinfo/nis3.cfm.

84. Eskin, *Child Abuse and Neglect*, 15.

85. Kempe et al., "The Battered-Child Syndrome," 145–46.

86. Etienne G. Krug et al., eds., "Child Abuse and Neglect by Parents and Other Caregivers," in *World Report on Violence and Health* (Geneva: World Health Organization, 2002), 67, 68.

87. Barbara Burns and Lewis P. Lipsitt, "Behavioral Factors in Crib Death: Toward an Understanding of the Sudden Infant Death Syndrome," *Journal of Applied Developmental Psychology* 12 (1991): 169.

88. Lewis P. Lipsitt, "Infants at Risk: Perinatal and Neonatal Factors," *International Journal of Behavioral Development* 2 (1979): 25.

89. Ibid., 36.

90. Burns and Lipsitt, "Behavioral Factors in Crib Death," 161.

91. Lipsitt connected his theory for SIDS to the Failure to Thrive Syndrome (FTTS). As its name suggests, the FTTS label was applied to young babies clinically documented as failing to thrive (measured especially in terms of physical growth rates). Lipsitt saw both SIDS and FTTS as the result of a "failure to produce adaptive reciprocating behaviors," where affected infants exhibited "diminished responses due to perinatal stresses, lack of opportunity for the responses present to be fully engaged by the environment, and inadequate learning experiences." In the 1970s, FTTS presented in an estimated 3 percent of children. Ibid., 178; Lewis P. Lipsitt, "Critical Conditions in Infancy: A Psychological Perspective," *American Psychologist* 34, no. 10 (October 1979): 977, 978.

92. Burns and Lipsitt, "Behavioral Factors in Crib Death," 175.

93. SIDS Joint Hearing 1985, 104.

94. Lipsitt, "Critical Conditions in Infancy," 976.

95. Arno Gruen, "Prior Themes of Rejection Among Parents of Sudden Infant Death Victims: Retrospective Accounts and a Theoretical Proposal Concerning Focusing, REM Sleep and the Failure to Arouse in Such Children" (Switzerland, November 1986), 7, 8, box no. 3843, folder no. 2, Willard E. Caldwell Papers, archives of the History of American Psychology, Center for the History of Psychology, University of Akron (hereafter, Caldwell Papers).

96. For example, two researchers stated, "It could be argued that victims of SIDS, who typically die quietly in their sleep, suffer more from a defect in arousal than in breathing." Eliot A. Phillipson and Colin E. Sullivan, "Arousal: The Forgotten Response to Respiratory Stimuli," *American Review of Respiratory Disease* 118 (1978): 807–9.

97. Gruen, "Prior Themes of Rejection," 11.

98. Gruen said his interviews revealed that SIDS parents had an overwhelming tendency towards a "preoccupation with death in dreams or fantasy or both prior to the infant's death,"

while near-miss parents did not exhibit any such preoccupations. Arno Gruen, "The Relationship of Sudden Infant Death and Parental Unconscious Conflicts," *Pre- and Peri-Natal Psychology* 2, no. 1 (Fall 1987): 52; Willard Caldwell, "Sudden Infant Death Syndrome: Toward an Integrated Theory of (ARSID) Apnea Relate [Sic] SIDS with Focus Upon 'Near Miss' Cases" n.d., 42, box no. 3849, folder no. 10, Caldwell Papers.

99. Gruen, "Prior Themes of Rejection," 18, 19, 21, 24, 31.

100. Ibid., 41, 80.

101. Gruen, "The Relationship of Sudden Infant Death and Parental Unconscious Conflicts," 53–54.

102. Ibid., 53.

103. Gruen, "Prior Themes of Rejection," 80.

104. More specifically, Gruen theorized that "the neurophysiological antecedents of SID[S] reside in a mothering that reinforces REM sleep, diminishes arousal through the thwarting of expectations and weakened sucking, and makes the infant's dream state too preoccupying." Under such conditions the occurrence of apnea can lead to death. Ibid., 83, 111a.

105. Ibid., 96.

106. Gruen, "The Relationship of Sudden Infant Death and Parental Unconscious Conflicts," 55.

107. "Mothers are also faulted when babies die of natural causes, especially when child care practices are identified as risk factors," they say. Molly Ladd-Taylor and Lauri Umansky, introduction to *"Bad" Mothers: The Politics of Blame in Twentieth-Century America*, ed. Molly Ladd-Taylor and Lauri Umansky (New York: New York University Press, 1998), 2, 6, 3, 4.

108. Rebecca Jo Plant, *Mom: The Transformation of Motherhood in Modern America* (Chicago: University of Chicago Press, 2010), 11, 13.

109. Paula J. Caplan, "Mother-Blaming," in *"Bad" Mothers: The Politics of Blame in Twentieth-Century America*, ed. Molly Ladd-Taylor and Lauri Umansky (New York: New York University Press, 1998), quote from 134, 139.

110. Lew Lipsitt, "Letter to the Network on Behavioral Factors in Unexpected Infant Death," July 6, 1988, box no. 3843, folder no. 5, Caldwell Papers.

111. Lew Lipsitt, "Letter to the 'SIDS and Behavior' Networkers," November 7, 1988, box no. 3843, folder no. 5, Caldwell Papers.

112. Ashley Montagu, "Sudden Infant Death Syndrome, Prenatal Breathing, and Maternal Care," letter to the editor, *New England Journal of Medicine* (May 13, 1985), 2, box no. 3843, folder no. 2, Caldwell Papers.

113. Steven Friedlander and Edward B. Shaw, "Psychogenic Factors in Sudden Infant Death: Some Dynamic Speculations," *Clinical Social Work Journal* 3, no. 4 (1975): 237–38.

114. Ibid., 241.

115. Ibid., 246.

116. Earl Ubell, "Crib Death: 10,000 Victims a Year, Cause Unknown," *New York Times*, January 30, 1972.

117. Gail Grenier Sweet, "Sudden Infant Death Syndrome: A Personal View," *Mothering*, Summer 1981, 106, box 3, folder 14, WSIDSP Records.

118. David Ralph, "Sudden Infant Death: Causes Remain Unknown," *Monroe Evening Times*, April 14, 1981, box 1, folder 6, WSIDSP Records.

119. Robinson, *SIDS 1974*, 341.

120. Ibid.

121. Jody W. Zylke, "Sudden Infant Death Syndrome: Resurgent Research Offers Hope," *JAMA* 262, no. 12 (September 1989): 1565; Marian Willinger, L. Stanley James, and Charlotte Catz, "Defining the Sudden Infant Death Syndrome (SIDS): Deliberations of an Expert Panel

Convened by the National Institute of Child Health and Human Development," *Pediatric Pathology* 11, no. 5 (1991): 677, 681.
122. Carol Gino, "SIDS Research That Causes Pain," *American Journal of Nursing* 88, no. 10 (October 1988): 1353.

CHAPTER 5   MOBILIZATION: SIDS ACTIVISM

1. United States Bureau of Investigation, "Uniform Crime Reports for the United States" (Washington, DC: Bureau of Investigation, U.S. Department of Justice, 1969), accessed at http://archive.org/stream/uniformcrimerepo1969unit/uniformcrimerepo1969unit_djvu .txt; Steven Pinker, "Decivilization in the 1960s," *Human Figurations: Long-Term Perspectives on the Human Condition*, from *The Better Angels of Our Nature: Why Violence Has Declined* (2011), 2, no. 2 (July 2013), accessed at http://quod.lib.umich.edu/h/humfig/11217607.0002 .206?view=text;rgn=main.
2. Carolyn Szybist Sodini, personal communication with the author, November 1, 2014; Edward M. Brecher, "What Doctors Now Know about 'Crib Deaths,'" *Redbook*, July 1968.
3. Szybist, personal communication, November 1, 2014.
4. Carolyn Szybist, "Resume," June 1979, 2.
5. Abraham Bergman, *The "Discovery" of Sudden Infant Death Syndrome: Lessons in the Practice of Political Medicine* (New York: Praeger, 1986), 5–7; "Foundation to Study Causes of Crib Deaths," n.d., box 132, folder 6, MCA Records; Michael P. Johnson and Karl Hufbauer, "Sudden Infant Death Syndrome as a Medical Research Problem since 1945," *Social Problems* 30, no. 1 (October 1, 1982): 69; Ralph F. Colin, "Appendix: The National Foundation for Sudden Infant Death," in *Sudden Infant Death Syndrome: Proceedings of the Second International Conference on Causes of Sudden Death in Infants* (Seattle: University of Washington Press, 1969), 226; Vivian Cadden, "Why Babies Die," *Redbook*, November 1968, 214–15.
6. "Rights of Children, Part 1: Examination of the Sudden Infant Death Syndrome," § Subcommittee on Children and Youth of the Committee on Labor and Public Welfare (1972), 59.
7. Carolyn Szybist, "A Study of the Organizational Structures of the National Sudden Infant Death Syndrome Foundation and Their Relationships to External Activity for Sudden Infant Death Syndrome in the United States" (National College of Education, 1980), 10.
8. "The National Foundation for Sudden Infant Death, Inc.," *Clinical Pediatrics* 11, no. 2 (1972): 83; Richard Raring, *Crib Death: Scourge of Infants, Shame of Society* (Hicksville, NY: Exposition Press, 1975), 120.
9. Bergman, *The "Discovery" of Sudden Infant Death Syndrome*, 18–19.
10. Ibid., 19–20; Mary S. Dore, "Appendix: Washington Association for Sudden Infant Study," in *Sudden Infant Death Syndrome: Proceedings of the Second International Conference on Causes of Sudden Death in Infants* (Seattle: University of Washington Press, 1969), 230.
11. Johnson and Hufbauer, "Sudden Infant Death Syndrome as a Medical Research Problem since 1945," 71.
12. Dore, "Appendix: Washington Association for Sudden Infant Study," 230.
13. Ibid., 234.
14. Saul Goldberg, "Appendix: The International Guild for Infant Survival," in *Sudden Infant Death Syndrome: Proceedings of the Second International Conference on Causes of Sudden Death in Infants* (Seattle: University of Washington Press, 1969), 228–29; Johnson and Hufbauer, "Sudden Infant Death Syndrome as a Medical Research Problem since 1945," 72.
15. Szybist, "A Study of the Organizational Structures of the National Sudden Infant Death Syndrome Foundation," 16.

16. "Sudden Infant Death Syndrome: Joint Hearing Before Certain Subcommittees of the Committee on Post Office and Civil Service and the Committee on Energy and Commerce and the Select Committee on Children, Youth, and Families," § House of Representatives, Congress (1985), 85.

17. Ralph F. Colin, "Appendix: The National Foundation for Sudden Infant Death," in *Sudden Infant Death Syndrome: Proceedings of the Second International Conference on Causes of Sudden Death in Infants* (Seattle: University of Washington Press, 1969), 226–27; Illinois Sudden Infant Death Syndrome Commission, *Infant Survival: "New Hope for the Family . . . ,"* Report and Recommendation of the Sudden Infant Death Syndrome (SIDS) Study Commission of the State of Illinois to the Members of the 78th General Assembly (Illinois, 1974), 9, Illinois SIDS Commission Records; The National Sudden Infant Death Syndrome Foundation, *Special Report to Senator Alan Cranston, Chairman, Sub-Committee on Child and Human Development, on the Implementation of the Sudden Infant Death Syndrome Acts, 1975—1979,* April 1979, 2, file E, Special Report to Sub Committee on Child and Human Development on Implementation of the Sudden Infant Death Syndrome Acts by National SIDS Foundation, April 1979, Illinois SIDS Commission Records.

18. National SIDS Foundation, Wisconsin Chapter, "NSIDSF, Wisconsin Chapter: Newsletter," Fall 1980, 3, box 2, folder 28, WSIDSP Records.

19. National Sudden Infant Death Syndrome Foundation, "1976 Annual Report," 1976, 3, William T. Grant Foundation Collection, Series 3, Sub-Series A, box 105, folder 1245, Rockefeller Archive Center (hereafter, NSIDSF Records); National Sudden Infant Death Syndrome Foundation, "1977 Annual Report," 1977, 6, 4, box 105, folder 1245, NSIDSF Records.

20. National Sudden Infant Death Syndrome Foundation, "Memorandum: Sudden Infant Death Syndrome Research Student and Training Fellowships," December 1, 1979, box 3, folder 1, WSIDSP Records; National Sudden Infant Death Syndrome Foundation, "Sudden Infant Death Syndrome Research: Student and Training Fellowships," 1982, box 1, folder 6, WSIDSP Records; National Sudden Infant Death Syndrome Foundation, "1976 Annual Report," 3.

21. Sudden Infant Death Syndrome: Joint Hearing Before Certain Subcommittees of the Committee on Post Office and Civil Service and the Committee on Energy and Commerce and the Select Committee on Children, Youth, and Families, 27, 30–31, 63; Szybist, "A Study of the Organizational Structures of the National Sudden Infant Death Syndrome Foundation," 6, 58.

22. Rights of Children, Part 1: Examination of the Sudden Infant Death Syndrome, 106.

23. Ana Maris Luker, letter to Dr. Edwin Larkin, February 21, 1979, box 1, folder 19, WSIDSP Records.

24. Carolyn Szybist, personal communication, October 30, 2014.

25. "The Tenth of July," *Pediatrics* 63, no. 4 (April 1979): 615.

26. National Sudden Infant Death Syndrome Foundation, Wisconsin Chapter, "National Sudden Infant Death Syndrome Foundation, Wisconsin Chapter: Newsletter," Fall 1979, box 2, folder 7, WSIDSP Records; Wisconsin Sudden Infant Death Syndrome Center, "Sudden Infant Death Syndrome Wisconsin Perspectives," vol. 1, no. 2, (September 1982), box 1, folder 6, WSIDSP Records.

27. National SIDS Foundation, Wisconsin Chapter, "NSIDSF, Wisconsin Chapter: Newsletter," Summer 1980, 2, box 2, folder 28, WSIDSP Records.

28. For an example of a poem, see National Sudden Infant Death Syndrome Foundation, Wisconsin Chapter, "National Sudden Infant Death Syndrome, Wisconsin Chapter: Newsletter," Spring 1981, 7, box 1, folder 6, WSIDSP Records.

29. Wisconsin Chapter NSIDSF, "Wisconsin Chapter NSIDSF Newsletter," Summer 1977, box 1, folder 19, WSIDSP Records.

30. National Sudden Infant Death Syndrome Foundation, Wisconsin Chapter, "Wisconsin Chapter, National Sudden Infant Death Syndrome Foundation Newsletter," Fall 1978, 2, box 1, folder 19, WSIDSP Records; National Sudden Infant Death Syndrome Foundation, Wisconsin Chapter, "National Sudden Infant Death Syndrome Foundation, Wisconsin Chapter: Newsletter," Fall 1979; National Sudden Infant Death Syndrome Foundation, Wisconsin Chapter, "National Sudden Infant Death Syndrome Foundation," Spring 1980, 3, box 2, folder 7, WSIDSP Records; National Sudden Infant Death Syndrome Foundation, Wisconsin Chapter, "National Sudden Infant Death Syndrome, Wisconsin Chapter: Newsletter," 1; National Sudden Infant Death Syndrome Foundation, Southeastern Wisconsin Chapter, "National Sudden Infant Death Syndrome Foundation, Southeastern Wisconsin Chapter: Newsletter," Summer 1982, 2, box 1, folder 6, WSIDSP Records; Wisconsin Sudden Infant Death Syndrome Center, "Sudden Infant Death Syndrome Wisconsin Perspectives," 8; National Foundation for Sudden Infant Death, "NFSID News Letter IV," Summer 1969, 8, box 12, file #1, Adams Papers.

31. Subcommittee on Health and Subcommittee on Child and Youth, "Sudden Infant Death Syndrome," § Committee on Labor and Public Welfare (1973), 148–49; Gerald D. LaVeck, letter to Saul Goldberg, November 4, 1970, box 12, file #1, Adams Papers.

32. Rights of Children, Part 1: Examination of the Sudden Infant Death Syndrome, 1972, 1, 42.

33. Merlin K. Duval, "Crib Deaths," *Vital Speeches of the Day* 38, no. 13 (April 1972): 396–98, quote on 396; Subcommittee on Health and Subcommittee on Child and Youth, "Sudden Infant Death Syndrome," § Committee on Labor and Public Welfare (1973), 31–34.

34. Rights of Children, Part 1: Examination of the Sudden Infant Death Syndrome, 1972, 22, 42.

35. Ibid., 59, 64; Subcommittee on Health and Subcommittee on Child and Youth, Sudden Infant Death Syndrome, 1973, 10, 143.

36. Wayne Welch, "Crib Death Tragedy: How Parents Adjust to Baby's Mysterious Disease," *San Francisco Chronicle*, October 5, 1971, box 12, file #1, Adams Papers.

37. Larry V. Lewman, "SIDS 1976 Update" (Oregon State Health Division Bulletin, 1976), 5, box 7, folder 10, Adelson Papers; Abraham Bergman and J. Bruce Beckwith, "Sudden Death Syndrome of Infancy," in *Ambulatory Pediatrics*, ed. Morris Green and Robert Haggerty (W. B. Saunders, 1968), 138.

38. Rights of Children, Part 1: Examination of the Sudden Infant Death Syndrome, 1972, 60.

39. "Lettergram to Theodore Curphey," July 6, 1961, box 16, folder 1, Curphey Papers.

40. Rights of Children, Part 1: Examination of the Sudden Infant Death Syndrome, 1972, 113.

41. This parent's name has been changed for confidentiality. Nancy Barton, letter to Theodore J. Curphey, March 25, 1966, box 17, folder 8, Curphey Papers.

42. Parent A, letter to Dr. Robert L. Austin, August 3, 1966, box 17, folder 8, Curphey Papers; Parent A, letter to the Children's Hospital, Research Division of the Virology Department, Washington, DC, July 12, 1966, box 17, folder 8, Curphey Papers; Parent A, letter to Theodore J. Curphey, July 1, 1966, box 17, folder 8, Curphey Papers; Parent A, letter to Theodore J. Curphey, October 5, 1966, box 17, folder 8, Curphey Papers; B. K. Tatschenko and E. Novikova, letter to Parent A from the Academy of Medical Sciences, Institute of Pediatrics, Moscow, August 17, 1966, box 17, folder 8, Curphey Papers.

43. Rights of Children, Part 1: Examination of the Sudden Infant Death Syndrome, 1972, 107, 110.

44. Ibid., 116.

45. Ibid., 20, 27.

46. Although a few SIDS parents indicated that prior knowledge of SIDS did not ease their experience, the majority expressed that it made their experience more tolerable. Ibid., 67, 62, 112.

47. Subcommittee on Health and Subcommittee on Child and Youth, *Sudden Infant Death Syndrome*, 1973, 141.

48. Raring specifically preferred the label of crib death to SIDS, calling medical acronyms "abominations" that "impede communication, lead to misunderstanding, [and] pollute our language." He also charged the HEW with adhering to an "official . . . policy of maintaining public ignorance on crib death." Raring, *Crib Death*, xi, 4, 5, 31.

49. Ibid., 37.

50. *Rights of Children, Part 1: Examination of the Sudden Infant Death Syndrome*, 1972, 76, 68.

51. Robert R. Robinson, ed., *SIDS 1974: Proceedings of the Francis E. Camps International Symposium on Sudden and Unexpected Deaths in Infancy* (Canada: The Canadian Foundation for the Study of Infant Deaths, 1974), 306, 347.

52. Subcommittee on Health and Subcommittee on Child and Youth, *Sudden Infant Death Syndrome*, 1973, 69; "Sudden Infant Death Syndrome," pub. L. no. 93–56, § Subcommittee on Public Health and Environment of the Committee on Interstate and Foreign Commerce (1973), 5–6; "Senate Backs Funds for Fight on Disease," *New York Times*, June 8, 1972.

53. Congress authorized the NICHD to allocate $2 million in SIDS research grants in 1975, $3 million in 1976, and $4 million in 1977. 93rd Congress, "Sudden Infant Death Syndrome Act of 1974," pub. L. no. 93–270 (1974); Eileen Hasselmeyer and Jehu Hunter, "The Sudden Infant Death Syndrome," *Obstetrics and Gynecology Annual* 4 (1975): 231–32.

54. Subcommittee on Health and Subcommittee on Child and Youth, *Sudden Infant Death Syndrome*, 1973, 12–19, quote on 13.

55. Ibid., 13.

56. In current U.S. dollars, about $27.00. Goldberg used the slightly elevated estimate that 12,500 cases occurred each year. Ibid., 148.

57. *Rights of Children, Part 1: Examination of the Sudden Infant Death Syndrome*, 1972, 101.

58. Ibid., 14; Johnson and Hufbauer, "Sudden Infant Death Syndrome as a Medical Research Problem since 1945," 75–76.

59. A. M. Jones and J. T. Weston, "Special Report: The Examination of the Sudden Infant Death Syndrome Infant: Investigative and Autopsy Protocols," *Journal of Forensic Sciences* 21, no. 4 (October 1976): 833.

60. Alan P. Cleveland, "Sudden Infant Death Syndrome (SIDS): A Burgeoning Medicolegal Problem," *American Journal of Law and Medicine* 1, no. 1 (March 1975): 68.

61. These are referred to interchangeably as SIDS centers, projects, and programs.

62. U.S. Department of Health and Human Services, "Information Exchange: National Sudden Infant Death Syndrome Resource Center" (U.S. Department of Health and Human Services, April 1994), 7, box no. 3843, folder no. 4, Caldwell Papers.

63. Beginning in 1979, amendments to the original SIDS Law of 1974 extended and increased SIDS center funding for another two years. "Ohio Chapter: National Sudden Infant Death Syndrome Foundation Newsletter," Spring 1980, 7, box 7, folder 2, Adelson Papers; Geraldine Norris, "New SIDS Legislation: SIDS Amendments of 1979 (P.L. 96–142)," February 25, 1980, box 2, folder 29, WSIDSP Records; "Second Annual Report on the Sudden Infant Death Syndrome Program under Title XI, Part B, Public Health Service Act," July 1981, 3, box 2, folder

18, WSIDSP Records; U.S. Department of Health and Human Services, "Sudden Infant Death Syndrome: Counseling and Information Program," n.d., box 2, folder 18, WSIDSP Records; John Niemitz, "Personal Notes, Fourth National SIDS Conference," June 2, 1980, box 2, folder 4, WSIDSP Records.

64. "Second Annual Report on the Sudden Infant Death Syndrome Program under Title XI, Part B, Public Health Service Act," 1981, 5.

65. Lewman, "SIDS 1976 Update," 2; Illinois Sudden Infant Death Syndrome Commission, "Infant Survival: 'New Hope for the Family . . . ,'" 1974, 42.

66. Subcommittee on Health and Subcommittee on Child and Youth, Sudden Infant Death Syndrome, 1973, 134; Randy Hanzlick and Debra Combs, "Medical Examiner and Coroner Systems," *JAMA* 279, no. 11 (March 1998): 870, 872.

67. Larry V. Lewman, "Oregon State Health Division Bulletin: SIDS," August 1973, 2–4, box 7, folder 7, Adelson Papers; Subcommittee on Health and Subcommittee on Child and Youth, Sudden Infant Death Syndrome, 1973, 131–34.

68. Geraldine Norris, letter to Donald Percy, August 21, 1978, box 1, folder 19, WSIDSP Records.

69. Mary Beckman, "Letter to All Interested Nursing Personnel," January 12, 1979, box 1, folder 7, WSIDSP Records; National Sudden Infant Death Syndrome Foundation, *1977 Annual Report*, 1977, 5, box 105, folder 1245, NSIDSF Records.

70. Illinois Sudden Infant Death Syndrome Commission, "Infant Survival: 'New Hope for the Family . . . ,'" Supplemental Report and Recommendations of the Sudden Infant Death Syndrome (SIDS) Study Commission of the State of Illinois (Illinois, April 1977), 1, A, Loose Materials, Illinois SIDS Commission Records.

71. Wisconsin Sudden Infant Death Syndrome Center, "Guidelines for Intervention: Hospital Emergency Room," n.d., 1, box 2, folder 18, WSIDSP Records.

72. National Sudden Infant Death Syndrome Foundation, "Facts about Sudden Infant Death Syndrome," 1979, box 2, folder 38, WSIDSP Records.

73. Wisconsin Sudden Infant Death Syndrome Center, "Guidelines for Intervention: Hospital Emergency Room," 1.

74. Abraham Bergman quoted in "Crib Deaths Linked to Normal Causes, Not Parental Neglect," *New York Times*, October 27, 1968.

75. Wisconsin Sudden Infant Death Syndrome Center, "Study Questions," 1981, box 2, folder 18, WSIDSP Records.

76. Wisconsin Sudden Infant Death Syndrome Project, letter to J. Stewart Burdick, chief of emergency medical services, Department of Health and Social Services, December 1, 1980, box 1, folder 1, WSIDSP Records.

77. "Sudden Infant Death Syndrome (SIDS) Information for Emergency Medical Technicians," n.d., EMT-3, EMT-6, box 2, folder 18, WSIDSP Records.

78. Ibid., EMT-4.

79. "Sudden Infant Death Syndrome (SIDS) Information for Police Officers," 1981, PO-4, PO-6, PO-7, box 2, folder 18, WSIDSP Records.

80. "Second Annual Report on the Sudden Infant Death Syndrome Program under Title XI, Part B, Public Health Service Act," 1981, 8.

81. Of the existing thirty-seven SIDS projects, twenty-four had autopsy rates higher than 80 percent, and some of those had rates broaching 100 percent. "Sudden Infant Death Syndrome Act Extension, 1978," § Subcommittee on Child and Human Development of the Committee on Human Resources (1978), 111, 121–22.

82. "Second Annual Report on the Sudden Infant Death Syndrome Program under Title XI, Part B, Public Health Service Act," 1981, 13, 14, 15.

83. "Federal Grant Application Materials," 1980, box 1, folder 1, WSIDSP Records.

84. Sandra Peterson, "Letter of Support, Wisconsin SIDS Project Progress Report," January 13, 1981, box 1, folder 1, WSIDSP Records.

85. For an example, see Lu Ann Ruby, January 29, 1982, box 1, folder 6, WSIDSP Records.

86. Some other SIDS projects did the same; one in California published pamphlets in "several" languages. "SIDS Regional Center, Loyola University of Chicago Stritch School of Medicine, Renewal Application," 1977, 18, 21, A, Loose Materials, Illinois SIDS Commission Records; "Sudden Infant Death Syndrome: Joint Hearing Before Certain Subcommittees of the Committee on Post Office and Civil Service and the Committee on Energy and Commerce and the Select Committee on Children, Youth, and Families," § House of Representatives, Congress (1985), 78.

87. "SIDS Progress Report," n.d., Exhibit XXXII, 2, C) Renewal Application for Ill. Dept. of Public Health Sudden Infant Death Syndrome Information and Counseling Center, Illinois SIDS Commission Records.

88. Welch, "Crib Death Tragedy: How Parents Adjust to Baby's Mysterious Disease."

89. Marilyn Schlice, letter to Bonnie Jackson, administrative secretary for the Washington State Chapter NSIDSF, August 1, 1978, box 1, folder 19, WSIDSP Records.

90. Johnson and Hufbauer, "Sudden Infant Death Syndrome as a Medical Research Problem since 1945," 77.

91. Szybist, "A Study of the Organizational Structures of the National Sudden Infant Death Syndrome Foundation," Q-12, Q-13, Q-14, Q-43, Q-46, 50.

92. Abraham Bergman, letter to Carolyn Szybist, March 22, 1979, E, Special Report to Sub Committee on Child and Human Development on Implementation of the Sudden Infant Death Syndrome Acts by National SIDS Foundation, April 1979, Illinois SIDS Commission Records.

93. John Niemitz, "Letter to Members of the Wisconsin SIDS Project Community Council and Other Friends of the Program," September 10, 1982, box 1, folder 6, WSIDSP Records; Sudden Infant Death Syndrome: Joint Hearing Before Certain Subcommittees of the Committee on Post Office and Civil Service and the Committee on Energy and Commerce and the Select Committee on Children, Youth, and Families, 1985, 68, 76, 78; Wisconsin Sudden Infant Death Syndrome Project, "Wisconsin Sudden Infant Death Syndrome Project Community Council Meeting," August 17, 1981, box 3, folder 14, WSIDSP Records; Jehu Hunter, "The Federal SIDS Support Network in Perspective," Annals of the New York Academy of Sciences 533 (August 1988): 156; "Information Sheet Regarding Maternal and Child Health Block Grant," n.d., 1, box 2, folder 45, WSIDSP Records; Sudden Infant Death Syndrome Clearinghouse, "Information Exchange," April 1981, 7, H, General Information on the Sudden Infant Death Syndrome Study Commission, Illinois SIDS Commission Records; Kenneth Finegold, Laura Wherry, and Stephanie Schardin, "Block Grants: Historical Overview and Lessons Learned," The Urban Institute, New Federalism: Issues and Options for States, A, no. 63 (April 2004): 2.

94. Sudden Infant Death Syndrome: Joint Hearing Before Certain Subcommittees of the Committee on Post Office and Civil Service and the Committee on Energy and Commerce and the Select Committee on Children, Youth, and Families, 1985, 68, 62–63, 22, 76.

95. US Department of Health, Education, and Welfare, "Maternal and Child Health Information: Seminar on SIDS," HSM 73–5050 (March 1973), 3, box 12, file #1, Adams Papers.

96. Subcommittee on Health and Subcommittee on Child and Youth, Sudden Infant Death Syndrome, 1973, 51.

97. Bradley H. Zebal, "Marketing Audit: The National SIDS Foundation" (M.B.A. program, Marketing for Non-Profit Organizations, University of Maryland, 1984), 5; National Sudden Infant Death Syndrome Foundation, Wisconsin Chapter, "National Sudden Infant Death Syndrome Foundation, Wisconsin Chapter: Newsletter," Fall 1980, 2.

98. Szybist, "A Study of the Organizational Structures of the National Sudden Infant Death Syndrome Foundation," 15; Stanford B. Friedman, letter to Robert Haggerty, November 2, 1979, box 105, folder 1245, NSIDSF Records; Stanford B. Friedman, letter to Robert Haggerty, September 14, 1981, box 105, folder 1247, NSIDSF Records.

99. Szybist, "A Study of the Organizational Structures of the National Sudden Infant Death Syndrome Foundation," 68; Zebal, "Marketing Audit: The National SIDS Foundation," 8.

100. Szybist, "A Study of the Organizational Structures of the National Sudden Infant Death Syndrome Foundation," 68.

101. Ibid., Q-21, Q-23, Q-24, Q-33, 44.

102. Zebal, "Marketing Audit: The National SIDS Foundation," 10.

103. Szybist, "A Study of the Organizational Structures of the National Sudden Infant Death Syndrome Foundation," 26.

104. Zebal, "Marketing Audit: The National SIDS Foundation," 4. (See also http://www.compassionatefriends.org/home.aspx; http://nationalshare.org/wp-content/uploads/2014/09/ShareHistory.pdf.)

105. US Department of Health and Human Services, "Information Exchange: National Sudden Infant Death Syndrome Resource Center," 7. (See also http://www.firstcandle.org/.)

106. "Evaluation of Nursing Seminar," June 14, 1979, box 1, folder 11, WSIDSP Records; "Evaluation of SIDS Nursing Seminar," January 17, 1978, box 1, folder 17, WSIDSP Records; "Evaluation of SIDS Nursing Seminar," October 11, 1978, box 1, folder 2, WSIDSP Records; "Evaluation of SIDS Nursing Seminar," April 18, 1979, box 1, folder 14, WSIDSP Records; "Evaluation of SIDS Workshop," October 3, 1979, box 1, folder 9, WSIDSP Records.

107. National Sudden Infant Death Syndrome Foundation, "1977 Annual Report," 2.

108. National Sudden Infant Death Syndrome Foundation, "Facts About Sudden Infant Death Syndrome," 1979, 10, box 105, folder 1247, NSIDSF Records.

109. Ibid.

110. "Presentation for Wisconsin SIDS Program," October 1979, 3, box 1, folder 9, WSIDSP Records; National Sudden Infant Death Syndrome Foundation, "1976 Annual Report," 2; Szybist, personal communication, November 26, 2014.

111. Szybist, personal communication, November 1, 2014.

112. Kathleen Wagner and Ethel Barron, "Crib Death: One Family's Nightmare," *Lady's Circle*, April 1971, 224.

113. Ari Goldman, "The Nightmare of Crib Death," *New York Times*, March 28, 1976.

114. Judy Klemesrud, "A Tragedy with an Aftermath of Guilt," *New York Times*, June 19, 1972.

115. "SIDS Regional Center, Loyola University of Chicago Stritch School of Medicine, Renewal Application," 17.

116. Hunter, "The Federal SIDS Support Network in Perspective," 156.

117. John Wanzenried, "'What to Say' and 'What Not to Say' to the Sudden Infant Death Syndrome Parent," n.d., 2, box 2, folder 26, WSIDSP Records.

118. David A. Baptiste, "Time-Elapsed Marital and Family Therapy with Sudden Infant Death Syndrome Families," *Family Systems Medicine* 1, no. 3 (1983): 57; Bradley H. Zebal and

Susan F. Woolsey, "SIDS and the Family: The Pediatrician's Role," *Pediatric Annals* 13, no. 3 (March 1984): 238.

119. Sudden Infant Death Syndrome: Joint Hearing Before Certain Subcommittees of the Committee on Post Office and Civil Service and the Committee on Energy and Commerce and the Select Committee on Children, Youth, and Families, 1985, 97.

CHAPTER 6   CAUSE FOR ALARM

1. "Obituary: Warren G. Guntheroth," *Seattle Times*, October 14, 2012; Ralph J. Wedgwood and Earl P. Benditt, eds., "Sudden Death in Infants: Proceedings of the Conference on Causes of Sudden Death in Infants," Public Health Service Publication No. 1412 (Conference on Causes of Sudden Death in Infants, Seattle, Washington: National Institute of Child Health and Human Development, 1963), 6–7; Abraham Bergman, J. Bruce Beckwith, and C. George Ray, eds., "Sudden Infant Death Syndrome: Proceedings of the Second International Conference on Causes of Sudden Death in Infants" (Second International Conference on Causes of Sudden Death in Infants, Children's Orthopedic Hospital and Medical Center and University of Washington School of Medicine, Seattle: University of Washington Press, 1969), 199, 201–2.

2. Warren G. Guntheroth, *Crib Death: The Sudden Infant Death Syndrome* (Mount Kisco, NY: Futura Publishing, 1989), 241, 274; "Alarming Babies," *Time*, February 5, 1979.

3. Cathleen Hoven Sparks, letter to executive director, Dane County Mental Health Center, April 23, 1981, box 1, folder 6, WSIDSP Records; National Sudden Infant Death Syndrome Foundation, Wisconsin Chapter, "National Sudden Infant Death Syndrome Foundation: Wisconsin Chapters, Newsletter," Spring 1981, 2, 5, box 1, folder 6, WSIDSP Records.

4. D. W. Hill, "Progress in Medical Instrumentation Over the Past Fifty Years," *Journal of Scientific Instruments* 2, no. 1 (1968): 697–701; Max Henry Weil and Wanchun Tang, "From Intensive Care to Critical Care Medicine: A Historical Perspective," *American Journal of Respiratory and Critical Care Medicine* 183, no. 11 (June 2011): 1452.

5. David Epstein and Judith E. Brill, "A History of Pediatric Critical Care Medicine," *Pediatric Research* 58, no. 5 (2005): 987–88, 994; Weil and Tang, "From Intensive Care to Critical Care Medicine," 1451–52.

6. Julie Fairman and Sarah Kagan, "Creating Critical Care: The Case of the Hospital of the University of Pennsylvania, 1950–1965," *Advances in Nursing Science* 22, no. 1 (September 1999): 63–77; Ronald Trubuhovich, "The Name of Our Specialty—With a Historical Perspective on 'Intensive Care,'" *Critical Care and Resuscitation* 10, no. 4 (December 2008): 328.

7. W.E.B. Edge, "An Electronic Neonatal Respiratory Monitor," *The Lancet* 275, no. 7138 (June 1960): 1330; W.E.B. Edge and W. L. Eaton, "An Electronic Neonatal Respiratory Monitor," *South African Medical Journal* 34 (September 1960): 781.

8. H. Wick and H. Schmidt, "Simple Warning System for Apnoea in Premature Infants," *The Lancet* 289, no. 7495 (April 1967): 880.

9. C.H.M. Walker and Phyllis Robbie, "Initial Experience with an Impedence Apnoea Monitor," *Archives of Disease in Childhood* 44, no. 233 (February 1969): 135.

10. Victor Chernick and Monte Raber, "Electrical Hazards in the Newborn Nursery," *Journal of Pediatrics* 77, no. 1 (July 1970): 143; J.F.L., "False Alarms in the Nursery," *Pediatrics* 61, no. 4 (April 1978): 666.

11. L. H. Stevens, "Sudden Unexplained Death in Infancy: Observations on a Natural Mechanism of Adoption of the Face Down Position," *American Journal of Diseases of Children* 110 (September 1965): 246–47.

12. David S. Bachman, "Prolonged Apnea, Vagal Overactivity, and Sudden Infant Death," *Pediatrics* 51, no. 4 (April 1973): 755.

13. Alfred Steinschneider, Steven L. Weinstein, and Earl Diamond, "The Sudden Infant Death Syndrome and Apnea/Obstruction During Neonatal Sleep," *Pediatrics* 70, no. 6 (December 1982): 858.

14. J. Geoff Gregory, "Citation Study of a Scientific Revolution: Sudden Infant Death Syndrome," *Scientometrics* 5 (1983): 316.

15. Marie Valdes-Dapena, *Current Status of SIDS Research*, Annual Report to the NSIDSF Board of Trustees (National Sudden Infant Death Syndrome Foundation, June 13, 1980), 1, box 7, folder 10, Adelson Papers.

16. "Alarming Babies."

17. Dorothy Kelly, Daniel C. Shannon, and Kathleen O'Connell, "Care of Infants with Near-Miss Sudden Infant Death Syndrome," *Pediatrics* 61, no. 4 (April 1978): 511.

18. As Steinschneider explained for his monitoring program in upstate New York, parents were asked to record details on any given alarm's timing, their child's behavioral state, respiratory activity, and skin color, as well as their own responses to the alarm. Parents also kept a daily log of any major changes in their baby's activities or any evident illnesses. Ibid., 512; John Favorito, Joan M. Orchado Pernice, and Patricia Ruggiero, "Apnea Monitoring to Prevent SIDS," *American Journal of Nursing* 79, no. 1 (January 1979): 102–3; Alfred Steinschneider, "Nasopharyngitis and Prolonged Sleep Apnea," *Pediatrics* 56, no. 6 (December 1975): 968.

19. The criteria for terminating monitor treatment were four weeks devoid of any prolonged apnea episodes (four weeks without any apneic events that triggered the alarm). Kelly, Shannon, and O'Connell, "Care of Infants with Near-Miss Sudden Infant Death Syndrome," 511, 512, 513, 514.

20. Ibid., 514.

21. Committee on Apnea, lead author Thomas Kowalski, *Physician Guidelines for Evaluation of Apnea in Infants* (Milwaukee, WI: Milwaukee Children's Hospital, April 9, 1981), box 1, folder 6, WSIDSP Records; National Sudden Infant Death Syndrome Foundation, "Position Statement on CBS 60 Minutes, March 8 1981: Segment on SIDS & Monitoring," April 1981, box 2, folder 7, WSIDSP Records; *Apnea, Monitoring, and Sudden Infant Death Syndrome* (Rockville, MD: U.S. Department of Health, Education, and Welfare, n.d.), box 2, folder 7, WSIDSP Records; "Wisconsin Sudden Infant Death Syndrome Project Community Council Meeting," February 16, 1981, 1, box 3, folder 10, WSIDSP Records; Kay Hendrix and Margaret Watkins, "Sudden Infant Death Syndrome: A Program for Assessment and Home Monitoring," *Journal of the Medical Association of the State of Alabama* 51, no. 9 (1982): 20; Saul Adler and W. Scott James, "A Community Program for the Prevention of Sudden Infant Death Syndrome," *Journal of the Medical Association of Georgia* 71, no. 6 (June 1982): 401, 404; D. P. Southall, "Role of Apnea in the Sudden Infant Death Syndrome: A Personal View," *Pediatrics* 80, no. 1 (January 1988): 76.

22. Favorito, Pernice, and Ruggiero, "Apnea Monitoring to Prevent SIDS," 102–4.

23. Beth Frawley Haight et al., *A Manual for Home Monitoring* (Chicago: National Sudden Infant Death Syndrome Foundation, 1980), 15.

24. Kit Bakke, "Apnea Monitoring Programs: Who Is a Candidate," *American Journal of Maternal Child Nursing* 8 (June 1983): 185.

25. Norman Lewak, Bradley H. Zebal, and Stanford B. Friedman, "Management of Infants with Apnea and Potential Apnea: A Survey of Pediatric Opinion," *Clinical Pediatrics* 23, no. 7 (July 1984): 369, 372.

26. "Sleep Studies and Sudden Infant Death: Apnea Discoveries Stir Optimism in the Etiologic Quest," *Medical World News*, October 5, 1973, 56, box 7, folder 7.

27. J.F.L., "False Alarms in the Nursery," 665–66.

28. Paul Duffty and M. Heather Bryan, "Home Apnea Monitoring in 'Near-Miss' Sudden Infant Death Syndrome (SIDS) and in Siblings of SIDS Victims," *Pediatrics* 70, no. 1 (July 1982): 73; Nicholas M. Nelson, "But Who Shall Monitor the Monitor?" *Pediatrics* 61, no. 4 (April 1978): 663.

29. Nelson, "But Who Shall Monitor the Monitor?" 663; "Home Monitoring for Crib Deaths?: Experts Disagree on Need to Watch Over SIDS Victims' Siblings," *Medical World News*, May 17, 1976, box 7, folder 6, Adelson Papers.

30. Lewak, Zebal, and Friedman, "Management of Infants with Apnea and Potential Apnea," 371.

31. Christian Guilleminault et al., "Apneas During Sleep in Infants: Possible Relationship with Sudden Infant Death Syndrome," *Science* 14, no. 190 (November 1975): 679; Marie Valdes-Dapena, "Sudden Unexplained Infant Death, 1970 Through 1975: An Evolution in Understanding," *Pathology Annual* 12, no. 1 (1977): 135; J.F.L., "False Alarms in the Nursery," 666; Ann Stark, Frederick Mandell, and H. William Taeusch, "Close Encounters with SIDS," *Pediatrics* 61, no. 4 (April 1978): 665; George Mendelson, "Letter to the Editor: Sudden Death in Infancy Syndrome in Western Australia," *Medical Journal of Australia* 1, no. 18 (May 1976): 677; Marie Valdes-Dapena, "Sudden Infant Death Syndrome: A Review of the Medical Literature 1974–1979," *Pediatrics* 66, no. 4 (October 1980): 603.

32. Gary H. Harding, "Apnoea Alarms," *The Lancet*, no. 8179 (May 1980): 1197.

33. Sandy Rovner, "SIDS: Debating the Value of Home Monitors," *Washington Post*, October 7, 1986; Dorothy Lipovenko, "Lifesaving Machine Rules Parents' Lives," *Globe and Mail*, January 14, 1982.

34. D. P. Southall, a pediatrician in Britain who became a central player in discounting the apnea theory, voiced similar concerns. "Sleep Studies and Sudden Infant Death," 57; D.P. Southall, "Home Monitoring and Its Role in the Sudden Infant Death Syndrome," *Pediatrics* 72, no. 1 (July 1983): 135.

35. "Warning on Apnea Monitors," *FDA Consumer*, November 1985, 2.

36. Joan E. Hodgman and Toke Hoppenbrouwers, "Home Monitoring for the Sudden Infant Death Syndrome: The Case Against," *Annals of the New York Academy of Sciences* 533 (August 1988): 173.

37. "Sleep Studies and Sudden Infant Death," 56; Abraham Bergman, J. Bruce Beckwith, and C. G. Ray, "The Apnea Monitor Business," *Pediatrics* 56, no. 1 (July 1975): 1–2.

38. For examples, see: Kaiser Institute of Princeton Inc., "Sudden Infant Death Syndrome (Crib Death)" (Information Distribution Center, 1981), box 1, folder 6, WSIDSP Records; Robin Palley, "For Sale: 'Misleading Booklet on Crib Death,'" *Philadelphia Inquirer*, August 1982, box 1, folder 6, WSIDSP Records; Richard C. Thompson, "A 'Complaint Department' for Medical Devices," *FDA Consumer*, March 1987.

39. "Sudden Infant Death Syndrome Act Extension, 1978," § Subcommittee on Child and Human Development of the Committee on Human Resources (1978), 368.

40. "Sleep Studies and Sudden Infant Death," 56.

41. Donald Eugene Theis, "Home Monitoring and Sudden Infant Death Syndrome: The Legal Implications," *University of Dayton Law Review* 5, no. 2 (1980): 245.

42. Alfred Steinschneider, "A Reexamination of the 'Apnea Monitor Business,'" *Pediatrics* 58, no. 1 (July 1976): 1; Warren G. Guntheroth, "Sudden Infant Death Syndrome (Crib Death)," *American*

Heart Journal 93, no. 6 (June 1977): 791; Lois Black, Leonard Hersher, and Alfred Steinschneider, "Impact of the Apnea Monitor on Family Life," *Pediatrics* 62, no. 5 (November 1978): 682–83.

43. Steinschneider, "A Reexamination of the 'Apnea Monitor Business,'" 2.

44. Favorito, Pernice, and Ruggiero, "Apnea Monitoring to Prevent SIDS," 104.

45. Black, Hersher, and Steinschneider, "Impact of the Apnea Monitor on Family Life," 685.

46. Dorothy Kelly and Daniel C. Shannon, "Sudden Infant Death Syndrome and Near Sudden Infant Death Syndrome: A Review of the Literature, 1964 to 1982," *Pediatric Clinics of North America* 29, no. 5 (October 1982): 1254.

47. Guntheroth, "Sudden Infant Death Syndrome (Crib Death)," 791.

48. Haight et al., *A Manual for Home Monitoring*, 13.

49. Hodgman and Hoppenbrouwers, "Home Monitoring for the Sudden Infant Death Syndrome: The Case Against," 356–57.

50. National Sudden Infant Death Syndrome Foundation, "The Infant at Risk: What Can We Do?" n.d., 2, box 2, folder 26, WSIDSP Records.

51. Anne Barr, "At Home with a Monitor" (National Sudden Infant Death Syndrome Foundation, 1980), 5, box 2, folder 7, WSIDSP Records; Favorito, Pernice, and Ruggiero, "Apnea Monitoring to Prevent SIDS," 103; Patricia Geary Dean, "Monitoring an Apneic Infant: Impact on the Infant's Mother," *Maternal-Child Nursing Journal* 15, no. 2 (1986): 72.

52. Abby L. Wasserman, "A Prospective Study of the Impact of Home Monitoring on the Family," *Pediatrics* 74, no. 3 (September 1984): 326.

53. Black, Hersher, and Steinschneider, "Impact of the Apnea Monitor on Family Life," 683, 682.

54. Rona Kavee, "Babies Tested for Sudden-Death Syndrome," *New York Times*, November 18, 1979; Eleanor Charles, "Drop Indicated in Crib-Death Rate," *New York Times*, July 26, 1981; Haight et al., *A Manual for Home Monitoring*, 6, 13, 20.

55. Black, Hersher, and Steinschneider, "Impact of the Apnea Monitor on Family Life," 684; Edwin Kiester, "The Black Box That Guards Debbie Whitney's Life," *Today's Health*, October 1974, 70, box 7, folder 7, Adelson Papers.

56. "'Miracle' Infant Lives by Monitor and Medication," *New York Times*, September 21, 1980.

57. Barr, "At Home with a Monitor," 5; Wasserman, "A Prospective Study of the Impact of Home Monitoring on the Family," 325.

58. Lipovenko, "Lifesaving Machine Rules Parents' Lives."

59. Black, Hersher, and Steinschneider, "Impact of the Apnea Monitor on Family Life," 684.

60. Barr, "At Home with a Monitor," 11.

61. Favorito, Pernice, and Ruggiero, "Apnea Monitoring to Prevent SIDS," 103; Wasserman, "A Prospective Study of the Impact of Home Monitoring on the Family," 326; Black, Hersher, and Steinschneider, "Impact of the Apnea Monitor on Family Life," 683, 685.

62. "Alarming Babies"; Kavee, "Babies Tested for Sudden-Death Syndrome"; Favorito, Pernice, and Ruggiero, "Apnea Monitoring to Prevent SIDS," 103; Jean Dietz, "Alarm Bell Helps Cut Crib Deaths," *Boston Globe*, January 16, 1979, box 7, folder 14, Adelson Papers; National Sudden Infant Death Syndrome Foundation, "Position Statement on CBS 60 Minutes, March 8 1981: Segment on SIDS and Monitoring," 5–6; Theis, "Home Monitoring and Sudden Infant Death Syndrome," 280; "Home Monitoring for Crib Deaths?"

63. Wasserman, "A Prospective Study of the Impact of Home Monitoring on the Family," 327.

64. Paul L. McGorrian, "Infant Who Stops Breathing Gets New Life-Saving Monitor," *St. Petersburg Times*, October 8, 1988.

65. Haight et al., *A Manual for Home Monitoring*, 14.

66. "'Miracle' Infant Lives by Monitor and Medication"; Walter Stevens, "8-Month-Old Girl Lives on Edge of Death," n.d., box 2, folder 23/24, WSIDSP Records.

67. D. P. Southall, "The Prevention of Sudden Infant Death Syndrome: Is There a Role for Home Monitoring?" *Journal of Medical Engineering and Technology* 9, no. 6 (1985): 259.

68. Lucinda Dykes, "The Whiplash Shaken Infant Syndrome: What Has Been Learned," *Child Abuse and Neglect* 10 (1986): 211, 219.

69. Dean, "Monitoring an Apneic Infant," 69.

70. Favorito, Pernice, and Ruggiero, "Apnea Monitoring to Prevent SIDS," 104; National Sudden Infant Death Syndrome Foundation, Wisconsin Chapter, "National Sudden Infant Death Syndrome Foundation, Wisconsin Chapter: Newsletter," Fall 1979, 2, box 2, folder 7, WSIDSP Records; Haight et al., *A Manual for Home Monitoring*, 19; "Wisconsin Sudden Infant Death Syndrome Project Community Council Meeting," May 18, 1981, 2, box 3, folder 12, WSIDSP Records; Wisconsin Sudden Infant Death Syndrome Center, "Sudden Infant Death Syndrome Wisconsin Perspectives," vol. 1, no. 2 (September 1982), 9, box 1, folder 6, WSIDSP Records, box 1, folder 6; "Meeting to Aid Parents of Apnea-Prone Children," *Omaha World-Herald*, August 8, 1985.

71. Other researchers similarly described that "the period of peak stress and anxiety for parents of infants on monitors is the first month at home, the so-called acute stage of home monitor use." Barr, "At Home with a Monitor," 6, 4; Joanne Riley Kilb, "Desensitization: A Process of Parents' Adjustment to the Home Apnea Monitoring of Their Infant" (master of science thesis, University of Arizona, 1985); footnote quote from Betty R. Vohr et al., "Mothers of Preterm and Full-Term Infants on Home Apnea Monitors," *American Journal of Diseases of Children* 142 (February 1988): 231.

72. Barr, "At Home with a Monitor," 8.

73. Black, Hersher, and Steinschneider, "Impact of the Apnea Monitor on Family Life," 681, 683; Favorito, Pernice, and Ruggiero, "Apnea Monitoring to Prevent SIDS," 104; Guntheroth, "Sudden Infant Death Syndrome (Crib Death)," 791; Barr, "At Home with a Monitor," 8.

74. Alan R. Spitzer and William W. Fox, "Sudden Infant Death Syndrome (SIDS): Guidelines for Averting Tragedy," *Postgraduate Medicine* 75, no. 5 (April 1984): 138; Dorothy Kelly, "Home Monitoring for the Sudden Infant Death Syndrome: The Case For," *Annals of the New York Academy of Sciences* 533 (August 1988): 161.

75. Sally L. Davison Ward et al., "Sudden Infant Death Syndrome in Infants Evaluated by Apnea Programs in California," *Pediatrics* 77, no. 4 (April 1986): 453.

76. The Western Massachusetts Apnea Evaluation Program had 211 patients involved in home monitoring. Thomas W. Rowland et al., "Home Infant Apnea Monitoring: A Five-Year Assessment," *Clinical Pediatrics* 26, no. 8 (August 1987): 383–84; Michael J. Light and Mary S. Sheridan, "The Home Apnea Monitoring Program for Newborns: The First 300 Patients," *Hawaii Medical Journal* 44, no. 11 (November 1985): 419–20.

77. David Z. Myerberg and Dennis L. Burech, "Home Monitoring of Infants in West Virginia: A Clinician's Viewpoint," *West Virginia Medical Journal* 79, no. 11 (November 1983): 246.

78. Margaret M. Andrews, Patricia R. Nuttall, and Dennis W. Nielson, "Home Apnea Monitoring in the Intermountain West," *Journal of Pediatric Health Care* 1, no. 5 (1987): 257.

79. Bakke, "Apnea Monitoring Programs," 185.

80. The Congressional Office of Technology's data worked out to between approximately 11 and 12.4 monitored infants per thousand live births, or just over 1 percent. Joseph Oren, Dorothy Kelly, and Daniel C. Shannon, "Identification of a High-Risk Group for Sudden Infant Death Syndrome Among Infants Who Were Resuscitated for Sleep Apnea," *Pediatrics* 77, no. 4 (April 1986): 495; Robert G. Meny et al., "Sudden Infant Death and Home Monitors," *American Journal*

of Diseases of Children 142 (October 1988): 1037 (also published in *JAMA*); Michael H. Malloy and Howard J. Hoffman, "Home Apnea Monitoring and Sudden Infant Death Syndrome," *Preventative Medicine* 25, no. 6 (November 1996): 645; Elizabeth Ahmann, Louise Wulff, and Robert G. Meny, "Home Apnea Monitoring and Disruptions in Family Life: A Multidimensional Controlled Study," *American Journal of Public Health* 82, no. 5 (May 1992): 719.

81. Joan Hollobon, "Officials Discourage Reliance on Breathing Monitor for Babies," *Globe and Mail*, July 31, 1981.

82. "Tragedy to Triumph: Helping Save Infants Became His Life Work," *Los Angeles Times*, December 1, 1986; "Sudden Infant Death Syndrome: Joint Hearing Before Certain Subcommittees of the Committee on Post Office and Civil Service and the Committee on Energy and Commerce and the Select Committee on Children, Youth, and Families," § House of Representatives, Congress (1985), 96.

83. Barr, "At Home with a Monitor," 3.

84. For examples, see Frances Patrick, "Crib Baby Is Saved Nine Times by Miracle Beeper That Alerts Parents," *The Star*, June 1, 1973, box 7, folder 6, Adelson Papers; Gail Grenier Sweet, "Sudden Infant Death Syndrome: A Personal View," *Mothering*, Summer 1981, 106, box 3, folder 14, WSIDSP Records.

85. Barr, "At Home with a Monitor," 8.

86. Black, Hersher, and Steinschneider, "Impact of the Apnea Monitor on Family Life," 683.

87. Norman Lewak, "Sudden Infant Death Syndrome in a Hospitalized Infant on an Apnea Monitor," *Pediatrics* 56, no. 2 (August 1975): 297.

88. Meny et al., "Sudden Infant Death and Home Monitors," 1037–38, 1039–40; Ward et al., "Sudden Infant Death Syndrome in Infants Evaluated by Apnea Programs in California," 453, 456.

89. H. Simpson, U. M. MacFadyen, and J. Y. Payton, "'Near-Miss' or 'Near-Myth' for Sudden Infant Death Syndrome?: Clinical Observations on 57 Infants," *Australian Paediatric Journal* 22, no. supplement 1 (1986): 47–51.

90. Bergman, Beckwith, and Ray, "Sudden Infant Death Syndrome: Proceedings of the Second International Conference on Causes of Sudden Death in Infants," 204.

91. J. Bruce Beckwith, *The Sudden Infant Death Syndrome* (Rockville, MD: U.S. Department of Health, Education, and Welfare, 1976), 26, box 7, folder 4, Adelson Papers.

92. A British physician similarly noted that "near-miss or aborted SIDS are undesirable terms because they imply more definite associations . . . than can be proved . . . In addition, they indicate with some certainty that the infant almost died." "Ohio Chapter: National Sudden Infant Death Syndrome Foundation Newsletter," Spring 1980, 5, box 7, folder 2, Adelson Papers; John G. Brooks, "Apnea of Infancy and Sudden Infant Death Syndrome," *American Journal of Diseases of Children* 136 (November 1982): 1015.

93. Nelson, "But Who Shall Monitor the Monitor?" 663; Dorothy Kelly and Daniel C. Shannon, "Periodic Breathing in Infants with Near-Miss Sudden Infant Death Syndrome," *Pediatrics* 63, no. 3 (March 1979): 355–60; Christian Guilleminault and Ronald Ariagno, "Why Should We Study the Infant 'Near Miss for Sudden Infant Death'?" *Early Human Development* 2, no. 3 (September 1978): 207–18; L. Speer, "Aborted Crib Death?" *JAMA* 223, no. 13 (1973): 1512; Christian Guilleminault et al., "Mixed Obstructive Sleep Apnea and Near Miss for Sudden Infant Death Syndrome: 2. Comparison of Near Miss and Normal Control Infants by Age," *Pediatrics* 64, no. 6 (December 1979): 882–91; Ehud Krongrad and Linda O'Neill, "Near Miss Sudden Infant Death Syndrome Episodes? A Clinical and Electrocardiographic Correlation," *Pediatrics* 77, no. 6 (June 1986): 811, 813–14; Ehud Krongrad, "Infants at High Risk for

Sudden Infant Death Syndrome??? Have They Been Identified???—A Commentary," *Pediatrics* 88, no. 6 (December 1991): 1274.

94. Christian Guilleminault, Margaret Owen Boeddiker, and Deborah Schwab, "Detection of Risk Factors for 'Near-Miss SIDS' Events in Full-Term Infants," *Neuropediatrics* 13, no. 1, supplement (1982): 29, 32; Ronald Ariagno et al., "'Near-Miss' for Sudden Infant Death Syndrome Infants: A Clinical Problem," *Pediatrics* 71, no. 5 (May 1983): 729.

95. Christian Guilleminault et al., "Abnormal Polygraphic Findings in Near-Miss Sudden Infant Death," *The Lancet* 307, no. 7973 (June 1976): 1326–27.

96. This is akin to Peter Kramer's coined term "diagnostic bracket creep," outlined in his book *Listening to Prozac.* Jeremy Greene illustrated the concept when he explained how statins transformed high cholesterol from a cardiovascular risk factor into a disease category in its own right. Peter Kramer, *Listening to Prozac: A Psychiatrist Explores Antidepressant Drugs and the Remaking of the Self* (New York: Viking Press, 1993); Jeremy Greene, "The Abnormal and the Pathological: Cholesterol, Statins, and the Threshold of Disease," in *Medicating Modern America: Prescription Drugs in History*, ed. Andrea Tone and Elizabeth Siegel Watkins (New York: New York University Press, 2007), 183–228.

97. Barry Gross, "Device Monitors Baby's Breathing: Crib-Sized Pad 'Senses' Problems," *Washington Post*, December 10, 1984.

98. Marie Valdes-Dapena and Alfred Steinschneider, "Sudden Infant Death Syndrome (SIDS), Apnea, and Near Miss for SIDS," *Emergency Medicine Clinics of North America* 1, no. 1 (April 1983): 35.

99. The NIH Consensus Statement described ALTE as a risk factor for SIDS. It strongly discouraged any over-the-counter monitoring sales, and stressed that the "overall fund of knowledge [on monitoring] is inadequate," but still acknowledged that monitoring was medically indicated for a very small group of high-risk infants. Its balanced conclusion asserted: "The literature on the effects of monitoring in families has serious flaws, but it suggests that monitoring can be *both* a source of stress and a source of support and reassurance for parents." Karen L. Hall and Barry Zalman, "Evaluation and Management of Apparent Life-Threatening Events in Children," *American Family Physician* 71, no. 12 (June 2005): 2302, 2303; National Institutes of Health, "Consensus Statement: National Institutes of Health Consensus Development Conference on Infantile Apnea and Home Monitoring, Sept. 29 to Oct. 1, 1986," *Pediatrics* 79, no. 2 (February 1987): 293, 294, 295, 299, 297.

100. Hodgman and Hoppenbrouwers, "Home Monitoring for the Sudden Infant Death Syndrome: The Case Against," 165.

101. William J. R. Daily, Marshall Klaus, and H. Belton P. Meyer, "Apnea in Premature Infants: Monitoring, Incidence, Heart Rate Changes, and an Effect of Environmental Temperature," *Pediatrics* 43, no. 4 (April 1969): 510.

102. Breath-holding spells can occur as often as multiple times per day or as infrequently as once in a year. Estimates of "severe" breath-holding spells were "reported to occur in approximately 0.1% to 4.6% of healthy children." The incidence of non-severe breath-holding was poorly documented, but one study recorded rates as high as 27 percent. Definitions from http://www.webmd.com/children/tc/breath-holding-spells-topic-overview and http://umm.edu/health/medical/ency/articles/breath-holding-spell; Francis DiMario, "Breath-Holding Spells in Childhood," *American Journal of Diseases of Children* 146 (January 1992): 125, 127.

103. L. H. Stevens, "Sudden Unexplained Death in Infancy," 245.

104. Ward et al., "Sudden Infant Death Syndrome in Infants Evaluated by Apnea Programs in California," 453, 456.

105. Joan E. Hodgman et al., "Respiratory Behavior in Near-Miss Sudden Infant Death Syndrome," *Pediatrics* 69, no. 6 (June 1982): 791–92.
106. A. N. Stanton, "'Near-Miss' Cot Deaths and Home Monitoring," *British Medical Journal* 285, no. 6353 (November 1982): 1441.
107. D. P. Southall et al., "Prolonged Apnea and Cardiac Arrhythmias in Infant Discharged from Neonatal Intensive Care Units: Failure to Predict an Increased Risk for Sudden Infant Death Syndrome," *Pediatrics* 70, no. 6 (December 1982): 844–51.
108. D. P. Southall, J. M. Richards, and M. De Wiet, "Identification of Infants Destined to Die Unexpectedly During Infancy: Evaluation of Predictive Importance of Prolonged Apnoea and Disorders of Cardiac Rhythm or Conduction," *British Medical Journal* 286, no. 6371 (April 1983): 1092–96; Mary McClain, "Sudden Infant Death Syndrome: An Update," *Journal of Emergency Nursing* 11, no. 5 (1985): 228; Barbara Burns and Lewis P. Lipsitt, "Behavioral Factors in Crib Death: Toward an Understanding of the Sudden Infant Death Syndrome," *Journal of Applied Developmental Psychology* 12 (1991): 167.
109. Ruth E. Little and Donald R. Peterson, "Sudden Infant Death Syndrome Epidemiology: A Review and Update," *Epidemiologic Reviews* 12 (1990): 242; Roger Byard, "Possible Mechanisms Responsible for the Sudden Infant Death Syndrome," *Journal of Pediatrics and Child Health* 27 (1991): 147; Committee on Fetus and Newborn, "Apnea, Sudden Infant Death Syndrome, and Home Monitoring," *Pediatrics* 111, no. 4 (April 2003): 914, 915.
110. American Academy of Pediatrics Committee on Infant and Preschool Child, "Home Monitoring for Sudden Infant Death," *Pediatrics* 55, no. 1 (1975): 144.
111. Task Force on Prolonged Apnea, "Prolonged Apnea," *Pediatrics* 61, no. 4 (April 1978): 651.
112. "Prolonged Infantile Apnea," *Pediatrics* 76, no. 1 (July 1985): 129.
113. Ibid.
114. Roy Meadow, "Munchausen Syndrome by Proxy," *Archives of Disease in Childhood* 57, no. 2 (1982): 92.
115. Roy Meadow, "Munchausen Syndrome by Proxy: The Hinterland of Child Abuse," *The Lancet* 310, no. 8033 (August 1977): 345.
116. The mothers in Meadow's 1982 report were engaged in quite revolting perpetrations, ranging from meddling with bodily fluid samples and dipping thermometers in hot substances to imply fevers to physically inducing rashes and administering sedatives or tranquilizers. Two of the nineteen children died. Meadow, "Munchausen Syndrome by Proxy," 92–93.
117. Meadow, "Munchausen Syndrome by Proxy: The Hinterland of Child Abuse," 345.
118. Roy Meadow, "Munchausen Syndrome by Proxy and Pseudo-Epilepsy," *Archives of Disease in Childhood* 57, no. 10 (October 1982): 812.
119. MSbP more generally was characterized by "(1) unusual or atypical symptoms, (2) symptoms that begin only in the parents' presence, (3) medically sophisticated parents, (4) 'exemplary' parent behavior, and (5) similar or unusual illness in a sibling or parent." For babies presenting with apnea, they specified, these features may translate to: "(1) history of multiple resuscitations (especially in the hospital setting), (2) no recognizable cardiorespiratory abnormalities between episodes, (3) resuscitations begun only in the parent's presence, (4) need for resuscitation documented by others; and (5) a sibling with a similar illness or death." Other studies drew similar connections between near-miss SIDS and MSbP using case report methodology. For example, see Richard M. Kravitz and Robert W. Wilmott, "Munchausen Syndrome by Proxy Presenting as Factitious Apnea," *Clinical Pediatrics* 29, no. 10 (October 1990): 587–92. Carol Lynn Rosen, James D. Frost, and Daniel G. Glaze,

"Clinical and Laboratory Observations: Child Abuse and Recurrent Infant Apnea," *Journal of Pediatrics* 109, no. 6 (December 1986): 1066.

120. D. P. Southall et al., "Apnoeic Episodes Induced by Smothering: Two Cases Identified by Covert Video Surveillance," *British Medical Journal* 294 (June 1987): 1637.

121. Southall became an extremely controversial figure. His unorthodox tactics constantly landed him in the middle of investigatory reviews and his medical license was challenged on multiple occasions (one of which resulted in a suspension and then his re-instatement). Regardless of one's personal opinions about Southall's methods, one thing he is not is careless. In all his projects, Southall consulted with superiors, supervisors, and police authorities, as well as convened (informal) ethical review committees. He continually defended his actions on the grounds that his primary responsibility as a pediatrician was to his own patients—children. M. P. Samuels et al., "Fourteen Cases of Imposed Upper Airway Obstruction," *Archives of Disease in Childhood* 67 (1992): 163–64, 168; "Profile: Professor David Southall," *BBC News*, April 14, 2005.

122. Roy Meadow, "Suffocation, Recurrent Apnea, and Sudden Infant Death," *Journal of Pediatrics* 117, no. 3 (September 1990): 355.

123. Ibid., 356.

124. Marian Willinger, L. Stanley James, and Charlotte Catz, "Defining the Sudden Infant Death Syndrome (SIDS): Deliberations of an Expert Panel Convened by the National Institute of Child Health and Human Development," *Pediatric Pathology* 11, no. 5 (1991): 681, 677, 680, 679; Jody W. Zylke, "Sudden Infant Death Syndrome: Resurgent Research Offers Hope," *JAMA* 262, no. 12 (September 1989): 1565.

125. One of the most notorious of these incidents was when Marybeth Tinning was convicted in 1986 of murdering her four-month-old daughter, Tami Lynne, and sentenced to twenty years in prison. Tinning was also suspected in the deaths of all eight of her other children between 1972 and 1985. Another well-known case was that of Stephen VanDerSluys, who was convicted of murdering two of his children whose deaths had been recorded as SIDS, also in the 1980s. James H. Leggett, "Tinning Sentence Is 20 Years to Life for Killing Baby," *Schenectady Gazette*, October 2, 1987; Terence Samuel, "Murder or Medical Mystery? Mother's Arrest Was Result of Hunch on Five Babies' Deaths," *The Inquirer*, April 3, 1994.

126. Samuel, "Murder or Medical Mystery?"

127. Ibid.

128. Quoted in Barry Bearak, "A Mother Who Lost Five Babies," *Los Angeles Times*, May 22, 1994.

129. Cynthia Sanz, "A Mother's Fatal Embrace," *People*, October 9, 1995; "N.Y. Mother Who Killed Her 5 Children for Crying," *Pittsburgh Post-Gazette*, August 18, 1998.

130. John F. Hick, "Sudden Infant Death Syndrome and Child Abuse," *Pediatrics* 52, no. 1 (July 1973): 147.

131. Alfred Steinschneider, "Response," *Pediatrics* 52, no. 1 (July 1973): 147.

132. Quoted in "Sudden Infant Death Syndrome," Pub. L. no. 93–56, § Subcommittee on Public Health and Environment of the Committee on Interstate and Foreign Commerce (1973), 56.

133. Richard Firstman and Jamie Talan, *The Death of Innocents: A True Story of Murder, Medicine, and High-Stake Science* (New York: Bantam Books, 1997), 73–74; Evelyn Nieves, "In Prison, a Mother Proclaims Innocence in Babies' Deaths," *New York Times*, May 19, 1995.

134. Carla Cantor, "SIDS: 'We Don't Know Why Your Baby Died,'" *New York Times*, March 13, 1988.

135. Many other parents amplified their alarms' volumes using microphones, and some even reported that they connected their apnea alarms to their home fire alarm systems. Kiester, "The Black Box That Guards Debbie Whitney's Life"; Robert R. Robinson, ed., *SIDS 1974: Proceedings of the Francis E. Camps International Symposium on Sudden and Unexpected Deaths in Infancy* (Toronto: Canadian Foundation for the Study of Infant Deaths, 1974), 316.

136. National Sudden Infant Death Syndrome Foundation, "Position Statement on CBS 60 Minutes, March 8, 1981: Segment on SIDS & Monitoring," 3. This was also intimated by parent Kathy Silvio in Kathy T. Silvio, "SIDS and Apnea Monitoring: A Parent's View," *Pediatric Annals* 13, no. 3 (March 1984): 234.

CHAPTER 7   SLEEP LIKE A BABY

1. J. P. Crozer Griffith, *The Care of the Baby: A Manual for Mothers and Nurses*, 5th ed. (Philadelphia: W. B. Saunders Company, 1911), 171.

2. A. C. Engelberts and G. A. de Jonge, "Choice of Sleeping Positioning for Infants: Possible Association with Cot Death," *Archives of Disease in Childhood* 65 (1990): 462.

3. Martin McKee et al., "Preventing Sudden Infant Deaths: The Slow Diffusion of an Idea," *Health Policy* 37 (1996): 117, 118; Ruth Gilbert et al., "Infant Sleeping Position and the Sudden Infant Death Syndrome: Systematic Review of Observational Studies and Historical Review of Recommendations for 1940 to 2002," *International Journal of Epidemiology* 34, no. 4 (August 2005): 877.

4. Germ theory was developed in the late-1800s and was "cemented" by the turn of the twentieth century; it explained disease as the result of germs, bacteria, and microbes instead of miasmas. Nancy Tomes, "Spreading the Germ Theory: Sanitary Science and Home Economics, 1880–1930," in *Women and Health in America: Historical Readings*, ed. Judith Leavitt, Second (Madison: University of Wisconsin Press, 1997), 598.

5. Peter N. Stearns, Anxious Parents: A History of Modern Childrearing in America (New York: New York University Press, 2003), 46; Peter N. Stearns, Perrin Rowland, and Lori Giarnella, "Children's Sleep: Sketching Historical Change," *Journal of Social History* 30, no. 2 (1996): 346, 348, quotes from 355, 349.

6. Pearl, "The Cradle," *Ladies' Home Journal*, November 1889; Stearns, Rowland, and Giarnella, "Children's Sleep: Sketching Historical Change," 348.

7. Louis Starr, "The Baby's 'Second Summer': Its Dangers and How They May Be Avoided," *Ladies' Home Journal*, September 1890; Griffith, *The Care of the Baby: A Manual for Mothers and Nurses*, 174–75; L. Emmett Holt and John Howland, *The Diseases of Infancy and Childhood*, Sixth Edition (New York: D. Appleton, 1912), 6.

8. R.Y.H., "Putting Baby to Sleep," *Ladies' Home Journal*, February 1892.

9. John Price Crozer Griffith, *The Diseases of Infants and Children*, vol. I (Philadelphia: W. B. Saunders, 1921), 74.

10. In 1906, Mildred K. Smith noted that even "aside from overlaying," it was also "no longer considered hygienic . . . for the infant to sleep with the mother." Willard Caldwell, "Conditioned Hyperventilation in Apnea" (Washington, DC, n.d.), 40, 41, box no. 3843, folder no. 1, Caldwell Papers; Mildred K. Smith, "In Motherland," *Pictorial Review*, April 1906, 37.

11. Emma J. Gray, "The Baby," *Godey's Lady's Book*, October 1890.

12. Lena Rivers, "Chat With Our Neighbors on Home Topics," *Godey's Lady's Book*, April 1890.

13. Americans' impetus to separate familial sleeping was fueled by concrete and abstract adjustments associated with modern living. Novel consumer goods such as radios introduced new noises in homes, and the spread of electricity meant homes could be well lit even after dark. Sex was increasingly elevated as a central component in marriage and was simultaneously treated as a private act that "must be kept secret from children." Stearns, Rowland, and Giarnella, "Children's Sleep: Sketching Historical Change," 357, 359, 360.

14. Quote from Edwin Graham, "Infant Mortality," *JAMA* 51, no. 13 (1908): 1048; Griffith, *The Care of the Baby: A Manual for Mothers and Nurses*, 173, 179; Griffith, *The Diseases of Infants and Children*, I:75; East Harlem Nursing Health Demonstration, "Lesson Outlines for Maternity Classes" (New York, NY, May 1926), 69, box 113, folder 5, MCA Records.

15. Holt and Howland, *The Diseases of Infancy and Childhood*, 10.

16. L. Emmett Holt and Henry L. K. Shaw, *Save the Babies* (Chicago: American Medical Association, 1915), 17.

17. Children's Bureau, *Infant Care*, 2, Children's Bureau Publication No. 8 (Washington, DC: Government Printing Office, 1921), 28; Children's Bureau, *Infant Care*, Bureau Publication No. 8 (Washington, DC: Government Printing Office, 1929), 38; Children's Bureau, *Infant Care*, Children's Bureau Publication No. 8 (Washington, DC: Government Printing Office, 1935), 38; Mrs. Max West, *Infant Care*, Care of Children Series No. 2, Bureau Publication No. 8 (Washington, DC: Government Printing Office, 1914), 56.

18. Norman E. Ditman, *Home Hygiene and Prevention of Disease* (New York: Duffield and Company, 1912), 18.

19. Helen Ball, Elaine Hooker, and Peter J. Kelly, "Where Will the Baby Sleep? Attitudes and Practices of New and Experienced Parents Regarding Cosleeping with Their Newborn Infants," *American Anthropologist* 101, no. 1 (March 1999): 144.

20. Griffith, *The Care of the Baby: A Manual for Mothers and Nurses*, 171.

21. Griffith, *The Diseases of Infants and Children*, 75.

22. Children's Bureau, *Infant Care*, Publication No. 8 (Government Printing Office, 1955), 17, 36, 37; Children's Bureau, *Infant Care* (Bronxville, NY: Child Care Publishers, 1962), 85.

23. The pamphlet also explained that parents could "do one another a service by spreading knowledge about this, and by urging, in their communities, that careful diagnosis be made of such sudden deaths." The subsequent edition of *Infant Care*, published in 1962, further noted that spreading the word about the safety of stomach sleeping and the fallacy of AMS reports in newspapers "would help to prevent the feelings of guilt that now crush those parents who would not otherwise understand that the loss of their baby was due to no fault of their own." Children's Bureau, *Infant Care*, 1955, 72; Children's Bureau, *Infant Care*, 1962, 163.

24. Children's Bureau, *Infant Care*, 11th ed., Children's Bureau Publication No. 8, 1963, 26.

25. Quoted in AAP Task Force on Infant Positioning and SIDS, "Positioning and SIDS: AAP Task Force on Infant Positioning and SIDS," *Pediatrics* 89, no. 6 (June 1992): 11.

26. Ibid., 1120; Christine Hiley, "Letter: Babies' Sleeping Position," *British Medical Journal* 305 (July 1992): 115.

27. Katherine Bain, "When a Baby Dies Unexpectedly," *The Child* 14, no. 9 (March 1950): 131.

28. This trend was not universal among western countries. In Britain, from the 1940s through the middle of the 1950s, pediatric literature favored back or side sleeping for babies. Starting in 1954, escalating in the 1960s, and lasting until the mid-1980s, a majority of texts (although not all) began to advocate for prone sleeping based on the supposition that it might be advantageous, particularly for premature infants. Engelberts and de Jonge, "Choice of Sleeping Positioning for Infants: Possible Association with Cot Death," 462; Gilbert et al., "Infant Sleeping

Position and the Sudden Infant Death Syndrome: Systematic Review of Observational Studies and Historical Review of Recommendations for 1940 to 2002," 876; McKee et al., "Preventing Sudden Infant Deaths: The Slow Diffusion of an Idea," 119.

29. Children's Bureau, *Infant Care*, 1955, 36; Children's Bureau, *Infant Care*, 1962, 85.

30. Children's Bureau, *Infant Care*, 1963, 25.

31. Children's Bureau, *Infant Care*, 1955, 71; Children's Bureau, *Infant Care*, 1962, 162.

32. Children's Bureau, *Infant Care*, 1963, 25, 71.

33. Caldwell, "Conditioned Hyperventilation in Apnea," 40, 41.

34. Evelyn Stern et al., "Sleep Cycle Characteristics in Infants," *Pediatrics* 43, no. 1 (January 1969): 68–69.

35. Ibid., 65; Susan Coons and Christian Guilleminault, "Development of Sleep-Wake Patterns and Non-Rapid Eye Movement Sleep Stages During the First Six Months of Life in Normal Infants," *Pediatrics* 69, no. 6 (June 1982): 797; M. B. Sterman and J. Hodgman, "The Role
of Sleep and Arousal in SIDS," *Annals of the New York Academy of Sciences* 533 (August 1988):
49–50.

36. M. Gabriel, M. Albani, and F. J. Schulte, "Apneic Spells and Sleep States in Preterm
Infants," *Pediatrics* 57, no. 1 (January 1976): 142–47; Jeffrey B. Gould et al., "The Sleep State
Characteristics of Apnea During Infancy," *Pediatrics* 59, no. 2 (February 1977): 190–91.

37. Jeffrey B. Gould, Austin F. S. Lee, and Suzette Morelock, "The Relationship between
Sleep and Sudden Infant Death," *Annals of the New York Academy of Sciences* 533 (August
1988): 74; Vicki L. Schechtman et al., "Sleep State Organization in Normal Infants
and Victims of the Sudden Infant Death Syndrome," *Pediatrics* 89, no. 5 (May 1992):
865, 868.

38. Harold Abramson, "Accidental Mechanical Suffocation in Infants," *Journal of Pediatrics* 25
(1944): 411, 412, 410.

39. Ibid., 412–13.

40. Jacob Werne and Irene Garrow, "Sudden Deaths of Infants Allegedly Due to Mechanical
Suffocation," *American Journal of Public Health* 37, no. 6 (June 1947): 684–85.

41. Keith Bowden, "Sudden Death or Alleged Accidental Suffocation in Babies," *Medical
Journal of Australia* 1, no. 3 (January 1950): 67.

42. Warren G. Guntheroth and Philip S. Spiers, "Review: Sleeping Prone and the Risk of
Sudden Infant Death Syndrome," *JAMA* 267, no. 17 (May 1992): 2359; "Sudden Death in
Infancy," box 7, folder 6, n.d., Adelson Papers.

43. This determination was retroactively calculated, not assessed by Curphey or his col-
leagues. For example, see "Lettergram to Theodore Curphey," July 6, 1961, box 16, folder 1,
Curphey Papers; "Lettergram to Theodore Curphey," February 6, 1962, box 16, folder 1, Cur-
phey Papers; "Lettergram to Theodore Curphey," January 15, 1962, box 16, folder 1, Curphey
Papers; "Lettergram to Theodore Curphey," January 8, 1962, box 16, folder 1, Curphey Papers;
National Foundation for Sudden Infant Death, "National Foundation for Sudden Infant
Death (SID) Epidemiological Investigation," March 1967, 3, box 17, folder 3, Curphey Papers.

44. McKee et al., "Preventing Sudden Infant Deaths: The Slow Diffusion of an Idea," 117,
118; Gilbert et al., "Infant Sleeping Position and the Sudden Infant Death Syndrome," 877;
Guntheroth and Spiers, "Review: Sleeping Prone and the Risk of Sudden Infant Death Syndrome," 2359.

45. Ralph J. Wedgwood and Earl P. Benditt, eds., "Sudden Death in Infants: Proceedings of
the Conference on Causes of Sudden Death in Infants," Public Health Service Publication
No. 1412 (Conference on Causes of Sudden Death in Infants, Seattle, Washington: National
Institute of Child Health and Human Development, 1963), 27, 28.

46. Abraham Bergman et al., "Studies of the Sudden Infant Death Syndrome in King County, Washington. III. Epidemiology," *Pediatrics* 49, no. 6 (1972): 866, 868.

47. Abraham Bergman, J. Bruce Beckwith, and C. George Ray, eds., "Sudden Infant Death Syndrome: Proceedings of the Second International Conference on Causes of Sudden Death in Infants" (Second International Conference on Causes of Sudden Death in Infants, Children's Orthopedic Hospital and Medical Center and University of Washington School of Medicine, Seattle: University of Washington Press, 1969), 52.

48. National Foundation for Sudden Infant Death, "National Foundation for Sudden Infant Death (SID) Epidemiological Investigation"; Wisconsin Sudden Infant Death Syndrome Project, "Home Visit Questionnaire," October 1979, box 1, folder 1, WSIDSP Records; Connie Guist, "Letter and Data Sheet Sent to Public Health Nurse Following a Telephoned SIDS Referral," November 1980, 2, box 1, folder 1, WSIDSP Records.

49. Michael P. Johnson and Karl Hufbauer, "Sudden Infant Death Syndrome as a Medical Research Problem since 1945," *Social Problems* 30, no. 1 (October 1, 1982): 66.

50. Stearns, *Anxious Parents*, 32.

51. Margaret Pomeroy, "The Nurse's Visit to SIDS Families," ed. J. Bruce Beckwith (National Foundation for Sudden Infant Death, n.d.), 2, box 2, folder 18, WSIDSP Records.

52. Subcommittee on Health and Subcommittee on Child and Youth, "Sudden Infant Death Syndrome," § Committee on Labor and Public Welfare (1973), 28–30.

53. Beverley J. Bayes, "Letter: Prone Infants and SIDS," *New England Journal of Medicine* 290, no. 12 (March 1974): 693, 694.

54. "Sudden Infant Death Case History" (L.A. County Health Department, Bureau of Maternal and Child Health, 1964), box 16, folder 4, Curphey Papers.

55. Eileen Hasselmeyer and Jehu Hunter, "The Sudden Infant Death Syndrome," *Obstetrics and Gynecology Annual* 4 (1975): 216; Ruth E. Little and Donald R. Peterson, "Sudden Infant Death Syndrome Epidemiology: A Review and Update," *Epidemiologic Reviews* 12 (1990): 242; Hiroshi Shiono et al., "Sudden Infant Death Syndrome in Japan," *American Journal of Forensic Medicine and Pathology* 9, no. 1 (1988): 7; Marie Valdes-Dapena, "Sudden Infant Death Syndrome: Overview of Recent Research Developments from a Pediatric Pathologist's Perspective," *Pediatrician* 15, no. 4 (1988): 223.

56. D. P. Davies, "Cot Death in Hong Kong: A Rare Problem?" *The Lancet* 14, no. 2 (December 1985): 1346–49.

57. M. Lee, D. P. Davies, and Y. F. Chan, "Prone or Supine for Preterm Babies?" *The Lancet* 331, no. 8598 (June 1988): 1332.

58. Jonathan Nicholl and Alicia O'Cathain, "Sleeping Position and SIDS," *The Lancet* 332, no. 8602 (July 1988): 106.

59. Susan Beal, "Sleeping Position and SIDS," *The Lancet* 332, no. 8609 (August 1988): 512.

60. The advantages claimed of prone sleeping were by and large unsubstantiated—they were not demonstrated using controlled studies, they related only to specific subsets of the population, or they "involve[d] unjustified extrapolation from physiological findings." G. A. de Jonge et al., "Cot Death and Prone Sleeping Position in The Netherlands," *British Medical Journal* 298 (March 1989): 722; Engelberts and de Jonge, "Choice of Sleeping Positioning for Infants: Possible Association with Cot Death," 465, 466, 462–63; McKee et al., "Preventing Sudden Infant Deaths: The Slow Diffusion of an Idea," 119.

61. A. C. Engelberts, G. A. De Jonge, and P. J. Kostense, "An Analysis of Trends in the Incidence of Sudden Infant Death in The Netherlands 1969–89," *Journal of Paediatrics and Child Health* 27, no. 6 (1991): 332–33; E. A. Mitchell, "Review Article: Cot Death: Should the Prone

Sleeping Position Be Discouraged," *Journal of Paediatrics and Child Health* 27, no. 6 (1991): 320; Roger Byard, "Possible Mechanisms Responsible for the Sudden Infant Death Syndrome," *Journal of Pediatrics and Child Health* 27 (1991): 150; Guntheroth and Spiers, "Review: Sleeping Prone and the Risk of Sudden Infant Death Syndrome," 2360.

62. S. M. Beal and C. F. Finch, "An Overview of Retrospective Case-Control Studies Investigating the Relationship Between Prone Sleeping Position and SIDS," *Journal of Paediatrics and Child Health* 27, no. 6 (1991): 337.

63. For example, see Adele C. Engelberts and Guus A. De Jonge, "Sleeping Position and Cot Death," *The Lancet* 332, no. 8616 (October 1988): 900.

64. David Southall, Valerie Stebbens, and Martin Samiels, "Letter: Bedding and Sleeping Position in the Sudden Infant Death Syndrome," *British Medical Journal* 301 (September 1990): 492.

65. T. Dwyer et al., "Prone Sleeping Position and SIDS: Evidence from Recent Case-Control and Cohort Studies in Tasmania," *Journal of Paediatrics and Child Health* 27, no. 6 (1991): 342; Terence Dwyer et al., "Prospective Cohort Study of Prone Sleeping Position and Sudden Infant Death Syndrome," *The Lancet* 337 (May 1991): 1244.

66. Susan R. Orenstein, "Throwing Out the Baby with the Bedding: A Commentary on the A.A.P. Statement on Positioning and SIDS," *Clinical Pediatrics* 31, no. 9 (September 1992): 546–47.

67. As Carl Hunt and Daniel Shannon expressed: "the families of recent SIDS victims may well have significant anger that the health care system did not alert them sooner to this 'effective' intervention." Shannon and Hunt also wondered about how the "new anxiety" regarding supine sleeping could "result in additional after-hours calls to the pediatrician," and translate into distress for physicians unable to help parents trying to implement supine sleeping. McKee et al., "Preventing Sudden Infant Deaths: The Slow Diffusion of an Idea," 129, 130; Carl E. Hunt and Daniel C. Shannon, "Sudden Infant Death Syndrome and Sleeping Position," *Pediatrics* 90, no. 1 (July 1992): 117, 118.

68. Hunt and Shannon, "Sudden Infant Death Syndrome and Sleeping Position," 115; F. J. Stanley and R. W. Byard, "The Association Between the Prone Sleeping Position and Sudden Infant Death Syndrome (SIDS): An Editorial Overview," *Journal of Paediatrics and Child Health* 27, no. 6 (1991): 325, 327; Orenstein, "Throwing Out the Baby with the Bedding: A Commentary on the A.A.P. Statement on Positioning and SIDS."

69. Mitchell, "Review Article: Cot Death: Should the Prone Sleeping Position Be Discouraged," 320–21.

70. McKee et al., "Preventing Sudden Infant Deaths: The Slow Diffusion of an Idea," 123–25.

71. Dwyer et al., "Prospective Cohort Study of Prone Sleeping Position and Sudden Infant Death Syndrome," 1244–46.

72. Guntheroth and Spiers, "Review: Sleeping Prone and the Risk of Sudden Infant Death Syndrome," 2359.

73. "The Second Month," *Ladies' Home Journal*, February 1903; West, *Infant Care*, 12; Stearns, Rowland, and Giarnella, "Children's Sleep: Sketching Historical Change," 358.

74. A brief piece in *The Lancet* from the 1930s specifically indicted soft pillows in cases of infant suffocation and recommended that "the feather pillow show be barred." Children's Bureau, *Infant Care*, 1962, 82–83; Children's Bureau, *Infant Care*, 1963, 25; Louise Bruner, "Babies Rarely Smother," *Today's Health*, July 1952, 72, box 7, folder 14, Adelson Papers; "The Dangers of the Feather Pillow," *The Lancet* 227, no. 5885 (June 1936): 1367–68.

75. "Death in the Crib," *Time*, July 6, 1970.

76. Richard Flaste, "Keeping the Children Safe, Signs of Hope, Voices of Concern: 1,500 Toys on Banned List," *New York Times*, March 25, 1974.

77. J. E. Smialek, P. Z. Smialek, and W. U. Spitz, "Accidental Bed Deaths in Infants Due to Unsafe Sleeping Situations," *Clinical Pediatrics* 16, no. 11 (November 1977): 1031, 1032, 1034–36.

78. Ramesh Ramanathan et al., "Sudden Infant Death Syndrome and Water Beds," *New England Journal of Medicine* 318, no. 25 (June 1988): 1700; Denise Cabrera, "Infant Pillows Linked to Deaths Being Recalled," *AP*, April 1990, box 7, folder 11, Adelson Papers; James S. Kemp and Bradley T. Thach, "Sudden Death in Infants Sleeping on Polystyrene-Filled Cushions," *New England Journal of Medicine* 324, no. 26 (June 1991): 1858.

79. Peter Fleming et al., "Interaction Between Bedding and Sleeping Position in the Sudden Infant Death Syndrome: A Population Based Case-Control Study," *British Medical Journal* 301 (July 1990): 85; S. A. Peterson and M. P. Wailoo, "Thermoregulation and Cot Death," *Current Paediatrics* 2, no. 4 (December 1992): 211–12; "Prone, Hot, and Dead," *The Lancet* 336, no. 8723 (November 1990): 1104.

80. Kemp and Thach, "Sudden Death in Infants Sleeping on Polystyrene-Filled Cushions," 1858, 1863.

81. "Correspondence: SIDS and Suffocation," *New England Journal of Medicine* 325, no. 25 (December 1991): 1807.

82. J. L. Luke, "Sleeping Arrangements of Sudden Infant Death Syndrome Victims in the District of Columbia: A Preliminary Report," *Journal of Forensic Sciences* 23, no. 2 (1978): 380, 382; Susan Okie, "Face to Face with the Toll of City Life," *Washington Post*, April 13, 1981.

83. A similar paper published in 1990 in the *Scandinavian Journal of Social Medicine* examined 1,480 SIDS cases over the course of almost two decades, and found that there were more cases on Saturdays and Sundays than any other days of the week, as well as a sizable number on holidays. More specifically, the authors registered a 26.7 percent increase in SIDS on weekends and holidays. J. A. Morris, "Increased Risk of Sudden Infant Death Syndrome in Older Infants at Weekends," *British Medical Journal* 293 (August 1986): 566; E. A. Mitchell and A. W. Stewart, "Deaths from Sudden Infant Death Syndrome on Public Holidays and Weekends," *Australian and New Zealand Journal of Medicine* 18, no. 7 (1988): 862–63; Birger Kaada and Erling Sivertsen, "Sudden Infant Death Syndrome During Weekends and Holidays in Norway 1967–1985," *Scandinavian Journal of Social Medicine* 18 (1990): 18.

84. "Obituary: Tine Thevenin," *Schleicher Funeral Homes and Cremation Services Obituaries*, June 2010, accessed at <http://www.schleicherfuneralhomes.com/fh/obituaries/obituary.cfm?o_id=651557&fh_id=11718>; "Remembering the Remarkable Lives Lost in 2010," *Talk of the Nation* (Boston: WBUR (NPR), December 30, 2010), accessed at <http://www.wbur.org/npr/132482172/remembering-some-remarkable-lives-lost-in-2010>.

85. Tine Thevenin, *The Family Bed*, 2nd ed. (Wayne, NJ: Avery Publishing Group, 1987), 3, 6.

86. "Sleeping in the parental bed was common in Cleveland families," the authors clarified, even though "none of the study participants was philosophically committed to the 'family bed' as an approach to child rearing." Betsy Lozoff, Abraham W. Wolf, and Nancy S. Davis, "Cosleeping in Urban Families with Young Children in the United States," *Pediatrics* 74, no. 2 (August 1984): 175, 176.

87. The debate to which Thevenin contributed was directed towards "normal" babies. Although American cultural and professional forces advanced separate sleeping, "near-miss" SIDS babies or "high-risk" babies constituted an entirely separate category of discussion. Thevenin, *The Family Bed*, quote from 131, 31–33.

88. Wenda Trevathan, *Ancient Bodies, Modern Lives: How Evolution Has Shaped Women's Health* (Oxford: Oxford University Press, 2010), 7; Randolph M. Nesse, "How Is Darwinian Medicine Useful?" *West Journal of Medicine* 174 (2001): 358–59.

89. Wenda Trevathan, E. O. Smith, and James McKenna, "Introduction and Overview of Evolutionary Medicine," in *Evolutionary Medicine and Health* (Oxford: Oxford University Press, 2007), 9, 26.

90. McKenna further suggested that solitary sleeping was far more beneficial for parents than for infants. James McKenna and Sarah Mosko, "Evolution and the Sudden Infant Death Syndrome (SIDS): Part 3: Infant Arousal and Parent-Infant Co-Sleeping," *Human Nature* 1, no. 3 (1990): 293, 315, 291–92; Trevathan, Smith, and McKenna, "Introduction and Overview of Evolutionary Medicine," 29.

91. Evelyn B. Thoman, "Co-Sleeping, An Ancient Practice: Issues of the Past and Present, and Possibilities for the Future," *Sleep Medicine Reviews* 10 (2006): 408–9.

92. Trevathan, Smith, and McKenna, "Introduction and Overview of Evolutionary Medicine," 28.

93. McKenna and Mosko, "Evolution and the Sudden Infant Death Syndrome (SIDS): Part 3," 292, 304–6.

94. Trevathan, Smith, and McKenna, "Introduction and Overview of Evolutionary Medicine," 27.

95. Roger Byard, "Is Co-Sleeping in Infancy a Desirable or Dangerous Practice?" *Journal of Paediatrics and Child Health* 30, no. 3 (1994): 199.

96. Marlene Zuk, *Paleofantasy: What Evolution Really Tells Us About Sex, Diet, and How We Live* (New York: W. W. Norton, 2013), 6.

97. Ibid., 213, 214.

98. James McKenna, "Evolution and Sudden Infant Death Syndrome (SIDS): Part I: Infant Responsivity to Parental Contact," *Human Nature* 1, no. 2 (1990): 149.

99. James McKenna, "An Anthropological Perspective on the Sudden Infant Death Syndrome (SIDS): The Role of Parental Breathing Cues and Speech Breathing Adaptations," *Medical Anthropology*, Cross-Cultural Studies in Health and Disease, 10, no. 1 (1986): 50.

100. McKenna and Mosko, "Evolution and the Sudden Infant Death Syndrome (SIDS): Part 3," 303.

101. McKenna did not neglect the hard sciences. He even relied on the budding epigenetics field to suggest that infants' prenatal environments began shaping their capabilities for survival before birth. Human fetuses were learning and "practicing" to breathe in the womb. McKenna, "An Anthropological Perspective on the Sudden Infant Death Syndrome (SIDS)," 28; James McKenna, "Evolution and the Sudden Infant Death Syndrome (SIDS): Part 2: Why Human Infants?" *Human Nature* 1, no. 2 (1990): 185, 199.

102. McKenna, "An Anthropological Perspective on the Sudden Infant Death Syndrome (SIDS)," 52, 37–38; McKenna, "Evolution and Sudden Infant Death Syndrome (SIDS): Part 1," 150–59.

103. Don Day, "Sleep with Tots to Avoid SIDS?" *Medical News*, December 4, 1985, box 7, folder 11, Adelson Papers; McKenna and Mosko, "Evolution and the Sudden Infant Death Syndrome (SIDS): Part 3," 292.

104. McKenna, "Evolution and Sudden Infant Death Syndrome (SIDS): Part 1," 148, 161–62.

105. McKenna, "An Anthropological Perspective on the Sudden Infant Death Syndrome (SIDS)," 53.

106. McKenna and Mosko, "Evolution and the Sudden Infant Death Syndrome (SIDS): Part 3," 291.

107. McKenna, "An Anthropological Perspective on the Sudden Infant Death Syndrome (SIDS)," 32, 52; McKenna, "Evolution and Sudden Infant Death Syndrome (SIDS): Part 1," 166.
108. James McKenna, Steve Mosco, and Claiborne Dungy, "Synchronous and Asynchronous Aspects of Sleep, Awake, and Arousal Patterns of Co-Sleeping Human Mother/Infant Pairs: A Preliminary Physiological Study with Implications for the Study of Sudden Infant Death Syndrome (Draft)," *Submitted to American Journal of Anthropology*, n.d., box no. 3844, folder 4, Caldwell Papers, 35.
109. McKenna, "Evolution and Sudden Infant Death Syndrome (SIDS): Part I," 148.
110. McKenna, "An Anthropological Perspective on the Sudden Infant Death Syndrome (SIDS)," 52, 37–38; McKenna, "Evolution and Sudden Infant Death Syndrome (SIDS): Part I," 150–59.
111. McKenna, "An Anthropological Perspective on the Sudden Infant Death Syndrome (SIDS)," 48; McKenna, "Evolution and Sudden Infant Death Syndrome (SIDS): Part I," 165; McKenna, "Evolution and the Sudden Infant Death Syndrome (SIDS): Part II," 198.
112. McKenna, "Evolution and Sudden Infant Death Syndrome (SIDS): Part I," 161–62.
113. McKenna, "An Anthropological Perspective on the Sudden Infant Death Syndrome (SIDS)," 51.
114. James McKenna and Thomas McDade, "Why Babies Should Never Sleep Alone: A Review of the Co-Sleeping Controversy in Relation to SIDS, Bedsharing and Breast Feeding," *Pediatric Respiratory Reviews* 6 (2005): 135; quote from Trevathan, *Ancient Bodies, Modern Lives*, 148.
115. McKenna and McDade, "Why Babies Should Never Sleep Alone," 135.
116. F.L.R. Williams, G. A. Lang, and D. T. Mage, "Sudden Unexpected Deaths in Dundee, 1882–1891: Overlying or SIDS?" *Scottish Medical Journal* 46, no. 2 (2001): 43; Byard, "Is Co-Sleeping in Infancy a Desirable or Dangerous Practice?" 199.
117. "Investigation of SIDS," *New England Journal of Medicine* 315, no. 26 (December 1986): 1677.
118. Kim A. Collins, "Death by Overlaying and Wedging: A 15-Year Retrospective Study," *The American Journal of Forensic Medicine and Pathology* 22, no. 2 (2001): 158.
119. Williams, Lang, and Mage, "Sudden Unexpected Deaths in Dundee, 1882–1891," 44, 45, quote on 46.
120. U.S. Department of Health and Human Services, "Information Exchange: National Sudden Infant Death Syndrome Resource Center" (U.S. Department of Health and Human Services, April 1994), 2, box no. 3843, folder no. 4, Caldwell Papers.
121. Christian F. Poets and David P. Southall, "Prone Sleeping Position and Sudden Infant Death," *New England Journal of Medicine* 329, no. 6 (August 1993): 425.
122. U.S. Public Health Services, "NICHD News Notes: Press Release—National Campaign to Reduce Risk of SIDS Launched: Infant Sleep Position Targeted" (U.S. Department of Health and Human Services, June 1994), 1–3, box no. 3843, folder 4, Caldwell Papers.
123. Between 1999 and 2001, SIDS declines appear to have been partly "offset by increased rates of cause unknown/unspecific and accidental suffocation and strangulation in bed" listings on death certificates. Fern R. Hauck and Kawai O. Tanabe, "International Trends in Sudden Infant Death Syndrome: Stabilization of Rates Requires Further Action," *Pediatrics* 122, no. 3 (September 2008): 660, 663.
124. Trevathan, *Ancient Bodies, Modern Lives*, 149.
125. He continued: "The full explanation as to why the supine infant sleep position is protective (infants arouse more and sleep lighter) might only be achieved by acknowledging complexity, that the infant sleep position is only one of many interactive behavioural and

physiological variables *each one of which changes in relation to the other when the breast feeding mother and infant sleep in close proximity.*" McKenna and McDade, "Why Babies Should Never Sleep Alone," 138, 140.

126. T. J. Mathews, Marian F. MacDorman, and Marie E. Thoma, "Infant Mortality Statistics From the 2013 Period Linked Birth/Infant Death Data Set," *National Vital Statistics Reports* 64, no. 9 (August 6, 2015): 9.

127. Fern R. Hauck et al., "Breastfeeding and Reduced Risk of Sudden Infant Death Syndrome: A Meta-Analysis," *Pediatrics* 128, no. 1 (July 2011): 1, 3.

128. Fern R. Hauck et al., "Evaluation of Bedtime Basics for Babies: A National Crib Distribution Program to Reduce the Risk of Sleep-Related Sudden Infant Deaths," *Journal of Community Health* 40, no. 3 (June 2015): 458.

129. Zuk, *Paleofantasy* 7, no. 9 (2014): 204.

130. As Zuk explains, McKenna's research-based conclusions "that babies evolved with immediate care, and might not thrive if that attentiveness was missing, differs from accepting that babies are the way they are because they evolved in the Pleistocene that way, and that change since that time would be bad for them and for us . . . Instead of assuming that babies from foraging societies are more natural and more accurately reflect our evolutionary past," Zuk continues, "McKenna and others like him test their ideas on real infants under modern-day circumstances." Ibid., 213, 218.

131. Trina C. Salm Ward, "Reasons for Mother-Infant Bed-Sharing: A Systematic Narrative Synthesis of the Literature and Implications for Future Research," *Maternal and Child Health Journal* (2014): 1.

132. As Fleming's article summarized, "it is clear that, for parents who smoke tobacco, drink alcohol or take recreational drugs, the risk of SIDS is significantly higher if they bedshare with their infant . . . and the risk is even higher for parents who fall asleep with their infants on the sofa. For mothers who breastfeed, do not smoke or drink alcohol, and do not use recreational drugs the evidence of an increased risk from bedsharing is very limited." Peter Fleming, Anna Pease, and Peter Blair, "Bed-Sharing and Unexpected Infant Deaths: What Is the Relationship?" *Paediatric Respiratory Reviews* 16 (2015): 63, 64, quote from 66; E. A. Mitchell, "Co-Sleeping and Sudden Infant Death Syndrome," *The Lancet* 348, no. 9040 (November 1996): 1466.

133. Helen Ball and Lane Volpe, "Sudden Infant Death Syndrome (SIDS) Risk Reduction and Infant Sleep Location—Moving the Discussion Forward," *Social Science and Medicine* 79 (2013): 84.

134. Roger W. Byard, "Overlaying, Co-Sleeping, Suffocation, and Sudden Infant Death Syndrome: The Elephant in the Room," *Forensic Science, Medicine, and Pathology,* 2014, 2.

135. Richard Naeye, "Sudden Infant Death Syndrome, Is the Confusion Ending?" *Modern Pathology* 1, no. 3 (1988): 171.

136. Jane Brody, "Personal Health," *New York Times,* March 29, 1978.

137. The same authors further posited that "the emerging evidence about sleeping position was seen by many professionals as threatening as it necessitated them to admit that what they did previously was wrong," and that this resistance played a significant role in "inhibiting dissemination of advice in the United States." McKee et al., "Preventing Sudden Infant Deaths: The Slow Diffusion of an Idea," 129.

CONCLUSION

1. Eileen Hasselmeyer and Jehu Hunter, "The Sudden Infant Death Syndrome," *Obstetrics and Gynecology Annual* 4 (1975): 221.

2. Lynn Barkley Burnett, "Sudden Infant Death Syndrome," ed. Kirsten A. Bechtel, *Medscape*, 2014, http://emedicine.medscape.com/article/804412-overview.

3. Helen Ball and Lane Volpe, "Sudden Infant Death Syndrome (SIDS) Risk Reduction and Infant Sleep Location—Moving the Discussion Forward," *Social Science and Medicine* 79 (2013): 85.

4. Fern R. Hauck and Kawai O. Tanabe, "International Trends in Sudden Infant Death Syndrome: Stabilization of Rates Requires Further Action," *Pediatrics* 122, no. 3 (September 2008): 662.

5. Ibid.

6. Ibid., 660; Fern R. Hauck et al., "The Contribution of Prone Sleeping Position to the Racial Disparity in Sudden Infant Death Syndrome: The Chicago Infant Mortality Study," *Pediatrics* 110, no. 4 (October 2002): 772, 773.

7. Ball and Volpe, "Sudden Infant Death Syndrome (SIDS) Risk Reduction and Infant Sleep Location," 88, 85; T. J. Mathews, Marian F. MacDorman, and Marie E. Thoma, "Infant Mortality Statistics from the 2013 Period Linked Birth/Infant Death Data Set," *National Vital Statistics Reports* 64, no. 9 (August 6, 2015): 9.

8. Burnett, "Sudden Infant Death Syndrome."

9. Fern R. Hauck et al., "Evaluation of Bedtime Basics for Babies: A National Crib Distribution Program to Reduce the Risk of Sleep-Related Sudden Infant Deaths," *Journal of Community Health* 40, no. 3 (June 2015): 457–63.

10. Michael H. Malloy and Marian MacDorman, "Changes in the Classification of Sudden Unexpected Infant Deaths: United States, 1992–2001," *Pediatrics* 115, no. 5 (May 2005): 1247, 1250; Rebecca Matthews and Andrea Moore, "Babies Are Still Dying of SIDS: A Safe Sleep Environment in Child-Care Settings Reduces Risk," *American Journal of Nursing* 113, no. 2 (February 2013): 60; Hauck and Tanabe, "International Trends in Sudden Infant Death Syndrome," 663.

11. Carrie K. Shapiro-Mendoza et al., "Recent National Trends in Sudden, Unexpected Infant Deaths: More Evidence Supporting a Change in Classification or Reporting," *American Journal of Epidemiology* 163, no. 8 (March 2006): 766, 767–68.

12. Michelle M. Carlberg, Carrie K. Shapiro-Mendoza, and Michael Goodman, "Maternal and Infant Characteristics Associated with Accidental Suffocation and Strangulation in Bed in US Infants," *Maternal and Child Health Journal* 16, no. 8 (November 2012): 1594–95.

13. SUID can be defined as "the death of a previously healthy infant <365 days old without an obvious cause before a medicolegal investigation." Carrie K. Shapiro-Mendoza et al., "The Sudden Unexpected Infant Death Case Registry: A Method to Improve Surveillance," *Pediatrics* 129, no. 2 (January 2012): e487; Mathews, MacDorman, and Thoma, "Infant Mortality Statistics," 11.

14. J. L. Emery, Sanita Chandra, and Enid F. Gilbert-Barness, "Findings in Child Deaths Registered as Sudden Infant Death Syndrome (SIDS) in Madison, Wisconsin," *Pediatric Pathology* 8, no. 2 (1988): 177.

15. Roger Byard, "Sudden Infant Death Syndrome: A 'Diagnosis' in Search of a Disease," *Journal of Clinical Forensic Medicine* 2 (1995): 121.

16. Charles Rosenberg, "Contested Boundaries: Psychiatry, Disease, and Diagnosis," *Perspectives in Biology and Medicine* 49, no. 3 (Summer 2006): 411.

17. Hasselmeyer and Hunter, "The Sudden Infant Death Syndrome," 221.

18. Leslie Reagan, *Dangerous Pregnancies: Mothers, Disabilities, and Abortion in Modern America* (Berkeley: University of California Press, 2010), 24.

INDEX

ABOUT THE AUTHOR

BRITTANY COWGILL has a Ph.D. from the University of Cincinnati.

Laura D. Hirshbein, *American Melancholy: Constructions of Depression in the Twentieth Century*

Laura D. Hirshbein, *Smoking Privileges: Psychiatry, the Mentally Ill, and the Tobacco Industry in America*

Timothy Hoff, *Practice under Pressure: Primary Care Physicians and Their Medicine in the Twenty-first Century*

Beatrix Hoffman, Nancy Tomes, Rachel N. Grob, and Mark Schlesinger, eds., *Patients as Policy Actors*

Ruth Horowitz, *Deciding the Public Interest: Medical Licensing and Discipline*

Powel Kazanjian, *Frederick Novy and the Development of Bacteriology in American Medicine*

Rebecca M. Kluchin, *Fit to Be Tied: Sterilization and Reproductive Rights in America, 1950–1980*

Jennifer Lisa Koslow, *Cultivating Health: Los Angeles Women and Public Health Reform*

Susan C. Lawrence, *Privacy and the Past: Research, Law, Archives, Ethics*

Bonnie Lefkowitz, *Community Health Centers: A Movement and the People Who Made It Happen*

Ellen Leopold, *Under the Radar: Cancer and the Cold War*

Barbara L. Ley, *From Pink to Green: Disease Prevention and the Environmental Breast Cancer Movement*

Sonja Mackenzie, *Structural Intimacies: Sexual Stories in the Black AIDS Epidemic*

Michelle McClellan, *Lady Lushes: Gender, Alcohol, and Medicine in Modern America*

David Mechanic, *The Truth about Health Care: Why Reform Is Not Working in America*

Richard A. Meckel, *Classrooms and Clinics: Urban Schools and the Protection and Promotion of Child Health, 1870–1930*

Alyssa Picard, *Making the American Mouth: Dentists and Public Health in the Twentieth Century*

Heather Munro Prescott, *The Morning After: A History of Emergency Contraception in the United States*

Andrew R. Ruis, *Eating to Learn, Learning to Eat: School Lunches and Nutrition Policy in the United States*

James A. Schafer Jr., *The Business of Private Medical Practice: Doctors, Specialization, and Urban Change in Philadelphia, 1900–1940*

David G. Schuster, *Neurasthenic Nation: America's Search for Health, Happiness, and Comfort, 1869–1920*

Karen Seccombe and Kim A. Hoffman, *Just Don't Get Sick: Access to Health Care in the Aftermath of Welfare Reform*

Leo B. Slater, *War and Disease: Biomedical Research on Malaria in the Twentieth Century*

Paige Hall Smith, Bernice L. Hausman, and Miriam Labbok, *Beyond Health, Beyond Choice: Breastfeeding Constraints and Realities*

Matthew Smith, *An Alternative History of Hyperactivity: Food Additives and the Feingold Diet*

Susan L. Smith, *Toxic Exposures: Mustard Gas and the Health Consequences of World War II in the United States*

Rosemary A. Stevens, Charles E. Rosenberg, and Lawton R. Burns, eds., *History and Health Policy in the United States: Putting the Past Back In*

Barbra Mann Wall, *American Catholic Hospitals: A Century of Changing Markets and Missions*

Frances Ward, *The Door of Last Resort: Memoirs of a Nurse Practitioner*